BARRON'S

HOW TO PREPARE FOR THE NEW MEDICAL COLLEGE ADMISSION TEST

MCAT

GEARED TO THE CURRENT EXAM!

FOURTH EDITION

by

HUGO R. SEIBEL
Professor of Anatomy
Curriculum Coordinator, School of Medicine — Year One, Director of Graduate Studies,
Director of Electron Microscopy, School of Basic Sciences,
Medical College of Virginia, Virginia Commonwealth University

and

KENNETH E. GUYER
Associate Professor of Biochemistry
School of Medicine, Marshall University

BARRON'S EDUCATIONAL SERIES, INC.
Woodbury, New York • London • Toronto • Sydney

All inquiries should be addressed to:
Barron's Educational Series, Inc.
113 Crossways Park Drive
Woodbury, New York 11797

Library of Congress Catalog Card No. 83-3778

International Standard Book No. 0-8120-2608-X

Library of Congress Cataloging in Publication Data
Seibel, Hugo R.
Barron's how to prepare for the new MCAT,
Medical College Admission Test.

"This book has been completely revised to
correspond with the new MCAT now being used."
Includes index.
1. Medicine—Examinations, questions, etc.
I. Guyer, Kenneth E. II. Title. III. Title:
How to prepare for the new MCAT, Medical College
Admission Test.
R838.5.B36 1983 610'.76 83-3778
ISBN 0-8120-2608-X

PRINTED IN THE UNITED STATES OF AMERICA

34567 056 987654321

Contents

Preface iv

Introduction v

Timetable for the New MCAT vii
Self-Scoring Charts vii
Test Preparation and Test-Taking Strategies Compiled with the Help of Successful Medical Students ix
A Positive Approach to Answering Questions and to Test Taking xi
Test-Taking Strategy for the Reading Portion of the Examination xiv

New MCAT Science Review 1

A Review of Key Subject Matter and Concepts 1

Model Examination A 89

Answer Key 133
Answer Explanations 135

Model Examination B 147

Answer Key 191
Answer Explanations 193

Model Examination C 207

Answer Key 253
Answer Explanations 255

Model Examination D 269

Answer Key 314
Answer Explanations 316

Appendix 327

Logarithms and Exponents 327
Table of Common Logarithms 329
Periodic Chart of the Elements 331
List of Elements with Their Symbols 332

Preface

Can you prepare for the Medical College Admission Test (MCAT)? Some students are hesitant to utilize a book of this sort to assist in preparation for the medical college admission test, perhaps believing there is something dishonest about this method of preparation. Other students may believe that they can utilize this book or a similar one just before the test to prepare themselves.

In our estimation both of these viewpoints are incorrect. These practice materials should provide experience in timed tests of this type and point out areas of weakness for additional study in appropriate textbooks. By proper and careful preparation utilizing all possible modes, the individual is simply presenting his or her true potential for the study of medicine. For maximum benefit we would suggest that students begin their preparation two or three months before the examination. This will allow time to take some of the practice examinations, review the areas of weakness, and retake some of the practice examinations without having the pressure of time to produce undue frustration and a feeling of hopelessness.

Obtaining admission to medical school is a very difficult task today. We hope that, in preparing this volume, we have been able to offer you a greater chance of success. Good luck!

We wish to acknowledge the help we have received from many of our colleagues; a special thank you should be extended to H. Meetz; G. D. Meetz; J. Gregorek; J. D. Reynolds; W. M. Reams; C. Kirksey; R. J. Krieg; J. H. Johnson; S. S. Craig; J. D. Povlishock; W. Seibel; L. Crane; L. P. Gartner; L. M. Sawyer; G. J. Somori; W. J. McIntyre; J. Washburn; J. L. Poland; S. L. Quattropani; M. P. Golka; F. M. Bush; R. L. Salisbury; M. M. Sholley; G. Miller; C. H. Fowlkes; R. B. Brandt; P. L. Szabo; N. Whisner; J. Wood; J. P. Guyer; and J. Kass. Particular gratitude is extended to Mrs. Marilyn P. Bertrand for her cheerful and spirited assistance and the typing of the manuscript. We are indebted to Mrs. Edith E. Seibel for her contributions and the proofreading of the book. Dr. Erwin E. Seibel deserves a special commendation since he contributed the bulk of the physics questions of this work.

Introduction

The New MCAT was first administered to prospective medical students in the spring of 1977. It represents an attempt to evaluate (1) the student's knowledge and ability to solve problems in the areas of biology, chemistry, and physics, and (2) the student's skill in analysis of paragraphs, tabular material, graphs, etc. Separate scores will be reported for Biology, Chemistry, Physics, Science Problems (mixed scientific disciplines), Skills Analysis: Quantitative, and Skills Analysis: Reading.

It is expected that those taking the test will have the equivalent of one year of college study in each of the following scientific areas: biology, general and/or inorganic chemistry, organic chemistry, and physics. Although advanced study in one or more of these disciplines may give a better understanding of concepts, it is not intended that the questions will require a knowledge of concepts not taught in basic courses.

A mathematics background including one year of college mathematics should suffice for this area of preparation; calculus is not required. Indeed, it has been suggested that high school courses including two years of algebra, use of trigonometric functions, memorization of sine and cosine of 0°, 90°, and 180°, facility in use of metric and English units and conversion from one set of units to another (when conversion factors are given); experimental error; statistics to include the concepts of arithmetic mean, range, variability, and significant figures; and vector addition and subtraction would represent adequate preparation in mathematics.

It is our suggestion that you begin preparation by studying the Science Review section of this book. Areas that are particularly difficult for you may require some review of your college texts. When you begin taking the practice tests, try to pace yourself to allow completion of each section within the allotted time. (If it is necessary to omit some questions because of time limitations, you may wish to go back after you have scored the test and try to answer them without the pressure of time.)

After taking your first practice test and correcting the answers, you should score your test as it will be done after the actual test. First count the number of correct answers in (1) Biology, (2) Chemistry, and (3) Physics. In each case this will represent the number of correct answers in that discipline in Science Knowledge and Science Problems.

The number of correct answers is the raw score and must then be converted into a 15-point scaled score *approximated by* the following tables.

Biology		Chemistry		Physics	
Raw Score	Scaled Score	Raw Score	Scaled Score	Raw Score	Scaled Score
0-2	1	0-3	1	0-2	1
3-4	2	4-6	2	3-4	2
5-7	3	7-10	3	5-7	3
8-10	4	11-13	4	8-10	4
11-13	5	14-17	5	11-13	5
14-16	6	18-21	6	14-16	6
17-19	7	22-25	7	17-19	7
20-22	8	26-29	8	20-22	8
23-25	9	30-31	9	23-25	9
26-28	10	34-37	10	26-28	10
29-30	11	38-41	11	29-30	11
31-32	12	42-43	12	31-32	12
33-34	13	44-45	13	33-34	13
35-36	14	46-47	14	35-36	14
37-38	15	48-49	15	37-38	15

Although individual medical schools will vary with respect to the scores they require, a standard score of 11 or greater will probably be considered to be quite competitive. A standard score of 7 or less would indicate an area requiring substantial additional preparation. Before taking the next practice test, you should concentrate on areas of low score.

You will also be scoring Science Problems; Skills Analysis: Reading; and Skills Analysis: Quantitative. These will also be converted to standard scores as *approximated by* the tables below.

Science Problems		Skills Analysis: Reading		Skills Analysis: Quantitative	
Raw Score	**Standard Score**	**Raw Score**	**Standard Score**	**Raw Score**	**Standard Score**
0-5	1	0-5	1	0-5	1
6-10	2	6-10	2	6-10	2
11-14	3	11-15	3	11-15	3
15-18	4	16-20	4	16-20	4
19-22	5	21-24	5	21-24	5
23-26	6	25-28	6	25-28	6
27-30	7	29-32	7	29-32	7
31-34	8	33-37	8	33-37	8
35-38	9	38-41	9	38-41	9
39-42	10	42-45	10	42-45	10
43-46	11	46-49	11	46-49	11
47-50	12	50-54	12	50-54	12
51-54	13	55-59	13	55-59	13
55-59	14	60-64	14	60-64	14
60-66	15	65-68	15	65-68	15

Before taking the next practice test, you should consider whether either of these latter three areas requires special attention. The Science Problems may be remediated by additional study and working problems. The two areas of Skills Analysis, however, may require a slightly different approach. Try going back over this part of the examination, reading carefully, and answering the questions again without a time limit. Read the paragraph again and try to determine why you missed certain questions. Be sure to use only the information in the paragraph. Then go on to additional practice examinations. One additional suggestion: Read the questions carefully before answering. Sometimes students answer the question they *expected* rather than the question that was asked. Try to avoid this pitfall.

If you are unable to read at the required rate and comprehension level, then your problem may be more serious. Probably one of the first approaches might be to review some of the reading sections of your Freshman course in English. If your grades in this course were low, you may need to take the course again or arrange for some tutoring.

As you progress through the other practice tests, you should develop facility in working faster to allow completion of each section. Although wild guessing is of no value, it is to your advantage to guess among a select number of answers if you have ruled out some answers.

Remember: we cannot hope to present everything you should have learned in years of study. We can only help you to identify areas of weakness, give some review of important concepts and provide experience and confidence in taking a test utilizing the format of the New Medical College Admission Test. We hope that this will allow you to reach your own potential on this test.

TIMETABLE FOR THE NEW MCAT*

TOTAL TIME: 6 hours, 30 minutes, plus 1 hour for lunch, 20 minutes for breaks

135 minutes	Science Knowledge (125 questions)	38 questions on biology 49 questions on chemistry 38 questions on physics
REST PERIOD		
85 minutes	Science Problems (66 questions)	18 questions on biology 30 questions on chemistry 18 questions on physics
LUNCH		
85 minutes	Skills Analysis: Reading (68 questions)	
REST PERIOD		
85 minutes	Skills Analysis: Quantitative (68 questions)	

*Format subject to change.

SELF-SCORING CHARTS

Model Examination A	Total Possible	Raw Score	MCAT Score
Science Knowledge:			
Biology	______	______	______
Chemistry	______	______	______
Physics	______	______	______
Science Problems	______	______	______
Skills Analysis:			
Reading	______	______	______
Quantitative	______	______	______

Model Examination B	Total Possible	Raw Score	MCAT Score
Science Knowledge:			
Biology	______	______	______
Chemistry	______	______	______
Physics	______	______	______
Science Problems	______	______	______
Skills Analysis:			
Reading	______	______	______
Quantitative	______	______	______

Model Examination C	Total Possible	Raw Score	MCAT Score
Science Knowledge:			
Biology			
Chemistry			
Physics			
Science Problems			
Skills Analysis:			
Reading			
Quantitative			

Model Examination D	Total Possible	Raw Score	MCAT Score
Science Knowledge:			
Biology			
Chemistry			
Physics			
Science Problems			
Skills Analysis:			
Reading			
Quantitative			

TEST PREPARATION AND TEST-TAKING STRATEGIES COMPILED WITH THE HELP OF SUCCESSFUL MEDICAL STUDENTS

During the last 18 years, we have been involved in the training of approximately 5000 medical students; we have explored and discussed with them their test-taking strategies, since prospective medical students, and particularly students who are already in medical school, are probably the best, most efficient, and skillful test takers in the world. They must be good to survive and to cope with the volume of detailed material. To do this, they have learned to recognize key elements and have trained themselves to be hard and cold in their determination to accomplish the task.

Over the years, we have found some common attitudes and methods, which we would like to mention to you. We have met in group discussion with several of our present students, and they have helped us compile their test preparation and test-taking strategies, which they recommend highly.

Test Preparation

A. Key elements in preparation
   1. Study!
   2. Fine-tune your knowledge reservoir!
   3. Be ready—mentally and physically!

B. Review
   Most students did a preliminary review of the material they expected to master before they undertook intensive study. They stressed:
   1. During the time of intensive study, none of the material should appear new. A sense of familiarity with the material being studied usually avoids a feeling of cramming.
   2. Set aside regular time periods for this specific task; do not squeeze it in here and there! Regular time periods increase efficiency and delineate purpose.
   3. Skip superfluous material and adjust to repetitious material.
   4. If you detect major gaps in your knowledge, fill these in. Otherwise, they will bother you and distract you from your effort. *Remember*, it's easier to remember a story than to remember isolated facts.
   5. Study, if you can, in a chronological order! You learn the material this way, and you will feel more comfortable because of the sequence, and you will enhance your recall.
   6. During your studying, vary your attack as required.
      a. Read the material.
      b. Speak out the material.
      c. Write out the material.
      d. Sketch some of the material.
      e. Underline some of the material.
      f. Outline some of the material.
      g. Resort, if necessary, to mnemonic devices.
   7. Understand the material before you commit it to memory.
   8. Organize the material, and learn it in parts rather than in isolated, single details. Try to build a framework of facts.
   9. Note and focus in on similar ideas from different subject matters. Put them meaningfully together, and keep them in association. Integrate your material.

Taking the Examination

1. Get a good night's rest before the examination.
2. Do not change your eating habits if possible.
3. Go through your normal pattern of physical exercises and routines, and take the test in stride, as if it were part of the routine. It's another day's work.
4. Follow directions.
5. Proportion your time.
6. Do not become interested in your surroundings.
7. Do not keep "one eye" on the proctor and the other on your material.
8. Divorce yourself from everything, and let no disturbance influence your concentration.
9. Your eyes should be fixed on the printed page, and your only objective should be to accomplish your task efficiently, with speed and accuracy.
10. Remember that distractions can be internal as well as external; come to the examination having a positive attitude and a sense of pride and accomplishment.
11. Do not become impatient or discouraged if you cannot start at once effectively—most of us need a little warm-up period for our concentration to reach peak level.
12. Be interested in yourself! Self-interest leads to motivation to concentrate; remember, you are working for yourself and for your own future.
13. Do not get annoyed. If you do and your concentration lapses, let up and relax and regroup for a minute—take a quick break.
14. If your annoyance persists, try looking over the material you have successfully completed. Some people recover quickly and remotivate themselves by doing so.
15. Do not become discouraged by an "off-the-wall" question. Skip it and forget it and proceed with vigor. You are not alone.
16. Do not decrease speed because of fear that you might miss something.
17. If you should draw a temporary blank, besides reading, recite the question to yourself, or even write it out—this might help recall—you are utilizing all your senses.
18. Try to visualize the place in the book where this material appeared—this might lead you to relate facts and increase chances of recall. Sometimes, taking your mind completely off the subject might calm your nerves and restore your concentration.
19. Read the complete question before answering it. Check your answers to catch careless mistakes.
20. Do not read into or think too much about a question you feel you have answered correctly—you may arrive at implications not intended by the examiner, and you may more likely change your answer from right to wrong.

Do Your Best, and Good Luck!

David Cohen—Class of 1983, MCV
Nancy Armstrong—Class of 1983, MCV
Alan R. Swajkoski—Class of 1983, MCV
John M. Ogren—Class of 1983, MCV
Nancy Ensley—Class of 1984, MCV
Michael G. Waters—Class of 1985, MCV
Michael S. Glock—Class of 1985, MCV
Linda S. Beahm—Class of 1985, MCV
Martha A. Riggle—Class of 1985, MCV
Joan B. Weber—Class of 1986, MCV

A POSITIVE APPROACH TO ANSWERING QUESTIONS AND TO TEST TAKING

A positive, competitive approach and attitude are qualities of a successful individual. Hand in hand, however, goes a fund in knowledge. Nothing succeeds like knowledge of the subject matter for test taking. Indeed, the suggestions on test taking are all built on knowledge, which is strongly reinforced by your confidence, it, in turn, being supported by an understanding of the process involved in the successful answering of questions.

In this section, several specific questions will be selected from the Model Tests and will be examined not only for content but also for the process involved in the selection of the correct answer.

General Key Rules for Answering Questions

1. Are there specific disclaimers? *Best*, *all*, *none*, or some variety of negatives that separate the correct answer from the multiplicity of possible answers are the types of disclaimers to look for.
2. Are there specific qualifying words or topics that can be underlined? Sometimes these are the same as the disclaimers in item #1.
3. Are there similarities of choices in the answers? These similarities may allow elimination of choices.
4. Can some choices, such as the choice *all of the above*, be eliminated? Sometimes opposite choices help in the selection and in the narrowing down of the answers to one out of two possibilities.
5. If you can, sometimes a quick drawing or a formula will clarify the questions and initiate and aid in recall.
6. Remember, and keep in mind at all times, that all multiple-choice questions are really TRUE or FALSE decisions on a statement. Sometimes, in some cases, when in a quandary, they can best be answered by "I don't know" and "I'll proceed to the next question and not disturb my pace and concentration."
7. *Be Positive!* If you have no good answers for several questions in a row, you positively *must forget them*. Do not dwell on failure, but have confidence in how much you know!

Application of Test-Taking Hints

We will use specific examples and apply our principles.

EXAMPLE: Model Examination B; Chemistry, Question 6

6. Glucose is NOT a (an)
   (A) aldose.
   (B) reducing sugar.
   (C) disaccharide.
   (D) sugar possessing optical activity.
   (E) monosaccharide.

ITEM 1: Note the specific disclaimer *NOT*. This is an obvious and common one in test questions. You should *underline* this word.

ITEM 2: Glucose is the topic of the question and should be *underlined*.

ITEM 3: Similarity or dissimilarity of choices! There is a strong *dissimilarity* between choice "C" (*di*saccharide) and choice "E" (*mono*saccharide). In fact, at this point, the answer is obvious to the knowledgeable individual. Since glucose is a *mono*saccharide, it cannot be a *di*saccharide; for the purpose of analyzation and this review, let us continue.

ITEM 4: Can choices be eliminated? Since both "C" and "E" cannot be true, *one* must be eliminated.

ITEM 5: A quick drawing to stimulate and help recall:

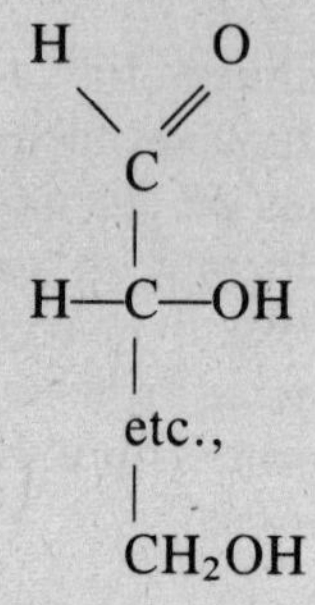

ITEM 6: All multiple-choice questions are TRUE or FALSE statements!

For statement (A): "Glucose is NOT an aldose."

FACT: An aldose is an aldehyde carbohydrate. Look at the structure in item 5! This is indeed an aldehyde:

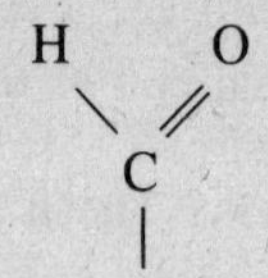

So, the choice is apparently true, but remember the disclaimer *NOT*. In this context, the answer for (A) is FALSE.

For statement (B): "Glucose is NOT a reducing sugar."

FACT: A reducing sugar is one that must be oxidized while reducing a metal ion ($Cu^{2+} \longrightarrow Cu^{+}$) (a gain of electrons is reduction). Remember the disclaimer *NOT*. In this context, the answer for (B) is FALSE.

For statement (C): "Glucose is NOT a disaccharide."

FACT: A disaccharide is a carbohydrate that may be hydrolyzed to a simpler carbohydrate. Carefully examine the sketch. Can this compound be hydrolyzed (split by water) into a smaller carbohydrate? Remember the disclaimer *NOT*. In this context, the answer for (C) is TRUE. During an examination with stress on speed and limited time, you would not wish to continue working on this question. Here, however, to continue the analysation of the process, please go on to the next statement.

For statement (D): "Glucose is NOT a sugar possessing optical activity."

FACT: An optically active compound requires an asymmetric carbon atom and no plane of symmetry. Examine the formula, and note carbon atom 2. Remember the disclaimer *NOT*. In this context, the answer for (D) is FALSE.

For statement (E): "Glucose is NOT a monosaccharide." Note the formula, and the opposite of choice (C). Remember the disclaimer *NOT*. In this context, the answer for (E) is FALSE.

In summary, we arrive at:

(A) FALSE
(B) FALSE
(C) TRUE
(D) FALSE
(E) FALSE

So, the answer is (C). Wow! That's easy if you know all the facts, but what if you don't? Suppose your array of answers was:

(A) FALSE
(B) I DON'T KNOW.
(C) TRUE
(D) FALSE
(E) FALSE

or a variation such as:

(A) I DON'T KNOW.
(B) I DON'T KNOW.
(C) TRUE
(D) I DON'T KNOW.
(E) I DON'T KNOW.

or:

(A) FALSE
(B) FALSE
(C) I DON'T KNOW.
(D) FALSE
(E) FALSE

The answer (C) is obvious in all three sets of answers above. However, what about:

(A) FALSE
(B) I DON'T KNOW.
(C) I DON'T KNOW.
(D) FALSE
(E) FALSE

Without additional information or a hunch or a gut feeling (which is a subliminal input), our advice would be to *let it go!* Pick one of the two, (B) or (C), and move on. You have a 50–50% chance of being right. The more "I don't know" answers for possible choices, the lower the probability of being right. So, for a particular examination, without additional information, decide to *always select* the first "I don't know" answer. This will cut through the random answer position on examinations. Remember that the answers on the key are randomly distributed. By adopting the above system, you put a degree of constancy into your pattern, and you don't float likewise. Your chances are drastically enhanced.

We will look at two more questions from the chemistry section of the first part of Model Examination B, using the same analytical techniques but in a less detailed way.

EXAMPLE: Model Examination B; Chemistry, Question 9

9. Alcohols have higher boiling points than do alkyl halides of the same chain lengths because
   (A) alcohols are more polar.
   (B) alcohols have higher molecular weights.
   (C) alcohols form ethers.
   (D) alcohols form intermolecular hydrogen bonds.
   (E) of all of the above.

KEY WORDS: Underline Alcohols, higher boiling points, alkyl halides, and same chain lengths.

(A) FALSE. Alkyl halides are more polar.
(E) "Of all of the above" can't be true if (A) is FALSE.
(B) FALSE. Halides have higher molecular weights than do alcohols.

(C) FALSE. The statement is true, but this is a chemical property not dealing with the physical property of a boiling point.
(D) TRUE. Compare CH_3OH(b.p.64.5) to CH_3Cl(b.p. −24)

In summary, we arrive at:

(A) FALSE
(B) FALSE
(C) FALSE
(D) TRUE
(E) FALSE

Let us quickly look at another example as we are solidifying our strategy.

EXAMPLE: Model Examination B; Chemistry, Question 38

38. All of the following are true EXCEPT
(A) $pH + pOH = 14$
(B) $(H^+)(OH^-) = 10^{-14}$
(C) $pH = \log \frac{1}{[H^+]}$
(D) the stronger acid has the larger pK_a
(E) the weaker acid has the larger pK_a

Note immediately that (D) and (E) are opposites. So, the focus should be on these.
FACT: $pK = -\log K$; a weaker acid has a smaller pK (i.e., a more negative exponent). Statement (D) is TRUE. Therefore, our answer is (E).

TEST-TAKING STRATEGY FOR THE READING PORTION OF THE EXAMINATION

As you practice, realize that the ability of mastering the reading material is a skill that you can learn and develop.

1. Even though scientific reading, unlike pleasure reading, involves word by word reading, you should coordinate speed and thought processes, and you should read as fast as you think. Backtracking usually interferes with efficient assimilation and processing of information.
2. Even though word by word reading is slower and more tedious, eliminate irrelevant thoughts. You don't want them to intrude just because you believe your mind must have something to think about. Usually, when you don't read fast enough, you preoccupy yourself. Henceforth, poor concentration is the unfortunate result.
3. Usually, poor concentration will lead to poor comprehension, and unnecessarily slow reading can lead to poor concentration and poor comprehension.
4. Don't hold back your thinking processes by unnecessary slow reading. Do not create a gap between reading and thinking.
5. Remember that it's a poor reader who stops too often and pauses too long at each stop.
6. Apply the same concentration whether a selection is long or short.
7. Look astutely for a general impression, main and central thoughts, and implications so that you may draw inferences.
8. Whether you are the original writer or the reader of a selection, you must approach it with the thought of a distinct design and technique used to present a specific subject matter and topic. Look for special effects and results.

9. You can usually identify the main topic of a paragraph by several key words that can be gleaned from the context. These key words could serve as possible titles. Concentrate on *why* certain words are used, and *how* they are used. By concentrating on *why* and *how*, you can establish and follow the main idea. During your reading, you should realize that the paragraph is merely a sum of its parts, as are the spokes that eventually fill the wheel.
10. Central thoughts are usually found in the lead sentence or in the summary sentence, but they may be located in other places and may, at times, be implied rather than stated. Read to understand by focusing on central ideas and units of thought.
11. Exhibit versatility, and adjust to the material.
12. Most of the material you will be confronted with will be familiar and understandable to you. In this context, you must focus on detail and read for specific comprehension and specific meanings. Try to determine the meaning of unfamiliar words as you reason through a selection.
13. Do not decrease speed because of fear that you might miss something, and do not fall into the trap of reading several sentences twice before you proceed.
14. Do not read each sentence as a distinct unit, but utilize each unit to build the paragraph and the selection to create the whole.
15. As you read a selection composed of several paragraphs, reflect whether succeeding paragraphs amplify the ideas or points raised in the preceeding paragraphs or whether they provide an example or illustration of them. If this is not the case, is a qualifier of a point introduced, or is another aspect of the same subject dealt with?
16. Before you answer the whole battery of questions, quickly review the selection again.
17. Under no circumstances should you get yourself involved more deeply than you need with the reading selection and with the task. Don't read into it; answer the questions on the basis of what is presented.

Key Words That Announce Conditions and Should Be Kept in Focus!

1. again, also, accordingly, just as
2. therefore, thus, hence, henceforth
3. for example, for instance, in other words
4. nevertheless, however, notice, but
5. always, at all times, under all circumstances, every time
6. finally, in conclusion, in brief, at last
7. never, not, no, none
8. only, specifically, significantly, importantly, decidingly
9. first, another, and, likewise, as well as, besides
10. despite, although, regardless

New MCAT Science Review

The purpose of this section is to help the student review some key material quickly, to place some of his or her information in perspective and to help identify areas of weakness and strength. No attempt has been made to cover all of the material in the subject matter; but it is hoped that after the student has worked through the practice examinations and has studied the explanations to the questions, this section will amplify for him the highlights and essentials that are expected baseline knowledge for all educated people. A brief presentation such as this cannot cover all areas in sufficient depth. Some areas will be omitted and others will be presented only in a simplified manner. The individual who is well prepared will sometimes recognize compromises that must be taken for the sake of brevity. This section should not be used as a substitute for a good general text in the areas but it should be used as a guide and in conjunction with a text so that the student may efficiently prepare for the MCAT. Again, we urge the student to begin preparation for the examination early and to be conscientious and thorough.

REVIEW OUTLINE

Biology

1. The Cell—Its Structure and Function
   A. Size
   B. Composition of Protoplasm
   C. Properties of the Cell and Protoplasm
   D. Components of a Typical Cell
   E. Cell Reduplication—Mitosis

2. Reproduction, Development, and Heredity
   A. Reproductive Organs
   B. Development
   C. Heredity

3. Nutrition and Digestion
   A. Carbohydrates
   B. Fats
   C. Vitamins
   D. Minerals
   E. Intestinal Tract
   F. Digestive Juices

4. The Endocrine System
   A. The Pituitary Gland
   B. The Thyroid Gland
   C. The Pancreas
   D. The Adrenal Glands

E. The Testes
F. The Ovaries
G. The Placenta
H. The Pineal
I. The Small Intestine

5. The Nervous System
A. Nervous Tissue
B. The Neuron
C. Classification of Neurons
D. Groups of Neurons
E. Organization of the C.N.S.—The Spinal Cord
F. The Spinal Nerves
G. Sensory Pathway
H. Voluntary Motor Pathway
I. Reflex Arc
J. Autonomic Nervous System
K. Cranial Nerves

6. Muscle
A. Classification
B. Structural Organization of a Muscle Fiber
C. Myofilaments
D. Excitation
E. Contraction
F. Muscle Twitch
G. Tetanus
H. Energy Sources

Chemistry

1. General Principles
A. Characteristics of Mixtures and Compounds
B. Reactions
C. Role of Enzymes in a Reaction
D. Molar and Normal Solutions
E. Temperature Conversion Factors
F. Formulas and Laws

2. Organic Chemistry
A. General Considerations
B. The Alkanes
C. The Cycloalkanes
D. The Alkenes
E. The Alkynes
F. Aromatic Compounds
G. The Grignard Reagent
H. Aldehydes and Ketones
I. Carboxylic Acids
J. Ethers

3. Biochemistry
A. Definition
B. Areas of Biochemistry

Physics

1. Accelerated Motion
   A. Falling Objects—Gravity Acceleration
   B. Uniform Velocity
   C. Nonuniform Motion
   D. Uniform Deceleration
   E. Free Fall

2. Forces and Motion
   A. Forces and Acceleration
   B. Weight and Acceleration
   C. Forces Acting Upon Each Other at Right Angles
   D. Forces Acting in the Same Direction

3. Projectile Motion

4. Friction

5. Work and Power
   A. Work and Energy
   B. Power—Units

6. Energy
   A. Potential Energy
   B. Kinetic Energy

7. Momentum

8. Uniform Circular Motion
   A. Centripetal Acceleration
   B. Circular Motion
   C. Centripetal Force
   D. Centrifugal Force

9. Fluids at Rest
   A. Pressure
   B. Density
   C. Specific Gravity

10. Gases
    A. Buoyancy
    B. Pressure and Volume of Gas

11. Temperature Calculations and Measurement

12. The General Gas Law

13. Heat
    A. Specific Heat
    B. Heat Lost = Heat Gained
    C. Heat of Vaporization

14. Thermodynamics
    A. Work and Heat
    B. Specific Heat of a Gas
    C. Efficiency of a Boiler

15. Magnetism

16. Electricity—Ohm's Law

17. Electric Circuits
    A. Emf and Internal Resistance
    B. Resistors in Series
    C. Resistors in Parallel
    D. Cells in Series
    E. Cells in Parallel

18. Electric Energy
    A. Joule's Law
    B. Power and Resistance

19. Machines and Mechanical Advantage
    A. Actual Mechanical Advantage
    B. Theoretical Mechanical Advantage

20. Wavelength

BIOLOGY

The Cell—Its Structure and Function

The cell is the basic unit of structure and function and basis of all life; all cells come from preexisting cells.

Size

Most cells are between 10 and 100μ (micra) in diameter. Measurements are made utilizing the following units:

1 cm = 10 mm
1 mm = 1000μ
1μ = 10,000 Å (angstrom units)

Average sizes of structures may be listed as follows:

cells about	10μ	(100,000 Å)
mitochondria about	1μ	(10,000 Å)
bacteria about	1μ	(10,000 Å)
viruses about	0.1μ	(1,000 Å)
macromolecules about	0.01μ	(100 Å)
molecules about	0.001μ	(10 Å)
hydrogen ion about	0.0001μ	(1 Å)

Resolution is commonly defined as the ability to discriminate two points and visualize them as two points, even though they are extremely close together. With the unaided eye these points might appear as one point, but the microscope can aid in resolving them as two. The resolution is dependent on the wavelength of the light source and can be calculated to be about one-half the wavelength. Examples of resolving power are:

human eye about 0.1 mm (100μ)
light microscope about 0.2μ (2000 Å)
electron microscope about 2–5 Å

Composition of Protoplasm

Protoplasm is made up mainly of proteins, carbohydrates, fats, salts and water; its average elemental composition is:

Oxygen 75+%
Carbon 10+%
Hydrogen 10%
Nitrogen 2+%
Sulfur about 0.2%
Phosphorus about 0.3%
Potassium about 0.3%
Chlorine about 0.1%
less than 0.1%—sodium
calcium
magnesium
iron, etc.

Properties of the Cell and Protoplasm

1. Irritability
2. Conductivity
3. Respiration
4. Absorption
5. Secretion
6. Excretion
7. Growth
8. Reproduction
9. Metabolism

Components of a Typical Cell

Cells are commonly recognized as having two major compartments: *cytoplasm*—includes all components within the cell membrane but outside the nucleus, ana *nucleoplasm*—includes everything within the nuclear membrane.

1. Cell Membrane: The cell membrane, or unit membrane, usually about 75 to 100 Å thick, is a trilaminar structure as observed with the electron microscope. Two protein layers sandwich a bimolecular lipid layer.

Danielli and Davson (1935) are responsible for the model described above; it has now been shown that the two electron dense protein layers (molecules) attach to the hydrophilic poles of the lipid molecules while the clear area is composed of the hydrophobic portion of the lipid molecules. The affinity of the outer layers of the unit membranes for heavy metals (lead salts) that are used as stains in electron microscopy imparts the electron density to them.

Cells must be held together and specialized structures are required. Adjacent cell membranes interdigitate and intercellular cement is utilized.

A desmosome is a specialized area of connection between adjacent cellular membranes (macula adherens).

A terminal bar is a dense area surrounding the apical cellular surface. It includes the tight junction (zona occludens) and the loose junction (zona adherens).

Layers of material (probably mucopolysaccharide) secreted by the cell are found on the surface of the cell. The most prominent layer is the basement membrane or basal lamina. The thick cellulose cell wall of plants falls within the above category. These structures are boundaries and must be traversed by material entering and leaving the cell. The cell membrane is semipermeable.

Microvilli are special adaptations at the apical border of the cell; they function in increasing the surface area and in absorption and resorption. Examples are the striated border and brush border.

2. Cytoplasmic Matrix: The cytoplasm of a cell appears homogeneous, translucent, and structureless; the homogeneous mass, which is also called cell-sap or hyaloplasm, contains inorganic substances and organic compounds of varying molecular sizes. The more peripheral layer of this matrix is also known as ectoplasm (plasmagel). It appears more rigid and seems to lack granules completely.

3. Cellular Inclusions: These may be composed of proteins, fats, carbohydrates, granules, pigments, and crystals.

a. *Secretion granules (products of cell activity).* These are usually membrane-bound products that await extrusion by the cell (exocrine secretion into ducts or endocrine secretion into the extracellular space and capillaries). Release of secretory product from the cells is via exocytosis. Under the general term endocytosis (taking into the cell), are the more specific terms, pinocytosis (taking in of fluid) and phagocytosis (taking in of solids).

b. *Lipid droplets.* These are globular accumulations synthesized by the cell. During periods of need they may serve as a source of energy.

c. *Glycogen granules.* These are small spherical units synthesized by the cell. They serve as storage reservoirs of carbohydrates.

d. *Pigment granules.* These may be of two types: endogenous pigments derived from cell metabolism or exogenous pigments taken in by the cell. Hemosiderin is an example of an exogenous pigment, while the lipochromes and the melanins are endogenous in nature.

e. *Vacuoles.* Under this general term may be classified any membrane-bound globular structure.

f. *Plastids.* The plastids are composed of leucoplasts, chromoplasts and chloroplasts. Leucoplasts resemble chloroplasts but have no chlorophyll; they manufacture starch, oil and protein. Chromoplasts possess pigments and are responsible for the color of flower petals. Chloroplasts possess chlorophyll, which is capable of capturing light energy to produce glucose from CO_2 and H_2O.

4. Mitochondria: Mitochondria are the best known of the cellular organelles. They had been described during the 19th century, notably by Kollicker and Fleming. Altman, using

Janus green, was able to stain them in 1890. Structurally, the mitochondrion is composed of an outer trilaminar membrane and an inner trilaminar membrane; the inner one folds and produces cristae.

Mitochondria are the biochemical powerplants of cells. They recover energy from foodstuffs (via Krebs cycle and respiratory chain) and convert it via phosphorylation into ATP (adenosine triphosphate). In this manner they produce the energy necessary for the metabolic processes. DNA has been found in the mitochondria of animals and the chloroplasts of plants. Mitochondria are capable of division.

5. Endoplasmic Reticulum—Smooth and Rough: This cellular organelle had not been observed by the light microscope; it was first described by Porter, Claude and Fallam in 1945. It is an extensive network of interconnecting channels; when ribosomes line the outer surface, it is designated as rough endoplasmic reticulum.

Rough ER seems to give rise to smooth ER. The endoplasmic reticular membranes are unit membranes (trilaminar).

The RER (rough endoplasmic reticulum) is the synthetic machinery of the cell; messenger RNA influences that machinery, but itself is manufactured in the nucleus. RER is mainly concerned with protein synthesis. SER (smooth endoplasmic reticulum) is mainly concerned with lipid or fat synthesis. In the liver, SER probably plays a significant role in the detoxification of potentially harmful substances.

6. The Golgi Complex: This structure was well known to light microscopists and was first described by Camillo Golgi in 1898.

The Golgi complex is prominent in glandular cells and is thought to function in the production, concentration, packaging, and transportation of secretory material. Important enzyme systems are associated with the membranes (flattened cisternae or round vesicles or sacs) of the Golgi complex. It is thought that substances manufactured by the endoplasmic reticulum are transferred to the Golgi vesicles, processed there, and then stored or released by the cell. The Golgi elaborates polysaccharide moieties.

7. Ribosomes: Ribosomes may be free or attached to the membranes of the endoplasmic reticulum, which is designated then as rough ER. Ribosomes are responsible for synthesis of proteins and other materials of the cell. If ribosomes appear in clusters in the cytoplasm, they are commonly termed polyribosomes or polysomes.

8. Lysosomes: Lysosomes contain acid phosphatase and other hydrolytic enzymes. These enzymes are enclosed by a membrane and are released when needed into the cell or into phagocytic vesicles, and so forth.

The enzymes found in lysosomes are probably manufactured by the endoplasmic reticulum.

9. Microtubules: These structures are usually associated with centrioles and basal bodies. They apparently function in the maintenance of the structural integrity (shape and rigidity) of the cell. Transport of material and movement of cilia and flagella are also ascribed to these organelles.

10. Nucleus: (described by Robert Brown in 1831)

a. *Nuclear envelope*. The nucleus is surrounded by a double-layered membrane which is pierced by small pores. The pores may be sealed by a fine diaphragm; the pores allow a communication whereby materials produced in the nucleus (notably messenger RNA) can pass into the cytoplasm to elicit their effects.

b. *Nuclear material*. Feulgen stained DNA; the nucleolus does not stain Feulgen positive and is composed of RNA. The combination of a purine or pyrimidine, a sugar, and phosphoric acid is called a nucleotide. A polymer of nucleotides is called a nucleic acid. There are two types of nucleic acids, differing mainly in their sugar molecule; DNA contains deoxyribose, and RNA contains ribose.

The nitrogenous bases can be listed as adenine, guanine, thymine, cytosine, and uracil. They pair in the following manner in DNA:

(1.) adenine and thymine
(2.) guanine and cytosine

There are four nitrogenous bases in RNA: adenine pairs with uracil and cytosine pairs with guanine.

The Watson and Crick model clearly illustrates the above pairings. Duplication of this material involves the splitting of the unions between purines and pyrimidines; each nucleotide then acquires a new complementary nucleotide and the phosphate and pentose moieties are then joined enzymatically and the duplication process has taken place.

RNA of the nucleolus provides the vehicle for the coded messages of the nuclear DNA to reach the machinery of the cell. Ribosomal RNA and RNA of the nucleolus are quite similar; ribosomal RNA probably is derived from RNA of the nucleolus. Messenger RNA from the nucleus brings the coded message for protein synthesis to ribosomal RNA. Ribosomal RNA imparts the message to transfer RNA, which carries the specific amino acids to the ribosomes, and protein synthesis is carried out.

Cell Reduplication – Mitosis

For purposes of convenience, mitosis is divided into prophase, metaphase, anaphase, and telophase; the process, however, is a continuous one. The major events during the phases are:

1. **Prophase:** Chromosomes become distinct and nucleolus (nucleoli) disappear(s); centriole(s) and asters and spindle appear; nuclear membrane disappears.

2. **Metaphase:** Chromosomes move to the equator of the cell and duplicate.

3. **Anaphase:** The two chromatids split apart and start migration toward the poles of the spindle; the spindle loses its definition.

4. **Telophase:** Chromosomes lengthen and become less distinct; nucleoli reappear.

The next period of growth and rest is known as *interphase*.

Reproduction, Development, and Heredity

Reproductive Organs

Male: Seminiferous tubules of the testis, epididymis, vas deferens, seminal vesicles, prostate, prostatic urethra, membranous urethra, penile urethra, glans penis.

Female: Ovaries, oviduct, uterus, vagina; the breasts (accessory organs).

Control (hormonal): For a detailed discussion of the hormonal interactions concerning the reproductive system, the reader is referred to the section dealing with the endocrine system. However, the cyclic activity of the female organism is briefly summarized since it is of the utmost importance and quite difficult.

The reproductive cycle is under hormonal regulation; gonadotropic hormones of the pituitary (anterior lobe) stimulate the ovaries to produce a mature egg. The pituitary and ovaries have a reciprocal effect upon each other. FSH (follicle stimulating hormone) from the pituitary elicits estrogen production from the developing follicle. When estrogen concentration reaches a certain blood level, it inhibits FSH production. At that time the egg is discharged and the cells lining the follicle come under the influence of another gonadotropin, LH (luteinizing hormone), which influences the development of the corpus luteum. The corpus luteum produces the hormone progesterone, which influences the wall of the uterus in preparation for implantation. As the concentration of progesterone rises, LH production is checked. If fertilization has occurred, the production of FSH is curtailed throughout the period of gestation through the production of estrogen by the placenta and ovary. If fertilization does not occur, the cycle begins anew.

Meiosis: Since an individual possesses an equal amount of genetic material from both his parents and the same number of chromosomes as either of his parents, a reduction to one half that number has to be accomplished in the development of the egg and sperm. Eggs and sperms are haploid; and a fertilized egg (zygote) possesses the diploid number of the parent again. The reduction occurs during meiosis.

The process of meiosis is best demonstrated in the following manner:

Haploid gametes; either sperm (spermatids) or egg (ova).

1,2 + 1a, 2a

The above unite in fertilization (form zygote) and the diploid adult somatic and primary germ cells are formed.

↓

1, 1a, 2, 2a

Primary germ cell in the adult undergoes gametogenesis (male) or oogenesis (female); the result eventually will be haploid cells.

Tetrad formation

↓

1, 1, 1a, 1a, 2, 2, 2a, 2a

The first meiotic or reduction division occurs next, and results in the following:

↓

1, 1a, 2, 2a + 1, 1a, 2, 2a

Meiosis II occurs now and four haploid cells are produced.

↓

1, 2 1a, 2a 1, 2 1a, 2a

Even though we have not indicated it, random assortment does take place during the process and chromosome combinations other than those illustrated are possible. In the human male four functional cells (sperms) are produced while in the human female one functional cell (egg) and three polar bodies are produced. This is the general gamut of the process of meiosis.

Types of Eggs: Isolecithal eggs are primitive and have a small amount of yolk that is distributed equally; examples are sea urchin eggs and amphioxus eggs. Telolecithal eggs have a large amount of yolk concentrated at one pole (lower or vegetal pole); examples are fish, amphibia, reptile, and bird eggs. Centrolecithal eggs show a concentration of yolk in their center; insect eggs are the prime example.

Semen: Semen is a fluid secreted by the male accessory sex glands, namely, the prostate, seminal vesicles, and bulbo-urethral glands. Fructose is added by the prostate, as are acid phosphatase, citric acid, calcium, and fibrinolysin. The seminal vesicles add phosphorylcholine. The vas deferens is just a tube through which sperm are transported from the testes to the urethra. Between 3 and 4 ml of semen comprise one ejaculation, which contains between 300 and 400 million sperm cells.

Chromosomes: Forty-four autosomal chromosomes are present in every diploid cell of the human body. Gametes, however, are haploid. The total chromosome number of the human being is 46 (male 44 plus X and Y; female 44 plus X and X).

Placenta: The placenta attached to the uterus of the female is the organ through which the fetus receives its nourishment, oxygen supply, certain immunological factors, and so forth, and rids itself of its waste products.

Fertilization: Fertilization can occur anywhere in the female reproductive tract and sometimes even in the peritoneal cavity. Usually, however, fertilization takes place in the upper one-third of the oviduct.

Hyaluronidase is an enzyme carried by sperm, capable of hydrolysis of hyaluronic acid, promoting fertilization (penetration of sperm). Hyaluronidase is medically used to promote the diffusion and absorption of many injected medications.

Twinning: Identical twins arise from the same egg. One egg is fertilized by one sperm and a splitting (separation) occurs during the early cleavage divisions. Fraternal twins arise from the fertilization of two eggs, each by one sperm. Identical twins always have the same sex. Fraternal twins may or may not have the same sex (50-50 proposition).

Other Modes of Reproduction: Budding, as in hydra, involves the multiplication of cells in one region of the organism and the organization of these cells into a new individual.

Binary fission or mitosis is a division of a cell into two equal parts and in this respect two new organisms (cells).

Parthenogenesis involves a mechanism in which a single cell is set apart for the purpose of reproduction. This cell has the capability to develop into a new organism.

A hermaphrodite possesses both male and female reproductive tissue.

Development

Development in animals results from the cleavage divisions of the zygote. The zygote divides first into two cells, then these divide into four, and so on, until it becomes a cell mass called the morula. Through more divisions the morula becomes a hollow ball of cells which is called the blastula. Cleavage has produced a single-layered blastula. Gastrulation is the next phase of development and in this phase the three-layered embryo is established. The next phase is the stage of organogenesis during which the various organ systems are formed. The basic derivatives of the three germ layers are listed below.

Embryonic membranes play a big role in the development of embryos of reptiles, birds, and mammals. The amnion surrounds the embryo; amniotic fluid fills the space between the embryo and the amnion and bathes and protects the fetus. The allantois serves to collect wastes in some cases; the yolk sac furnishes nutrients in some cases (they are outgrowths from the intestinal tract); and the chorion envelopes all the membranes discussed.

Derivatives of Germ Layers: In general the major derivatives of the germ layers are as follows:

1. *mesoderm* gives rise to connective tissue, bone and cartilage; both striated and smooth muscle; blood and lymph cells and the walls of the vascular channels; kidneys; gonads; and spleen.

2. *ectoderm* gives rise to the epidermis, the hypophysis, the central and peripheral nervous system, the epithelium of the sense organs, and the epithelial lining of some other organs.

3. *endoderm* gives rise to tonsils, thyroid, parathyroids, thymus, liver and pancreas; epithelial lining of gut; respiratory tract; and urinary bladder.

Blue Baby: A blue baby has a blue hue of the skin due to the mixing of oxygenated and non-oxygenated blood in the circulation. This mixing comes about because either the foramen ovale or the ductus arteriosus or both have failed to close. The foramen ovale is the opening between the right and left atria; the ductus arteriosus is a connection between the left pulmonary artery and the arch of the aorta.

Heredity

Chromosomes within the nucleus of the cells are the source of the inheritable material; chromosomes contain specific units called genes which are arranged in linear order on the chromosomes. Genes are paired elements, held together in a specific linkage arrangement. One member of each pair of genes separates during germ cell production; therefore, each germ cell contains only one set. An allele is one of a pair of genes that occupies the same locus on homologous chromosomes. Genotype refers to the genetic make-up of the organism. The genotype is expressed via phenotypic characteristics that are visible and observable under normal circumstances.

Mendel is responsible for the discovery of several intriguing phenomena:

1. He showed that each member of a pair of genes will be found in a different gamete; they were contributed to that individual by his parents and underwent no change such as blending while they were associated. This is Mendel's first law (law of segregation) which affirms that *allelomorphs segregate*.

2. Mendel also documented that the distribution of members of one pair has absolutely no bearing on the distribution of another pair. For example, if an individual possesses one pair of alleles Y and y, and another pair Z and z, the individual will produce approximately equal numbers of gametes of the four possible chance combinations of one member from each pair (YZ; Yz; yZ; yz). This law is known as independent assortment; the law does not apply to linked genes but only to genes located on different chromosomes. Independent behavior of chromosomes during meiosis is essential.

Mendel also showed that certain characteristics mask other traits; this phenomenon is known as dominance.

Genetic phenomena are best explained and demonstrated by problem solving, and it will be attempted in this manner.

Dominance: Dominance is expressed in terms of a pair of alleles. A gene which produces and expresses the same characteristic whether it is present alone (in the heterozygous state matched to a gene not possessing the same trait) or with a gene possessing the same trait (in the homozygous state) is said to be dominant to the allele with which it is paired. The allele which is ineffective in the expression of its trait in the heterozygote is said to be recessive to the dominant. Let us illustrate with the following example.

The trait of green eyes did not occur in the F_1 (offspring from parents) but made its appearance in the F_2 (offspring of F_1 or offspring of offspring from the parents) generation. We are dealing with a recessive trait that is being masked by a dominant one. AA (brown eyes) bred with aa (green eyes) results in all F_1, Aa (genotypically heterozygous but phenotypically A; all brown eyes). Breeding of the offspring Aa with Aa results in 1 AA 2 Aa 1aa genotype and 3:1 phenotype. The above demonstrates a one factor cross.

Let us now demonstrate several typical two factor crosses:

1. Crossing of two types of organisms yields the classical 9:3:3:1 ratio. The cross would be considered an expression of phenotypic ratio.

The example calls for a cross between individuals possessing a genetic makeup of RrSs × RrSs. Construct the Punnett square below and see the results in a 9:3:3:1 phenotypic ratio.

	RS	Rs	rS	rs
RS	RRSS	RRSs	RrSS	RrSs
Rs	RRSs	RRss	RrSs	Rrss
rS	RrSS	RrSs	rrSS	rrSs
rs	RrSs	Rrss	rrSs	rrss

R_S_ or RS = 9
R_ss or Rss = 3
rrS_ or rrS = 3
rrSS or rrss = 1

2. In rabbits, rough coat is dominant over smooth coat. Brown is dominant over grey fur color. A rough, brown male is mated to a couple of smooth, grey females. The offspring are counted as: 18 rough, brown; 21 rough, grey; 16 smooth, brown; 24 smooth, grey. If this male had been mated to a female of his own genotype, what proportion of the offspring would have exhibited rough, grey coats? The answer is 3 out of 16 and is obtained in the following manner.

Basic genetic knowledge is applied.

rough	=	(dominant)
smooth	=	(recessive)
brown	=	(dominant)
grey	=	(recessive)

The male is crossed to several smooth grey females; they had to be homozygous recessive genotype. Since all four combinations appeared, we can assume that the male was genotypically heterozygous even though he appeared phenotypically dominant. If first we crossed this heterozygous male RrBb × rrbb, the result would be RrBb; Rrbb; rrBb; rrbb; in other words the four combinations given. Now let us cross the RrBb male × RrBb female; the following combinations would have to be considered in both male and female: RB; Rb; rB; rb. If these are crossed, we find 3 out of 16 possess rough grey coats (namely RRbb; Rrbb and Rrbb).

Incomplete Dominance: Seeds from a self-pollinated gold flowering plant produce 56 charcoal, 130 gold and 61 beige flowering plants. The plant is heterozygous with incomplete dominance of its traits.

The phenomenon illustrated here is incomplete dominance (blending of two traits). Let us assume:

		charcoal C
		beige B
		gold BC
Cross:	→	BC × BC
Result:		1 BB (beige)
		2 BC (gold)
		1 CC (charcoal)

Backcross: A backcross consists of crossing a dominant phenotype with a pure homozygous recessive. In this manner a breeder can determine if the phenotype is heterozygous or homozygous. The backcross is used, therefore, to determine if a line is genotypically pure.

Probability Ratios: Genetic ratios are probability ratios. If, for example, we mate (B = black dominant; b = grey recessive) two heterozygous black squirrels (Bb) and 4 offspring are produced, the ratio of 3 black and 1 grey should be probable. However, what are the chances of all black and all grey litters?

Many crosses of heterozygous (Bb) animals will result in a fairly close 3:1 ratio. We, therefore, can see that we have 3 chances out of 4 to produce an individual exhibiting the dominant trait, and 1 chance out of 4 to show the recessive trait.

Therefore, to produce black squirrels (BB or Bb, 3 out of 4) we multiply $\frac{3}{4} \times \frac{3}{4} \times \frac{3}{4} \times \frac{3}{4} = 81/256$; to produce grey squirrels (bb, 1 out of 4) we multiply $\frac{1}{4} \times \frac{1}{4} \times \frac{1}{4} \times \frac{1}{4} = 1/256$.

Polygenic Traits: In morning glories, genes C and P are necessary for pink flowers. In the absence of either (ccP__ or C__pp) or both (ccpp) of these genes, the flowers are blue. What will be the result of the following crosses as far as flower color of the offspring and proportion of the offspring are concerned? Cross a. Ccpp × ccPp = 1 pink : 3 blue; b. ccpp × CcPp = 1 pink : 3 blue.

In essence the expression of pink requires C__ P__, and all others will be blue. The offspring may be Cc or cc with equal probability (i.e., 50%); the same is true for Pp and pp (50%). If the chance of C__ is 0.5 and the chance of P__ is 0.5, then the chance of C__ P__ is $0.5 \times 0.5 = 0.25$. Thus, ¼ will be pink and ¾ will be blue.

Sex Determination: A male carries a XY and a female a XX complement of chromosomes. If a male embryo were to result, the sperm that fertilizes an egg would have to possess a Y chromosome.

Sex Linked Traits: Both sexes carry a complete complement of sex-linked genes. A female, however, with the XX arrangement will only exhibit a recessive gene if it has received it from both parents (a rare event if we are dealing with an uncommon gene of the population) while in the male with the XY arrangement the recessive gene cannot be masked since there is no partner X chromosome and, therefore, a larger number of recessive genes are expressed (examples are hemophilia and color blindness). A man receives his X chromosome from his mother and passes it on to his daughters not his sons. His daughters in this respect are the carriers of his sex-linked traits and their sons will be the affected ones. Let us illustrate with an example. The normal czarinas of Russia produced sons suffering from hemophilia, a disease that is caused by a sex-linked recessive gene, h. The more dominant gene, H, produces normal blood clotting. Genotypically, these women must have carried Hh (X_H and X_h). A daughter, depending on the father (X_HY or X_hY), could have carried X_HX_h or X_HX_H while a son could have been born with either an X_HY or an X_hY (hemophilic) chromosomal complement.

Another way of expressing a sex-linked or, strictly speaking, sex-limited phenomenon is shown in the example below.

A cattle breeder has in his herd a y-linked trait which produces white stockings. A calf sired by a white-stockinged bull is born. The breeder determines that the chances of white stockings by this inheritance are 50%. If the calf born had been a female, the chances of exhibiting the trait (or serving as a carrier) were zero. The explanation is that the male may contribute gametes containing either X or Y chromosomes, but the female can contribute only gametes containing X chromosomes. If the X chromosome is contributed by the male, an unaffected female offspring will result; if the Y chromosome is contributed by the male, an affected male offspring will result. These two possibilities are of equal probability (i.e., 50%). If the sex of the offspring is known, there is no doubt about whether it has the trait. All males (100%) and no females (0%) would have the trait. Females could not even be carriers for a Y-linked trait.

Mutation: A mutation may be thought of as a sudden change in the genetic makeup of the organism. It may be beneficial or harmful. It may occur spontaneously or may be experimentally produced with chemicals, X-rays, cosmic rays, and so forth. It may or may not be passed on to the next generation because, for example, it may be lethal or otherwise preclude reproduction.

Blood Types: The ABO blood grouping system is explained on the basis of a single triallelic system with genes A, B, and O operating at a single genetic locus. Phenotypic and genotypic characteristics may be expressed as follows:

Phenotype	Genotype
A	A/A; A/O
B	B/B; B/O
O	O/O
AB	A/B

The A and B genes appear to be codominant; they are dominant over O, which is recessive.

As can be seen from the above table, there are four major blood types and the explanation as to universal donor and recipient is based on the following:

Type	Agglutinogens on Cells	Agglutinins in Serum and Plasma
AB—can receive A, B, AB or O (universal recipient)	A, B	none
A —can receive A, O	A	anti b
B —can receive B, O	B	anti a
O —can receive only O, but can give to all; therefore, O is the universal donor	O	anti ab

Rh Factor: Rhesus (Rh) agglutinogen is present in humans and is represented by a dominant gene R. The agglutinogen of an Rh positive fetus passes across the placenta, enters the maternal blood stream, and elicits the production of an agglutinin (antibody) by the mother. The agglutinin passes into the circulation of the fetus and if present in sufficient concentration can produce agglutination, at times fatal to the developing fetus.

Nutrition and Digestion

The environment must supply its organisms with adequate nutrients via the food supply. Organisms require the basic elements making up protoplasm, the enzymes that catalyze and control the metabolic activity, and vitamins and hormones that have profound effects on the overall function of the system. Elements that are needed in very small quantities are called trace elements. No organism is independent of the environment, but on nutritional self-sufficiency we can classify organisms into autotrophs and heterotrophs. Heterotrophs include all animals; autotrophs include all those that carry out photosynthesis and can manufacture organic constituents from inorganic material. Although all organisms require intake of nutrients, we shall confine this discussion to nutrition and digestion in higher animals (particularly humans).

Few free amino acids are available in the diet. Amino acid intake is primarily in the form of proteins (high molecular weight heteropolymers of amino acids). Amino acids are necessary for the production and maintenance of protoplasm. Certain amino acids are denoted as essential in all higher animals; these are: L-leucine; L-methionine; L-phenylalanine; L-valine; L-lysine; L-isoleucine; L-threonine and L-tryptophan. In the rat, however, all of the above eight plus histidine and arginine are essential. Among the nonessential amino acids (synthesized by the organism) are glycine, alanine, serine, cystine, tyrosine, and proline. Not all proteins have a complete complement of all amino acids; therefore, dietary intake must be adjusted to meet the needs of the organism.

Unit for Measuring Value of Foods: The calorie is the unit of heat used in measuring the value of foods for producing heat and energy in the human body. It is equivalent to the amount of heat that is required to raise the temperature of one kilogram of water one degree Celsius.

Carbohydrates

Of primary importance in human nutrition are the monosaccharides, disaccharides, and polysaccharides. Monosaccharides ordinarily are simple 5- or 6-carbon sugars; they cannot be broken down into smaller units. Common examples are glucose and fructose.

Disaccharides are formed by the union of two 6-carbon monosaccharides and thus contain 12 carbons; they can be broken down by hydrolysis into their component hexose sugars. Common examples are sucrose (containing glucose and fructose) and lactose (containing glucose and galactose). Polysaccharides are large molecules formed by the union of many monosaccharides; they can be broken down into their respective monosaccharides. Common examples are glucose polymers, starch, and glycogen.

Fats

Fats may be grouped into simple lipids, compound lipids, and lipids derived from simple and compound lipids by hydrolysis. Fats are composed of three fatty acid molecules joined to a molecule of glycerol. Simple lipids are esters of fatty acids with various alcohols. Waxes possess alcohols other than glycerol. Cholesterol esters are a combination of fatty acids and sterol alcohols such as cholesterol. Compound lipids are composed of esters of fatty acids and glycerol; they also incorporate other chemical groups. Derived lipids are obtained by hydrolysis of simple and compound lipids and can be grouped into free fatty acids, alcohols, and sterol alcohols. Fatty acids may be either saturated or unsaturated. The unsaturated fatty acids may contain cis or trans double bonds, but cis double bonds are more common.

Vitamins

Vitamins are organic substances which are needed in minute quantities; vitamins often play a role as part of an enzyme system. Vitamins are used up in the metabolic activities and must be constantly replaced; the organism, however, is not capable of synthesizing a vitamin (at least in sufficient quantities) and must obtain it from the outside. Autotrophs have no requirement like heterotrophs for vitamins. Deficiency of a vitamin reduces the metabolic efficiency of the process which depends on it and symptoms arise for the deficiency diseases. Most deficiency diseases in the young will lead to stunting. Vitamins can be grouped into fat-soluble and water-soluble substances.

Fat-soluble Vitamins:

1. *Vitamin A*. This vitamin is formed from the carotenoid provitamins (yellow pigments of most vegetables and fruits). Deficiency in man causes poor dark vision adaptation, conjunctivitis and keratinization of the cornea.
2. *Vitamin D*. This vitamin does not occur naturally and is manufactured in the animal body by the utilization of ultraviolet light. Deficiency in humans mainly affects bones and teeth; in the child, rickets and in the adult, osteomalacia are consequences. The vitamin enhances the absorption of calcium and phosphorus from the intestinal tract.
3. *Vitamin E*. This vitamin is essential for normal reproduction in a variety of animals. Deficiency causes non-motility of sperm (sterility) and general loss of sexual instincts in the male. In the female, while conception and early embryological development are not impaired, about halfway through the pregnancy the fetus will abort. In the human the need for this vitamin is unclear.
4. *Vitamin K*. This vitamin is necessary for the production of prothrombin and thus for normal blood clotting to occur. Deficiency causes abnormally long clotting times and hemorrhage.

Water-soluble Vitamins:

1. *Thiamine (Vitamin B_1)*. This vitamin is essential for the proper functioning of the nervous system; it is an antagonist to acetylcholine. Deficiency will result in beriberi in humans and polyneuritis in birds.
2. *Riboflavin (Vitamin B_2)*. Riboflavin functions in the conversion of tryptophan to nicotinic acid. No recognized disease is associated with a deficiency. General problems with vision, skin, coordination and growth do occur.
3. *Niacin (Nicotinic acid)*. Niacin is the functional group of the coenzymes NAD and NADP. Deficiency results in blacktongue in canines and pellagra in humans. Dermatitis and neurological lesions are manifestations of pellagra. As noted above, tryptophan may be converted to nicotinic acid.

4. *Pyridoxine (Vitamin B_6)*. This vitamin is essential for the complete metabolism of tryptophan. The most common symptom of a deficiency is a seborrheic dermatitis.

5. *Cobalamin (Vitamin B_{12})*. This vitamin is essential for normal development of red blood cells. Anemia is a sign of deficiency.

6. *Ascorbic acid (Vitamin C)*. This vitamin is essential for the formation of intercellular substances in the animal body. Scurvy is the classical deficiency disease attributed to lack of this compound in the diet.

Minerals

Minerals are also utilized by the tissues of the body. Among the most common ones found on the label of a bottle of vitamin and mineral supplements are calcium, phosphorus, potassium, sodium, magnesium, chlorine, manganese, iodine, iron, zinc, copper, cobalt, bromine and fluorine. Except in unusual circumstances, of course, these will be in the normal diet and need not be taken in pills.

Intestinal Tract

The parts of the human intestinal tract may be listed in the following order:

1. oral cavity (receives salivary gland secretions)
2. esophagus
3. cardiac sphincter
4. stomach
5. pyloric sphincter
6. duodenum (receives bile and pancreatic secretions)
7. jejunum (absorption of nutrients)
8. ileum (absorption of nutrients)
9. cecum
10. ascending colon (water absorption takes place in the colon)
11. transverse colon
12. descending colon
13. sigmoid colon
14. rectum
15. anal sphincter

Digestive Juices

1. Ptyalin or salivary amylase is produced by the parotid glands, the submandibular glands, and the sublingual glands (salivary glands). Starch, its substrate, is broken up into molecules of the disaccharide maltose and eventually into glucose.

2. The gastric mucosa secretes hydrochloric acid, mucin and the enzymes rennin, pepsin and lipase. An average of 2 to 3 liters is secreted within a 24-hour time period. The pH of gastric juice usually varies from 0.9 to 1.5. This acidity allows pepsin to act while it inhibits ptyalin (salivary amylase). Food usually remains in the stomach for 3 to 4 hours.

Rennin is secreted by the stomach. This enzyme splits some peptide bonds in casein to produce a calcium-precipitable paracasein.

Pepsin is a proteinase of gastric juice derived from its precursor pepsinogen, which is secreted by the chief cells of the gastric mucosa. Pepsin acts upon protein substrates, breaking them down to amino acids, proteoses, and peptones.

3. Pancreatic juice contains proteolytic, lipolytic, and amylolytic enzymes. Pancreatic amylase is an enzyme which hydrolyzes starch to maltose.

Steapsin or pancreatic lipase facilitates the digestion of fats.

Trypsinogen is secreted by the pancreas and converted to the active enzyme trypsin, by enterokinase. Trypsin's substrates are proteins but specifically it further disintegrates proteoses and peptones.

Chymotrypsinogen is the precursor in pancreatic juice of the enzyme chymotrypsin. Trypsin is active in this conversion. Chymotrypsin acts with trypsin to hydrolyze proteins and protein products to polypeptides and amino acids.

4. Bile is secreted by the liver, stored and concentrated in the gall bladder and poured into the duodenum. It primarily contains bile salts, cholesterol, lecithin, pigments, and mucin. It aids in the emulsification, digestion, and absorption of fat. It also contributes to the alkalinization of the intestines.

Lacteals are found in the villi of the small intestines; they are part of the lymphatic system and function to take up chyle containing fat in lipoproteins.

5. Enzymes have been mentioned in the digestive process; although no detailed discussion is contemplated, the reader should be aware that enzymes are proteins and are influenced by:

a. *Temperature:* They are inactivated usually above 60°C. Rate of reaction is controlled as in any chemical reaction; the rate is approximately doubled by each 10°C increase. Low temperatures slow the reaction.

b. *pH:* There is an optimum pH (or pH range) for every reaction.

c. *Poisons:* Some enzymes themselves can be harmful to the organism, but they are also susceptible to compounds like cyanide, which inactivate them.

d. *Concentration:* The rate of reaction is directly proportional to the amount of enzyme present in relation to substrate. If a coenzyme or specific activator is required, that substance may also control the overall rate of the reaction.

The Endocrine System

Two systems modulate, integrate, and control the activities of the body; they are the nervous and endocrine systems. The response in nervous control is rapid while control via the endocrine system is fairly slow and longer lasting. The endocrine glands are ductless glands and secrete their products, called hormones, into the capillaries (bloodstream). Hormones are substances that are secreted into the bloodstream and travel to their target organs to elicit their effects. The product of the target organ may also feed back upon the organ that stimulated its activity and production and manipulate in this respect its cycle of function. It may shut off the supply of stimulating hormone; this activity is called a negative feedback. The controlling mechanism can be thought of as a neuro-endocrine-somatic tissue relationship, or the brain affecting the pituitary gland, which in turn affects the target organs, which then elicit their effect upon the body tissues and cells. Hormones cannot be classified into one chemical class; they are, however, all organic substances and may be proteins, peptides, amino acids (or amino acid derivatives), and steroids, or prostaglandins (derivatives of essential fatty acids). Generally the glands which produce protein hormones embryologically originate from the alimentary tract; they are the anterior pituitary, thyroid, parathyroids, and pancreas. Glands which produce steroid products are derived from the celomic mesothelium and are the testes, ovaries, and adrenal cortex. Glands whose products are small molecular weight amines arise from cells of nervous tissue derivation and are the neurohypophysis and the adrenal medulla.

It is the purpose of this chapter to give the student a brief description of each endocrine organ, its products, and the results of hypo- and hypersecretion.

The Pituitary Gland

The pituitary gland is commonly divided into an anterior and a posterior lobe according to origin. The anterior lobe (adenohypophysis) originates from the oral epithelium of the roof of the mouth in the embryo (Rathke's pouch) while the posterior lobe (neurohypophysis) is a downgrowth of the floor of the brain (in relation to the third ventricle and the hypothalamic areas).

Three cell types are found in the anterior lobe: chromophobes 50%; acidophils 40%; basophils 10%. Chromophobes are considered to be resting cells.

Hormones Secreted by Acidophils (Alpha Cells):

1. *Somatotropic hormone (STH)*
   a. Stimulates general body growth
   b. Hypersecretion—before ossification is complete, giantism
   —after ossification is complete, acromegaly
   c. Hyposecretion—dwarfism
2. *Lactogenic hormone* or luteotrophic hormone (LTH) or prolactin
   a. Promotes growth of breast which was already stimulated by estrogen and progesterone, especially during the last trimester of pregnancy
   b. Promotes and maintains lactation
   c. Helps in the maintenance of the corpus luteum
   d. Promotes maternal instinct

Hormones Secreted by Basophils (Beta and Delta Cells):

1. *Beta cells*
   a. Thyroid stimulating hormone (TSH)
      (1.) Stimulates the thyroid gland to produce its hormones T_3 (triiodothyronine) and T_4 (tetraiodothyronine or thyroxin)
      (2.) Modulates the iodide trapping mechanisms
      (3.) Hypersecretion—goiter, exophthalmos
      (4.) Hyposecretion—diminished thyroid function and lethargy
   b. Adrenocorticotropic hormone (ACTH)
      (1.) Stimulates the adrenal cortex to produce glucocorticoids (cortisol, etc.)
      (2.) Does *not* stimulate mineralocorticoid activity (aldosterone production)
      (3.) Affects production of adrenal androgens
   c. Melanocyte stimulating hormone (MSH) or intermedin
      (1.) Function poorly understood in humans
      (2.) This hormone causes the dispersion of pigment in the chromatophores of the skin of cold-blooded vertebrates and a darkening of the skin results; the action of MSH allows for quick changes in the skin color in response to changes in the external environment.
2. *Delta cells*
   a. Luteinizing hormone (LH) in female
   Interstitial cell stimulating hormone (ICSH) in male
      (1.) In the female this hormone is necessary for preovulatory development of the ovarian follicle, ovulation, and formation of the corpus luteum.
      (2.) In the female it modulates the production of estrogen and progesterone.
      (3.) In the male this hormone stimulates the interstitial cells of the testes, which results in a secretion of testicular androgens.
   b. Follicle stimulating hormone (FSH)
      (1.) In the female this hormone stimulates the growth of the ovarian follicle.
      (2.) In the male FSH stimulates the testes to produce sperm (spermatogenesis).

Hormones of the Neurohypophysis:

The posterior lobe or neurohypophysis develops from the floor of the third ventricle of the brain. The function of this portion of the pituitary gland is to store and release the hormones oxytocin (produced by the paraventricular nucleus of the hypothalamus) and vasopressin or antidiuretic hormone (ADH, produced by the supraoptic nucleus of the hypothalamus).

1. *Oxytocin*

a. Stimulates the contraction of the smooth muscle of the uterus and may play some role in the initiation of labor

b. Stimulates the ejection of milk by affecting the myoepithelial cells of the breast tissue (mammary gland)

2. *Vasopressin; antidiuretic hormone (ADH)*

a. Acts upon the renal tubules to aid water resorption and thereby restricts diuresis; a lack of hormone results in the condition known as diabetes insipidus.

The Pituitary Portal System: In humans the pituitary gland receives its blood supply via the right and left superior and the right and left inferior pituitary arteries from the internal carotid artery system. These vessels supply the hypothalamic areas, the pituitary stalk, and the posterior lobe. The anterior lobe, however, receives no arterial blood supply. The entire blood supply to the anterior lobe is derived from the pituitary portal veins. These veins arise from the capillary network of the median eminence and the infundibular stem. The vascular tufts of the primary capillary system are in close relationship with the nerve endings of the hypothalamo-hypophyseal tract. It is hypothesized that upon excitation these nerve fibers liberate their secretory products into this system, which then, via the portal veins, transports these neurosecretory products to the sinusoids of the anterior lobe. It is in this manner that the activity of the anterior lobe is governed by the hypothalamic areas.

The Thyroid Gland

The thyroid gland is derived from the pharynx (the foramen cecum of the tongue). Its structural unit is the follicle; the follicle is composed of a unit of epithelial cells that surround a colloid space. Colloid is located extracellularly and contains thyroglobulin. The function of the thyroid gland is to produce colloidal material which contains the thyroid hormones (T_3—triiodothyronine and T_4—thyroxin) which affect the rate of metabolism of all the tissues of the body.

The iodides consumed in our food and water are absorbed and carried to the iodide pool in the extracellular fluid via the circulatory system. Five basic events can be identified in thyroid hormone production: a. trapping iodide; b. oxidation of iodide to organic iodine; c. synthesis of hormone; d. storage of hormone as the thyroglobulin moiety in the follicle; and e. release of the hormone into the circulation. TSH from the anterior pituitary influences greatly the trapping mechanism; thiocyanates block this mechanism while thiouracil blocks the oxidation and synthetic steps. These compounds are classified as antithyroid agents.

The production of the hormone thyrocalcitonin has just recently been implicated with the parafollicular cells of the thyroid gland. This hormone is an antagonist of parathyroid hormone and its functions are to lower the serum calcium level and to enhance the deposition of calcium in bone.

Action of Thyroid Hormone:

1. *Controls the rate of metabolism.*
2. *Controls the growth, maturation, and differentiation of the organism.*
3. *Influences nervous system activity.*

Problems Associated with Thyroid Function:

1. *Cretinism.* Congenital failure of proper development of the thyroid gland. The cretin is a dwarf physically and mentally.

2. *Myxedema.* Acquired thyroid deficiency in the adult. This deficiency can be of two types:

a. Thyroid deficiency due to thyroidectomy, neoplasms, thyroiditis, and so forth.

b. A pituitary deficiency in the secretion of TSH.
The thyroid in these cases appears atrophic, hard, and fibrous. The clinical picture is the presentation of a patient who is fairly heavy, phlegmatic, and devoid of expression; his skin is rough and dry and sensitive to cold. The patient is sluggish mentally and physically. Laboratory tests would show a low basal metabolic rate, low protein bound iodine, and a high serum cholesterol level.

3. *Goiter*. Any enlargement of the gland not due to neoplasm or inflammatory disease. Endemic goiters are due to lack of intake of iodine caused by deficiency in the soil and water. This results in increased TSH production, thyroid compensatory hypertrophy, and eventual exhaustion of the gland.

4. *Hyperthyroidism*. Increased activity by the organ. The patient exhibits loss of weight, nervousness, irritability, increased metabolic rate, rapid heart rate, sweating, and so forth. Exophthalmos, a protrusion of the eyeballs, is exhibited and thought to be due to an increased production of TSH. Hyperthyroidism may be an adjunct to the development of a goiter or may arise *de novo*.

The Parathyroid Glands: There are usually four parathyroid glands which are in relation to the thyroid gland. The parathyroid glands produce parathyroid hormone, which governs the metabolism of calcium and phosphorus. The parathyroids are essential to life; their removal will result in cramps, convulsions, tremors, and death due to tetany. The condition is due to the increased irritability of the muscular and nervous system caused by the decrease of calcium levels in the blood and body fluids. The activity of the parathyroids depends on the level of ionized calcium in the serum.

Problems Associated with Parathyroid Function:

1. *Hypoparathyroidism*. This condition will result in a decrease of urinary excretion of phosphorus and its concomitant rise in the serum; this results in a shift in the calcium-phosphorus serum levels and a decline in calcium resorption from bone. The fall in serum calcium will produce tetany. Low serum levels of calcium may also be influenced by deficient intake of calcium, deficiency of vitamin D in the diet, problems with intestinal absorption or increased demand for calcium during pregnancy.

2. *Hyperparathyroidism*. Tumor is the most frequent cause of this condition. In this condition urinary phosphorus excretion is elevated and serum levels are decreased. Calcium resorption from bone is increased and serum levels rise. The glomerular filtrate is saturated and stones may form. Secondary renal disease may occur.

The Pancreas

The pancreas is both an endocrine and exocrine gland. The endocrine portion to be discussed is located in the islets of Langerhans. The function of the islets of Langerhans is to produce insulin by the beta cells and glucagon by the alpha cells. A deficiency of insulin production results in the disease known as diabetes mellitus (elevated blood sugar level). The beta cells do not seem to depend upon any outside trophic influences and the primary physiologic stimulus for insulin production seems to be the level of the blood sugar.

Insulin promotes the removal of glucose from the blood and also the conversion of glucose to glycogen in muscle and liver. It increases the rate of oxidation of glucose in the tissues, the conversion of carbohydrates into fats, the mobilization of fatty acids from adipose tissue, and the rate of protein synthesis.

Glucagon is the glycogenolytic hormone produced by the alpha cells of the pancreas; its principal action is to stimulate the conversion of glycogen to glucose by the liver. Glucagon also increases the peripheral utilization of glucose; therefore, it should not be referred to as simply the antagonist of insulin. Its secretion is controlled by the concentration of blood glucose and blood insulin level. If insulin levels rise and blood glucose levels drop, glucagon secretion increases.

The Adrenal Glands

The adrenal is divided into a cortex and a medulla. The cortex is derived from mesoderm of the Wolffian ridge in conjunction with the sex glands, while the medulla is of ectodermal, neural crest origin in conjunction with the anlage of the sympathetic nerve cells. In fetal life the adrenal is composed almost completely of cortex, but after birth the entire fetal cortex rapidly degenerates and is replaced by the adult cortex and medulla. The cortex, which produces the mineralocorticoids and glucocorticoids, is divided into three zones: a. the most peripheral zona glomerulosa; b. the intermediate zona fasciculata; and c. the zona reticularis bordering the medulla. The function of the adrenal cortex is to produce the sex hormones: androgens, estrogens, and progesterone, and the corticosteroids: glucocorticoids and mineralocorticoids.

The zona glomerulosa is rich in lipids, especially cholesterol, from which the mineralocorticoids are formed. Aldosterone is the most powerful mineralocorticoid. Mineralocorticoids function in the retention of water, sodium, chloride, and increase urinary loss of potassium and phosphorus by action on the renal tubules. This regulation of the electrolytes is essential to life. No pituitary control is present.

The zona fasciculata and reticularis are the sources of the glucocorticoids; i.e., 17-hydroxycorticosteroids. Corticosterone (hydroxycorticosterone), cortisone (compound E), and hydrocortisone (cortisol or compound F) are the most widely known compounds. The levels of these hormones are increased by ACTH; they are gluconeogenic in nature. They convert amino acids into sugar instead of protein and in this way increase blood sugar and liver glycogen levels. Cortisone—in addition to influencing protein, carbohydrate, and fat metabolism— a. affects the permeability of cell membranes; b. interferes with the antigen-antibody response by inhibiting antibody formation; and c. suppresses the inflammatory response. Cortisone, however, only relieves the symptoms of disease without influencing the cause.

The zona reticularis is responsible for the production of the sex hormones or 17-ketosteroids. The action of these hormones is no different from the action of the estrogens, androgens, and progesterone (the regular sex hormones produced by the testes and ovaries); i.e., they masculinize the body and increase the synthesis of amino acids and protein from nitrogen; they favor the retention of nitrogen, phosphorus, potassium, sodium, and chloride. ACTH has some control of these hormones.

Problems Associated with Adrenal Cortex Function:

1. *Hypofunction or chronic adrenal insufficiency.* Addison's disease. This condition is due to inadequate amounts of steroid hormones. Deficiency of glucocorticoids makes the patient easily susceptible to stress; deficiency or mineralocorticoids leads to a fall in serum sodium and rise in serum potassium. These patients lack proper resistance to infection and are easily dehydrated. Patients exhibit general languor and debility, a very weak heart, irritability of the stomach, and a peculiar change in skin color due to the deposition of melanin; this feature is highly characteristic.

2. *Hyperadrenalism*
   a. Overfunction of zona glomerulosa—aldosteronism (Conn's syndrome).
   b. Overfunction of zona fasciculata—(Cushing's syndrome).
   c. Overfunction of zona reticularis—adrenal virilism (Adreno-genital syndrome).

Primary Aldosteronism—Conn's Syndrome:

Characterized by:

1. Periodic severe muscular weakness or paralysis.
2. Intermittent tetany and paresthesia.
3. Hypertension.
4. Renal disfunction.

Cushing's Syndrome:

Characterized by:

1. Painful adiposity of face, neck, and trunk (full moon face).
2. Hirsutism in the female and preadolescent males.
3. Peculiar body striations.
4. Sexual dystrophy.
5. Muscular weakness and atrophy.
6. Hypertension.

Adrenal Virilism—Adrenogenital Syndrome:
Characterized by:

1. Hirsutism.
2. Virilism.
3. Excessive muscularity.

The adrenal medulla is intimately connected with the nervous system and develops from the neural crest. The cells of the adrenal medulla are modified ganglion cells and receive stimulation from the preganglionic fibers whose cell bodies are located in the intermedio-lateral cell columns of the spinal cord in the thoraco-lumbar segments dealing with the sympathetic outflow of the autonomic nervous system. Sectioning of the splanchnic nerves to the adrenal medulla will result in cessation of secretion, while stimulation of these nerves enhances secretion markedly. The function of the adrenal medulla is to secrete adrenalin (epinephrine) and nor-adrenalin (nor-epinephrine).

In general we can say that these hormones help the body in frightful and stressful situations. They affect the vascular system, the heart, respiration, carbohydrate metabolism, the pupillary dilators, the intestines, and uterine musculature.

A clinical picture of nor-adrenalism during which these pressor amines are produced in excess will show: a. hypertension; b. headache; c. palpitation; d. dyspnea; e. weakness; and f. chest and/or abdominal pain, etc.

The Testes

The testes function in the production of sperm and also contain interstitial cells, which produce the male sex hormone testosterone. Testosterone promotes and maintains the development of the male accessory genital organs (prostate and seminal vesicles) and secondary sex characteristics, i.e., beard growth, hair growth (pubic, axilla, trunk and limbs), and scrotal growth. It maintains spermatogenesis, is responsible for the deepening of the voice, the greater muscular development of men, sex urge, and acne at puberty. It also exerts an influence upon nitrogen, electrolyte and water balance within the system. Both males and females produce estrogens and androgens and it is the ratio of the two which determines male and female characteristics.

The Ovaries

Like the testes, the ovaries are endocrine glands; they have three functions: a. they produce the female gamete (ovum); b. they produce estrogens, which function in the preparation for fertilization of the egg and in the production of secondary female sex characteristics; and c. they produce progesterone, which prepares the uterus for implantation. FSH from the pituitary initiates the development of the follicle and the production of estrogen; when the level of estrogen rises above a certain point, it shuts off FSH production, ovulation occurs, and LH and prolactin production take over in the development of the corpus luteum, which secretes progesterone. This hormone prepares the uterus for implantation of the fertilized egg; it promotes mammary gland development and prohibits additional ovulation. If fertilization does not occur, the corpus luteum regresses, progesterone production falls, and since maintenance of the lining of the uterus depends on progesterone, menstruation is the next phase of the cycle. If fertilization has occurred, the corpus luteum is maintained and secretes progesterone almost to the termination of the pregnancy.

The Placenta

While the placenta is mainly concerned with support and nourishment of the developing embryo, it secretes estrogens, progesterone, and chorionic gonadotropin. Excess chorionic gonadotropin (similar to luteinizing hormone) is excreted in the urine and is the basis of most pregnancy tests. The estrogen production by the placenta inhibits FSH production and in this manner inhibits follicle development during pregnancy.

The Pineal

The pineal organ is a diencephalic outgrowth. It has been linked to photoperiodism and seasonal breeding; experimental evidence now suggests that it produces an antigonadotropic substance. How the pineal influences the reproductive organs remains to be established.

The Small Intestine

Food materials stimulate the secretion of certain hormones by the gastrointestinal mucosa and they may be summarized as follows:

1. **Secretin:** from duodenal mucosa—stimulates pancreatic juice secretion which is low in enzymatic content.
2. **Pancreozymin:** from duodenal mucosa—stimulates pancreatic juice secretion rich in enzymes.
3. **Cholecystokinin:** from duodenal mucosa—stimulates the contraction and emptying of the gall bladder.
4. **Enterogastrone:** from duodenal mucosa—inhibits motility and depresses the acid secretion by the stomach.
5. **Gastrin:** from pyloric region of stomach—enhances acid secretion by the stomach.

The Nervous System

The nervous system is usually divided into: a. central nervous system (brain and spinal cord) and b. peripheral nervous system (peripheral nerves and ganglia). The peripheral nervous system is divided into a somatic system and visceral (autonomic) system.

Nervous Tissue

Nervous tissue consists of neurons (nerve cells and their processes) and supportive elements. Neuroglia in the central nervous system and Schwann cells in the peripheral nervous system are the supportive elements.

The Neuron

The neuron is a cellular element and as a highly specialized cell, it carries out the function of nervous transmission. The neuron is like many other cells within the body in that it consists of a nucleus with an associated nucleolus and a cytoplasm which is rich in organelles, the most prominent of which are the rough-surfaced endoplasmic reticulum (Nissl substance), mitochondria, and the Golgi apparatus. In addition to the above characteristics, it should be noted that neurons possess numerous cytoplasmic processes or appendages. In almost all of the many varieties of neurons, there are two kinds of processes: the *dendrites* and the *axon*.

The Dendrites:

1. are direct extensions of the cytoplasm.
2. are generally multiple.
3. provide an increased surface area, the dendritic zone, to allow for synaptic interaction.

The Axon:

1. There is only one per neuron.

2. This process arises from a conical elevation of cytoplasm which is devoid of rough-surfaced endoplasmic reticulum (Nissl) and this area is called the *axon hillock*.

3. It is usually thinner and longer than the dendrites of the same neuron.

4. It may be surrounded by a *myelin sheath* which is produced by the *oligodendrocytes* in the CNS and by the *Schwann cells* in the PNS. Discontinuities in this myelin sheath occur at intervals known as the *nodes of Ranvier*. Though many axons are myelinated and are referred to as myelinated nerve fibers, numerous others possess no myelin ensheathment and thus are referred to as unmyelinated nerve fibers.

5. At its ending, the axon transmits impulses: a. to other neurons—the site of this impulse transmission being called a *synapse*; and, b. to effector cells such as muscle fibers or gland cells. This junction with skeletal muscle fibers constitutes a *motor end plate*.

The Synapse: The synapse is the site of contact between two neurons; it may be, and most commonly is, between an axon and a dendrite; however, contacts between an axon and the cell body and between axons and axons have also been observed. A typical synapse seen between an axon and dendrite (axodendritic synapse) has the following properties:

1. As the axon terminal reaches the synaptic site, it forms a bulbous head called a *bouton*. This bouton, which constitutes the presynaptic element of the synapse, contains numerous mitochondria and specialized vesicles, the synaptic vesicles, which contain the various neurotransmitters (acetylcholine is the primary one).

2. The dendrite, which constitutes the postsynaptic element of the synapse, is separated from the bouton by a cleft which varies in width from 150 to 200 Å.

3. This axo-dendritic synapse is *not* a site where cytoplasmic continuity is established between the axon and the dendrite, as both the pre- and postsynaptic elements are separated by a cleft. However, via the process of synaptic vesicle release, this axo-dendritic synapse establishes a functional (chemical) continuity across the expanse of the cleft.

Classification of Neurons

Multipolar Neurons: Most abundant; somatic and visceral motor, and associational.

Unipolar Neurons: Somatic and visceral *sensory* neurons; cell bodies are located in cranial sensory and dorsal root ganglia; peripheral process goes out to receptor and central process travels into the central nervous system.

Bipolar Neurons: These are special *sensory* neurons; cell bodies are located in special sense organs; i.e., eye (retina), ear (spiral and vestibular ganglia), and nose (olfactory epithelium).

Groups of Neurons

Nucleus: cluster of nerve cell bodies *within* the central nervous system.

Ganglion: cluster of nerve cells bodies *outside* the central nervous system.

Cortex: layered arrangement of nerve cells bodies on the surface of the cerebrum and cerebellum (gray matter).

Organization of the C.N.S.–The Spinal Cord

Before one can appreciate the organization of the cerebral mass and brain stem, it is necessary to understand the basic structural organization found throughout the extent of the spinal cord. If one were to examine a cross section through any level of the spinal cord, the following would be seen:

1. A centrally located H-shaped mass which contains the cell bodies of neurons. This H-shaped mass is divided into dorsal and ventral columns or horns in which are located those cell bodies that are responsible for sensory and motor phenomena respectively. This H-shaped mass is collectively referred to as the gray matter.

2. Peripheral to this H-shaped mass is white matter, which is made up primarily of myelinated nerve fibers.

3. Entering the spinal cord at the apex of the dorsal horn or column is the dorsal root of the spinal nerve. The cell bodies of these fibers are unipolar and are located in the dorsal root ganglion. The ventral root exits from the ventral horn of the gray matter. The cell bodies of these fibers are multipolar and located in the ventral horn.

The Spinal Nerves: Recall that these are part of the peripheral nervous system.

1. A spinal nerve, like any nerve, is composed of nerve fibers (axons and their sheaths) coursing together outside the C.N.S., surrounded by well-organized, protective connective tissue sheaths.

2. Functional Components of Spinal Nerves—contain both sensory and motor fibers.

a. Sensory: a. from receptors in skin and skeletal muscle; b. from receptors in smooth muscle in walls of organs and blood vessels.

b. Motor: a. to skeletal muscle; b. autonomic fibers to smooth muscle, cardiac muscle, and glands.

Sensory Pathway

A *typical sensory pathway* contains three neurons in a chain from the receptor on the surface of the body to *consciousness* in the *cerebral cortex* (Primary: 1°; Secondary: 2°, and Tertiary: 3° neurons).

1° neuron: has its unipolar cell body in the dorsal root ganglion; its peripheral process goes out to the receptor through the spinal nerve; its central process follows the dorsal root and synapses in the C.N.S. with a second order (2°) neuron.

2° neuron: has its cell body in the C.N.S.; its axon *crosses the midline* and ascends to the thalamus where it synapses with a third order (3°) neuron.

3° neuron: has its cell body in the thalamus; its axon ascends to the *cerebral cortex.*

Voluntary Motor Pathway

A typical voluntary motor pathway contains two neurons from the cerebral cortex to the *effector organ* in skeletal muscle.

Neuron 1: (upper motor neuron) has its cell body in the cerebral cortex; its axon descends and terminates in the ventral horn, synapsing on the cell body of a *motor* neuron, Neuron 2.

Neuron 2: (lower motor neuron) has its cell body in the ventral horn of the spinal cord; its axon (efferent fiber) leaves the spinal cord through the ventral root and follows the spinal nerve to the skeletal muscle where it terminates as a motor end plate.

Reflex Arc

The typical pathway of a reflex may be outlined as follows: sensory receptor on dendrite of dorsal root ganglion cell ⟶ ganglion cell ⟶ axon of cell ⟶ dorsal root ⟶ dorsal horn of spinal cord ⟶ either directly to motor cell in ventral horn or via internuncial (association) neuron to ventral horn motor cell ⟶ axon via ventral root ⟶ spinal nerve ⟶ effector organ (e.g., muscle).

Autonomic Nervous System

The autonomic nervous system innervates all smooth muscle, cardiac muscle, and glands. The autonomic nervous system is divided into a sympathetic (flight and fight) component and parasympathetic (maintains homeostasis) component. The autonomic nervous system exerts important influences on the intrinsic eye musculature, skin glands, the cardiovascular, respiratory, endocrine, and reproductive systems.

Fear, rage, pain, and the like, evoke sympathetic activity which mobilizes the resources of the body. Gastrointestinal activity is curtailed; heart rate and blood pressure increase and coronary arteries and bronchioles dilate.

Cranial Nerves

The cranial nerves are so named to describe those peripheral nerves which leave the brain stem and to distinguish these nerves from the spinal nerves which take their origin from the spinal cord and supply the neck, trunk, and extremities. It is customary to subdivide the cranial nerves into twelve pairs and to number and name these pairs as follows:

I. The olfactory nerve
II. The optic nerve
III. The oculomotor nerve
IV. The trochlear nerve
V. The trigeminal nerve
VI. The abducens nerve
VII. The facial nerve
VIII. The vestibulocochlear (auditory nerve)
IX. The glossopharyngeal nerve
X. The vagus nerve
XI. The spinal accessory nerve
XII. The hypoglossal nerve

No.	Nerve	General Components	Peripheral Termination and Modality Supplied	Damage to Nerve Results in
I	Olfactory	Sensory	Nasal mucosa—olfaction	Anosmia; Parosmia
II	Optic	Sensory	Rods and cones of retina—vision	Visual field defects
III	Oculomotor	Motor	Superior, inferior and medial rectus muscles and inferior oblique muscle—rotate eyeball	Strabismus or squint—deviation of the eyeball; Diplopia—double vision
		Motor	To a muscle which constricts pupil To ciliary muscle whose contraction thickens lens	Dilated pupil; Loss of light reflexes Loss of accommodation

No.	Nerve	General Components	Peripheral Termination and Modality Supplied	Damage to Nerve Results in
IV	Trochlear	Motor	Superior oblique muscle—rotates eyeball	Strabismus and diplopia
V	Trigeminal	Motor	Muscles of mastication—mastication	Paralysis of the muscles of mastication
		Sensory	Skin of face and mucosa of mouth and nose—supplies sensation	Loss of sensation over the distribution of V; Loss of reflex; Tic douloureux—pain over the distribution of V
VI	Abducens	Motor	Lateral rectus muscle—moves eyeball laterally	Loss of the ability to abduct eyeball
VII	Facial	Motor	Muscles of facial expression	Facial paralysis (Bell's palsy); Expressionless face with a drooping mouth
		Sensory	Taste buds on the anterior ⅔ of the tongue	Loss of taste on the anterior ⅔ of the tongue
VIII	Vestibulocochlear	Sensory (Vestibular portion)	Cristae of semicircular canals—provides for equilibrium	Vertigo, nystagmus and nausea
		Sensory (Cochlear portion)	Hair cells in the organ of Corti—provides for hearing	Deafness
IX	Glossopharyngeal	Motor	Parotid gland—provides for glandular secretion	Loss of secretion
		Sensory	Taste buds in the posterior ⅓ of the tongue	Loss of taste in the posterior ⅓ of the tongue
		Sensory	Epiglottis, root of tongue, soft palate	Loss of gag reflex
X	Vagus	Motor	Palate and pharyngeal constrictors and intrinsic muscles of larynx	Aphonia and dysphonia
		Motor	Via the cardiac and pulmonary ganglia to the cardiac muscle and to the smooth muscle and the glands of the pulmonary and gastrointestinal systems—provides for autonomic regulation of the above named organs	Autonomic disturbances
XI	Spinal Accessory	Motor	Trapezius and sternomastoid muscles	Difficulty in rotating head or raising chin
XII	Hypoglossal	Motor	Muscles of the tongue	Paralysis of tongue

Muscle

Classification

A muscle cell not only has the ability to propagate an action potential along its cell membrane, as does a nerve cell, but also has the internal machinery to give it the unique ability to contract.

Most muscles in the body can be classified as striated muscles in reference to the fact that when observed under a light microscope the muscular tissue has light and dark bands or striations running across it. Although both skeletal and cardiac muscles are striated and therefore have similar structural organizations, they do possess some characteristic functional differences. Skeletal muscle contraction, for example, is made up of the contraction of many motor units. A motor unit consists of a single motor neuron coming from the spinal cord of the CNS and all the muscle fibers which it innervates (3 to 150).

In contrast to skeletal muscle, cardiac muscle is a functional syncytium. This means that although anatomically it consists of individual cells the entire mass normally responds as a unit and all of the cells contract together. In addition, cardiac muscle has the property of automaticity which means that the heart initiates its own contraction without the need for motor nerves. Motor nerves may alter this inherent rhythm but the resource for initiating the contraction lies within the special cardiac cells called pacemaker cells. Here an action potential is initiated and spreads to the cardiac cells.

Non-striated muscle consists of multi-unit and unitary (visceral) smooth muscle. Visceral smooth muscle has many of the properties of cardiac muscle. To some extent it acts as a functional syncytium. For example, large areas of intestinal smooth muscle will contract as a unit.

The basic contractile mechanism is probably the same in all muscle types although the structural organization of smooth muscle is very different from that of striated muscle. We will concentrate on skeletal muscle, knowing that what we discuss can be applied to cardiac muscle and to some extent to smooth muscle.

Structural Organization of a Muscle Fiber

A muscle fiber is a single muscle cell. If we look at a section of a fiber we see that it is complete with a cell membrane called the sarcolemma and has several nuclei located just under the sarcolemma—it is multinucleated. Each fiber is composed of numerous cylindrical fibrils running the entire length of the fiber.

The fibril exhibits light and dark bands—the "I" and "A" bands respectively. The "I" band is bisected by the "Z" line and the "A" band by the "M" line. There is a somewhat lighter band within the "A" band that is called the "H" band. An even lighter area in the middle of the "H" zone on either side of the"M" line is called the "pseudo-H" band.

These striations are produced by the arrangement within the fibril of myofilaments which make up the contractile machinery. A sarcomere, the area between two "Z" bands, is the functional unit of muscle.

Myofilaments

1. The thick and thin myofilaments form the contractile machinery of muscle and are made up of proteins. Approximately 54% of all the contractile proteins (by weight) is myosin. The thick myofilament is composed of many myosin molecules oriented tail-end to tail-end at the center with myosin molecules staggered from the center to the myofilament tip.

2. The second major contractile protein is actin. Actin is a globular protein. The thin myofilament contains two chains of F-actin arranged in a twisted fashion. This configura-

tion gives the thin myofilament a certain periodicity. Associated with the thin myofilament along its entire length is the globular protein troponin. The presence of troponin along with tropomyosin-B inhibits myosin and actin interaction—it represses actomyosin formation. Calcium ions released following an action potential in the fiber membrane and T-tubules bind with tropinin, making it the Ca^{++} binding site. Calcium-troponin binding removes the inhibition of actomyosin formation.

Excitation

Contraction in a skeletal muscle is triggered by the generation of an action potential in the muscle membrane. Each motor neuron upon entering a skeletal muscle loses its myelin sheath and divides into branches with each branch innervating a single muscle fiber, forming a *neuromuscular junction*. Each fiber normally has one neuromuscular junction which is located near the center of the fiber. A *motor unit* consists of a single motor neuron and all the muscle fibers innervated by it. The *motor end plate* is the specialized part of the muscle fiber's membrane lying under the nerve.

The impulse arriving at the end of the motor neuron causes liberation of *acetylcholine* from vesicles in the nerve terminal. The acetylcholine acts at specific sites normally found only on the motor end plate section of the fiber membrane and increases the permeability of the motor end plate. The resulting Na^+ influx produces a depolarizing potential called the end-plate potential. This in turn depolarizes adjacent areas of the fiber membrane, triggering an action potential which is propagated in both directions from the central neuromuscular junction toward the fiber ends. Normally the magnitude of the end-plate potential is sufficient to discharge the muscle membrane, so that each impulse in the nerve ending produces a response in the muscle. The acetylcholine is rapidly destroyed by the enzyme *acetylcholinesterase* which is found in high concentrations at the neuromuscular junction.

Contraction

If we want to describe the characteristics of muscular contraction we should start by describing the sarcomere response during contraction. According to the sliding filament theory the sarcomere response to excitation involves the sliding of thin and thick myofilaments past one another. Neither the thick nor thin myofilaments change in length. If we could imagine observing this contraction under a light microscope we would see the narrowing of the "H" and "I" bands during contraction while the width of the "A" band would remain constant.

The word *contraction* refers to those processes which are manifested externally by either a *shortening* of a muscle or by *tension development* in a muscle. If the muscle length is held constant, the contraction is referred to as an *isometric contraction*. In an isometric contraction the passive tension remains constant with the *active tension* being added to it to produce the *total tension* of the muscle.

If the muscle shortens during contraction, it is called an *isotonic contraction* and the total tension remains constant.

Muscle Twitch

A muscle's response to a single maximal stimulus is a *muscle twitch*. The beginning of muscular activity is signalled by the record of the *electrical activity* in the sarcolemma. The *latent period* is the delay between imposition of the stimulus and the development of tension.

Tetanus

The response to a volley of stimuli is called *tetanus* if the frequency of stimulation is fast enough that the contractile responses will undergo summation. If the frequency of stimulation is very fast, the result is *complete tetanus*. In complete tetanus the frequency of stimulation is fast enough that the "active state" is maintained.

Energy Sources

In any phenomenon including muscular contraction the energy input to the system and the energy output from the system are equal. Let us consider first the energy sources for muscular contraction. The immediate energy source for contraction is ATP which can be hydrolyzed by actomyosin to give ADP, P_i, and the energy which is in some way associated with cross-bridge motion.

The ultimate source of this ATP is the ATP produced by the intermediary metabolism of carbohydrates and lipids. Skeletal muscle has the biochemical machinery to utilize both. With mild exercise oxygen availability after an initial period of adjustment is sufficient so that the aerobic pathways for ATP production can keep pace with the ATP utilization during the exercise—a new equilibrium is reached. During short-term, violent exertion, however, aerobic energy production cannot keep pace with energy utilization and even during the onset of mild exercise aerobic energy production initially lags behind energy utilization. Yet the ATP concentration remains constant. The reason is that there are stores of CP (creatine phosphate) in muscles and ATP levels can be maintained at the expense of CP levels. In these cases of insufficient oxygen availability, anaerobic pathways can produce enough additional ATP to permit those short-term bursts of exercise but in so doing lactic acid is generated. This incomplete oxidation produces substantially less energy than the complete aerobic oxidation to carbon dioxide and water.

CHEMISTRY

General Chemistry

The Atom

John Dalton's theories—still accepted

a. An element is composed of atoms. All atoms of an element possess the same chemical properties.

b. Atoms of different elements have different properties.

c. During a chemical reaction (nuclear reactions excepted, of course) atoms and elements are not created nor do they disappear.

d. Atoms of more than one element may react to form compounds. In a pure compound the number of atoms of each element is constant.

Components of the Atom

1. **Nucleus:** The nucleus—found at the center of an atom—contains neutrons and protons.

a. Neutrons—no charge—mass of about 1 dalton

b. Protons—charge of +1—mass of about 1 dalton. Number of protons in an atom determines the atomic number and the identity of the element.

2. **Electrons:** Electrons—charge of −1—mass of about 0.0005 dalton. Number of electrons circling the nucleus is equal to the number of protons in the nucleus.

Placement of Electrons—Energy Levels

1. Quantum numbers:

a. Principal quantum number, n, determines the shell. It may be 1, 2, 3, 4, etc., in increasing distance from the nucleus and increasing energy. The K shell has a principal quantum number of 1.

b. Angular momentum quantum number, l, determines the subshell. $l = 0, 1, 2, \ldots, (n - 1)$.

c. Magnetic quantum number, m_l, determines the orbital: $m_l = l, l - 1, \ldots, 0, \ldots, 1 - l, -l$. The energies are virtually identical.

d. Spin quantum number, m_s, describes the spin of an electron. Allowed values are $+\frac{1}{2}$ and $-\frac{1}{2}$.

2. Pauli exclusion principle: No two electrons in an atom may have exactly the same quantum number (i.e., all four).

3. Total number of electrons in a shell: The total number of electrons in a shell is $2n^2$.

4. Order of filling orbitals: Orbitals are filled from lower to higher energy levels. They may be designated in shorthand form. For example, the following oxygen atom may be designated as $1s^22s^22p^4$. Within the $2p$ orbitals, it is possible for an electron to be in $2p_x$, $2p_y$, or $2p_z$. Hund's rule states that one electron of parallel spin will go into each of these until each has one electron; additional electrons of antiparallel spin will then be added as necessary until all are filled.

	$1s$	$2s$	$2p_x$	$2p_y$	$2p_z$
			$2p$		
Oxygen	(⇅)	(⇅)	(⇅)	(↑)	(↑)

5. The excited state: The situation described above is that of the ground state. By input of energy it is possible to raise electrons to higher energy levels. When electrons drop back from these higher energy levels (excited state) to the levels required by the ground state, there is emission of radiation (emission spectrum).

Gases

1. Ideal gas law: Although early laws were formulated by Boyle, by Charles, and by Gay-Lussac to explain parts of the interrelationships between temperature, pressure, and volume of a gas, one simple formula sums it up:

$$\frac{P_1V_1}{T_1} = \frac{P_2V_2}{T_2} = nR$$

where P = pressure
V = volume
T = absolute temperature in convenient units
n = moles of the gas
R = universal gas constant in appropriate units

2. Partial pressures:

$$P_T = P_1 + P_2 + \cdots + P_n$$

(i.e., the total pressure of a mixture of gases is equal to the sum of the partial pressures)

3. Diffusion—Graham's Law:

$$\frac{v_1}{v_2} = \sqrt{\frac{m_2}{m_1}}$$

where v = velocity
m = molecular weight

Thus, a gas of twice the molecular weight will diffuse one-fourth as fast.

Liquids and Solids

Ideal gases are assumed to have negligible intermolecular interactions. Within a homologous series of organic compounds, the boiling point increases with increasing molecular weight. The same relationship may be seen within the halogens.

There are, however, forces in some compounds that cause them to be liquids or even solids at temperatures at which their molecular weights would suggest that they should be gases.

1. **Dipole forces:** In certain asymmetrical molecules the electrons become unevenly distributed between regions, and there results a partial positive charge in one region (and a partial negative charge in another). Molecules become arranged so that there is electrostatic attraction between adjacent molecules.

2. **Hydrogen bonds:** Hydrogen in one molecule may bond to oxygen, nitrogen, or fluorine in another molecule. The energy required to break this bond is about 10 kcal.

3. **London-van der Waals dispersion forces:** These forces involve interaction between molecules on the basis of their polarizability. They may be important in polar or nonpolar compounds.

4. **Ionic forces:** Oppositely charged ions exhibit coulombic attraction.

Phase Changes

1. **Nature of the solid, liquid, and gaseous phases:**

$$\text{Solid} \underset{B}{\overset{A}{\rightleftharpoons}} \text{Liquid} \underset{D}{\overset{C}{\rightleftharpoons}} \text{Gas}$$

where *A* is melting or fusion
B is freezing
C is vaporization or boiling
D is condensation

2. **Energy of phase transition:**
   a. The energy involved in conversion from the solid to the liquid phase is H_f.
   b. The energy involved in conversion from the liquid to the gaseous phase is H_v.
   c. All molecules in one phase do not have the same energy—there is a range. A liquid at a temperature below its boiling point is subject to some of its molecules being vaporized by virtue of the fact that some molecules are sufficiently energetic to be converted into the gaseous state. The temperature of the liquid, however, is a measure of the average energy.

3. **Phase diagram:** The phase diagram allows the visualization of possible phases at particular temperatures and pressures.

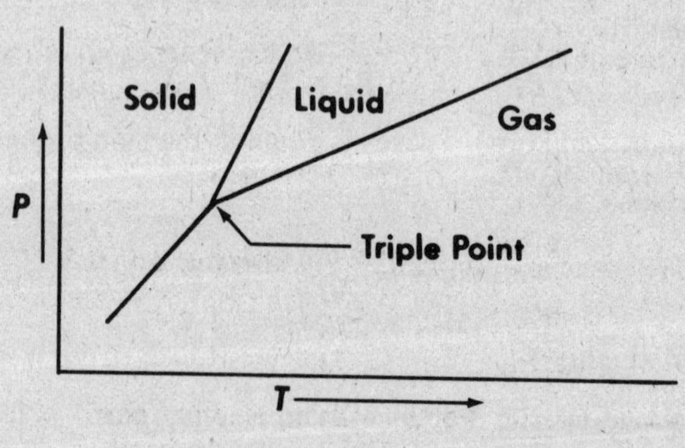

Note that the lines between phases in the phase diagram represent those conditions of pressure and temperature at which the phases indicated on the two sides of the lines may coexist. The point of intersection of the three lines is designated as *the triple point*; at this temperature and pressure all three phases may coexist.

Solutions

1. Concentration units:

a. Molarity

moles/liter = grams/molecular weight/liters of solution

b. Molality = moles of solute/kilograms of solvent

c. Normality = equivalents of solute/liters of solution

d. Equivalents = grams/equivalent weight

2. Colligative properties: Based on the number of dissolved particles, without regard to their nature.

a. Boiling point elevation

Boiling point elevation = $K_b m$

where K_b is a constant for the specific solvent and m = molarity of solute.

Note, however, that a 1 molal solution of NaCl would have twice the calculated effect since it would be 1 molal each in Na^+ and Cl^- (i.e., 2 molal total).

b. Freezing point depression

Freezing point depression = $K_f m$

where K_f is a constant for the specific solvent and m = molality of solute particles (see comment above regarding ionizable solutes).

c. Osmotic pressure. When an aqueous solution is placed on one side of a semi-permeable membrane and pure water on the other side, there is net movement of water across the membrane. The applied pressure required to produce a net movement of zero is called the osmotic pressure.

$$\pi V = nRT$$

where π = osmotic pressure
V = volume
n = moles of particles in solution
R is the universal gas constant
T is the temperature, °K

3. Solubility: A comparatively insoluble inorganic compound in water is in equilibrium with its soluble ions.

$$Al(OH)_3 \downarrow \rightleftharpoons Al^{3+} + 3OH^-$$

The solubility product constant is K_{sp}.

$$K_{sp} = 5 \times 10^{-33} = [Al^{3+}][OH^-]^3$$

Thus, in the specific case of $Al(OH)_3$, if the product of the molar concentration of OH^- raised to the third power and Al^{3+} exceeds 5×10^{-33}, precipitation will occur.

Acids and Bases, pH and Buffers

1. Acids:

a. Bronsted-Lowry acid—a material that donates a proton:

$$\underset{\text{(acid)}}{HCl} + H_2O \longrightarrow H_3O^+ + Cl^-$$

b. Lewis acid—a material that accepts an electron pair

2. **Base:**

a. Brönsted-Lowry base—a material that accepts a proton:

$$H_3O^+ + \underset{\text{(base)}}{NaOH} \rightleftharpoons 2H_2O + Na^+$$

b. Lewis base—a material that donates an electron pair

3. **Strength of acids and bases:**

a. Strong acids and bases. A strong acid or base is assumed to be completely ionized. Therefore the concentration of acid is equal to the concentration of hydrogen ions (or hydronium ions).

$$HCl + H_2O \longrightarrow H_2O^+ + Cl^- \quad \textit{or} \quad HCl \longrightarrow H^+ + Cl^-$$

b. Weak acids and bases

(1) $HF \rightleftharpoons H^+ + F^-$

$K_a = \dfrac{[H^+][F^-]}{[HF]} = 7 \times 10^{-4}$ (in this specific case)

Consider a $1M$ solution of HF for example:

$[H^+] = [F^-]$

So, $K_a[HF] = [H^+][F^-] = [H^+]^2$

and $[H^+] = \sqrt{K_a[HF]} = \sqrt{7 \times 10^{-4}} = 2.6 \times 10^{-2}$

(2) Bases

$NH_3 + H_2O \rightleftharpoons NH_4^+ + OH^-$

$K_b[NH_3] = [NH_4^+][OH^-]$

$K_b = 1.8 \times 10^{-5}$ for this particular base.

Computation similar to that for acid would allow one to determine the $[OH^-]$ for a 1 molar NH_3 solution.

4. **pH, pOH, and pK_w:**

a. $pH = -\log[H^+]$

The pH of pure water is 7.

b. $pOH = -\log[OH^-]$

The pOH of pure water is 7.

c. $pK_w = pH + pOH = 14$

d. Changes in pH and hydrogen ions. Remember that pH is a logarithmic scale. A decrease of one unit in pH (e.g., from 7 to 6) indicates an increase in hydrogen ions by a factor of 10.

5. **Solutions of salts:**

a. A solution of the salt of a strong acid and a strong base is highly ionized and neutral.

b. A solution of the salt of a strong acid and a weak base is acidic.

c. A solution of the salt of a weak acid and a strong base is basic.

6. **Buffers:** A buffer is a solution containing a weak acid or a weak base *and* a salt of that weak acid or weak base.

a. $HA \rightleftharpoons H^+ + A^-$

For an acid HA, we may use the formula above. A^-, the anion formed by the acid ionization, is the salt (also referred to as a conjugate base). Little buffering would be noted unless more A^- is present. (This could be accomplished by adding the sodium salt Na^+A^-).

b. Henderson-Hasselbalch equation:

$$pH = pK_a + \log \frac{[\text{salt}]}{[\text{acid}]}$$

For a buffer of the acid HA and its sodium salt:

$$pH = pK_a + \log \frac{[NaA]}{[HA]}$$

It may be noted that when the concentrations of the salt and the acid are equal, pH = pK_a.

In what pH range would maximum buffering occur? Try the calculations with different ratios of the buffer pair and the addition of small amounts of acid or base. You will find that maximum buffering occurs at or near the pK_a of the buffer pair.

7. Volumetric calculations with acids and bases:

a. Molarity = grams acid or base/molecular weight/liters

b. Normality = grams acid or base/equivalent weight/liters

For a monoprotic acid such as HCl, the normality equals the molarity. For a diprotic acid such as H_2SO_4, the normality is twice the molarity.

c. Number of equivalents in neutralization:

$$L_{acid} \times N_{acid} = L_{base} \times N_{base} = \text{number of equivalents}$$

Thermodynamics

1. Laws:

a. *First law*. Energy can neither be created nor destroyed.

b. *Second law*. The spontaneous flow of heat is always unidirectional from the higher to the lower temperature.

c. *Third law*. The entropy of all pure crystalline solids may be taken as zero at the absolute zero of temperature.

2. Change in enthalpy: The change in enthalpy is ΔH. Changes in heat content indicate spontaneity of a reaction. A negative ΔH for a reaction indicates that the products have a lower heat content than the reactants; therefore, heat is evolved. Since enthalpy is independent of the route of a reaction, it is possible to algebraically add reactions.

	$Pb(s) + O_2(g)$	$\longrightarrow PbO_2(s)$	$\Delta H = -66.1$
	$2H_2O(g)$	$\longrightarrow 2H_2(g) + O_2(g)$	$\Delta H = +115.6$
Sum	$Pb(s) + 2H_2O(g)$	$\longrightarrow PbO_2(s) + 2H_2(g)$	$\Delta H = +49.5$

In this example the overall reaction input of heat would be required.

3. Change in entropy: The change in entropy is ΔS. Entropy may be described as the degree of disorder of a system. It is also seen as unrecoverable energy. Without the addition of energy to a system, entropy increases to a maximum.

4. Changes in Gibbs free energy: Changes in Gibbs free energy are ΔG. Some of the energy of a reaction is unavailable for useful work. The term ΔG indicates the energy that is available for useful work.

$$\Delta G = \Delta H - T\,\Delta S$$

where T = absolute temperature, °K

A negative ΔG indicates a reaction that is thermodynamically favorable.

General Principles

Characteristics of Mixtures and Compounds

Mixture	Compound
1. Physical union	Chemical union
2. No new substances are formed	New substances are formed
3. Can be separated by physical means	Can be separated by chemical means
4. Elements form no definite proportions	Elements form definite proportions

Reactions

1. Single Replacement Reaction: In a single replacement reaction a more active element reacts with a compound to replace a less active one. A new element and a new compound are the result.

Examples: $Fe + CuSO_4 \longrightarrow FeSO_4 + Cu$
$Zn + CuSO_4 \longrightarrow ZnSO_4 + Cu$

2. Double Replacement Reaction: Double replacement reactions involve a double exchange; compounds react chemically to form two new compounds.

Examples: $NaCl + AgNO_3 \longrightarrow NaNO_3 + AgCl$
$HCl + NaOH \longrightarrow NaCl + H_2O$

In the first example a precipitate (AgCl) is formed and in the second example a weakly ionized compound (H_2O) is formed. In the other cases (e.g., $NaCl + KNO_3$) a double replacement reaction could be written, but the equilibrium would involve all possible combinations of cations and anions since neither a precipitate, nor a gas, nor a weakly ionized compound is formed.

3. Synthesis Reaction: In a synthesis reaction two or more elements can unite to form a single compound.

Examples: $Fe + S \xrightarrow{\Delta} FeS$
$CO_2 + H_2O \longrightarrow H_2CO_3$

4. Decomposition Reaction: In a decomposition reaction a compound is broken down into simpler compounds or into its elements.

Examples: $2KClO_3 \longrightarrow 2KCl + 3O_2$
$2HgO \longrightarrow 2Hg + O_2$

Role of Enzymes in a Reaction

Consider the following reaction:

$$\underset{1}{A + B + C} \xrightarrow[2]{\text{E (enzyme)}} \underset{3}{ABCE} \longrightarrow \underset{4}{D + F} + \underset{2}{E}$$

Substrate(s) or reactant(s) (1) react(s) with the enzyme (2) to form an enzyme–subtrate complex (3). This complex breaks down into product(s) (4), and free enzyme (2) ready for the formation of a new enzyme–substrate complex is available again.

An enzyme speeds up the rate of the reaction but is not used up itself in the reaction.

Molar and Normal Solutions

Normality and molarity are useful concepts that you should be able to define. A 1-molar solution contains 1 gram molecular weight per liter. A 1-normal solution contains

1 equivalent per liter. For a monoprotic acid such as HCl, the normality equals the molarity.

Temperature Conversion Factors

On the Celsius scale (°C) the freezing point of water is 0°, and the boiling point is 100°. On the Fahrenheit scale (°F) they are respectively 32° and 212°.

The absolute Kelvin scale lists as absolute zero a temperature of −273°C, and therefore the Kelvin and Celsius scales differ only in the choice of point zero. Kelvin temperature is, therefore, 273 plus the Celsius temperature. Let us illustrate and work two examples:

1. 104°F is how many degrees on the Kelvin scale? The answer is 313° and is obtained in the following manner:

First we must convert Fahrenheit to Celsius by using the following formulas:

$$\text{Celsius equals } \frac{5}{9} \times (\text{Fahrenheit} - 32)$$

$$\text{Fahrenheit equals } \frac{9}{5}\, C + 32$$

$$\text{Celsius} = \frac{5}{9} \times (104 - 32)$$

$$C = \frac{5}{9} \times 72$$

$$C = 40°$$

Now we take Kelvin 273° and add 40° and obtain a Kelvin temperature of 313°.

2. 45°C will equal how many degrees F?

We utilize the conversion factors:

$$°F = \frac{9}{5} C° + 32$$

or

$$°C = \frac{5}{9} (F° - 32)$$

$$°F = \frac{9}{5} (45) + 32$$

$$°F = 81 + 32$$

$$°F = 113°$$

Formulas and Laws

1. Specific Gravity: Specific gravity is usually expressed as the weight of an object in air divided by the loss of weight when weighed in water.

Example: A ball of steel weighs 300 grams in air and 250 grams when submerged in water; its specific gravity is 6.

$$\text{Specific Gravity} = \frac{\text{Weight in Air}}{\text{Loss of Weight}}$$

$$\text{Specific Gravity} = \frac{300}{50} = 6$$

2. **Density:** Density is expressed as $\frac{W \text{ (weight)}}{V \text{ (volume)}}$.

Example: A piece of iron 60 inches long, 12 inches wide and 2 inches high weighs 2000 lb. The density of this piece is 1.39 lb./in.^{3} and was obtained as follows:

$$D = \frac{W}{V} = \frac{2000 \text{ lb.}}{60 \text{ in.} \times 12 \text{ in.} \times 2 \text{ in.}}$$

$$D = \frac{2000 \text{ lb.}}{1440 \text{ in.}^3} = 1.39 \text{ lb./in.}^3$$

Organic Chemistry

It is not possible to present a course in organic chemistry in the limited space we have allotted. All we can hope to do is to help you review some of the high points.

General Considerations

1. **Definition:** Organic chemistry is the chemistry of compounds of carbon. Historically, it has been the study of chemical compounds from living or dead organisms. Until 1828, it was believed that these compounds could not be synthesized from "inorganic" compounds outside living organisms. This theory was first breached by Friedrich Wöhler in 1828; he was successful in synthesizing urea from the inorganic compound, ammonium cyanate.

2. **Bonds:** In general, the bonds in the stable organic compounds are covalent bonds, formed by the sharing of electrons between atoms. If the electrons are shared unequally between two atoms, the bond is said to be a polar bond (e.g., C—Br or C—O).

3. **Electronic Configuration of the Carbon Atom:** It is generally true that the orbital electrons in the outer unfilled shell are the most important in predicting the metal/non-metal character of the compound as well as the expected valence. The carbon atom has two electrons in the *K* shell and four in the *L* shell ($1s^2\,2s^2\,2p_x^{\,1}\,2p_y^{\,1}$). It might be expected to lose four electrons to produce the electronic configuration of the noble element helium, or gain four electrons to produce the electronic configuration of the noble element neon. For the most part it shares electrons to complete the *L* shell. Thus it may be said to have a valence of 4 (see below).

4. **Bond Hybridization:** The orbital electrons of the carbon atom consist of two electrons in the $1s$ orbital, two electrons in the $2s$ orbital and one electron each in the $2p_x$ and $2p_y$ orbitals. (This may be written as $1s^22s^22p_x^{\,1}2p_y^{\,1}$.) It exhibits a valence of 4. In simple compounds such as methane, four equivalent covalent bonds are formed. This may be considered to occur by raising one of the $2s$ orbital electrons to the $2p_z$ orbital and then forming four hybridized orbitals from the three $2p$ orbitals and the one remaining $2s$ orbital. These hybridized orbitals are sp^3 orbitals. The four covalent bonds in methane are the result of overlap of the one orbital electron of each of four hydrogen atoms with one sp^3 hybridized orbital electron of the carbon atom. These four bonds are called sigma bonds.

In a compound such as ethylene (ethene), however, there are pi as well as sigma bonds. Two of the three $2p$ orbital electrons are hybridized with the remaining $2s$ orbital electron. Thus there are three equivalent sp^2 hybridized orbital electrons for each carbon atom. These participate in the covalent sigma bond between the two carbon atoms and in the covalent sigma bonds between the carbon atom and the hydrogen atoms. The remaining $2p$ orbital electron in each carbon atom participates in the weaker second bond between the two carbon atoms (a pi bond).

Compounds such as acetylene (ethyne) have a triple bond, consisting of one sigma bond and two pi bonds. In each carbon atom participating in a triple bond, there is contribution of two hybridized *sp* orbital electrons to produce two pi bonds. The stronger sigma bond between the carbon atoms is produced by the contribution of one 2*p* electron from each carbon atom. In acetylene itself there is another sigma bond between the carbon atom and a hydrogen atom; this bond is produced by the overlap of a 2*p* orbital from the carbon atom and the sole electron from the hydrogen atom.

The Alkanes

Alkanes are saturated noncyclic compounds of carbon and hydrogen. If carbon atoms are arranged in a straight chain sequence

C–C–C–C

and hydrogen atoms are added to account for each carbon atom's valence of four, we produce a compound like this:

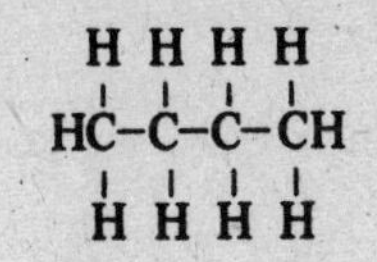

This compound is *n*-butane. The *n* designates the straight chain character. Another compound with the same numbers of carbon and hydrogen atoms is isobutane (or 2-methylpropane).

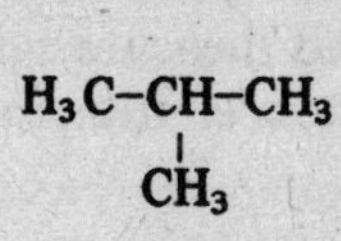

It is useful to learn the names of many of the alkanes. With modification these names are an integral part of the names of the derivatives of alkanes.

Chain Length	Name	Chain Length	Name
1	Methane	11	Undecane
2	Ethane	12	Dodecane
3	Propane	13	Tridecane
4	Butane	14	Tetradecane
5	Pentane	15	Pentadecane
6	Hexane	16	Hexadecane
7	Heptane	17	Heptadecane
8	Octane	18	Octadecane
9	Nonane	19	Nonadecane
10	Decane	20	Eicosane

The IUPAC rules for nomenclature require that a compound that is not a straight chain be named on the basis of its longest chain. Thus, the following compound is 2-methyl-4-ethylheptane:

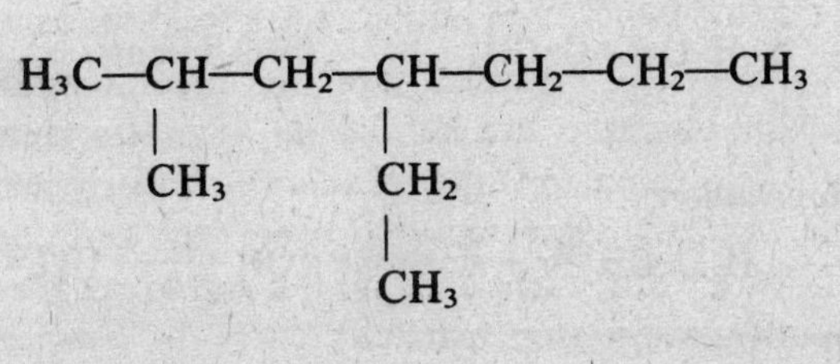

1. Synthesis—Wurtz Reaction:

$$2RBr + 2Na \longrightarrow RR + 2NaBr$$

(R will often be used to refer to an unspecified alkyl group.) More specifically:

$$2CH_3Br + 2Na \longrightarrow CH_3 - CH_3 + 2NaBr$$

If a mixture of two alkyl bromides is used, a mixture of three possible products is expected.

2. Reactions:

The alkanes are not very reactive, but they will undergo some reactions.

a. *Halogenation*

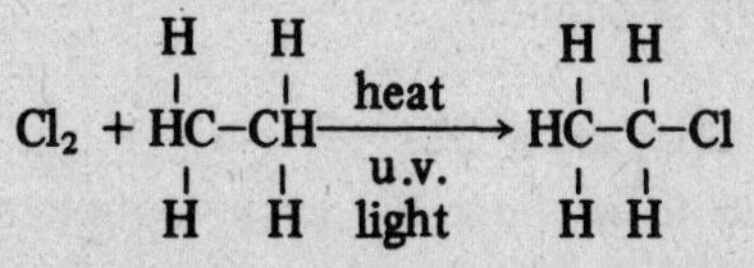

Reaction may continue and produce a more highly chlorinated product.

b. *Oxidation*

Alkanes may be oxidized to produce CO_2, water and energy.

The Cycloalkanes

The small ring cycloalkanes (cyclopropane and cyclobutane) are strained and are more reactive. Cyclopropane is planar, and the bond angles must be 60°. The normal bond angle is 109°28′. Five- and six-membered rings are not appreciably strained. Larger rings were once thought to be unstable because of the strain (Baeyer), but puckering allows relative freedom from strain.

Example:

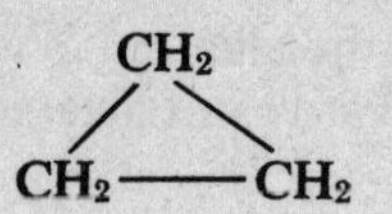

cyclopropane

The Alkenes

The alkenes may be considered as alkanes from which hydrogen has been removed, producing a carbon-to-carbon double bond. The simplest example of this series is ethene (ethylene).

$H_2C{=}CH_2$	ethene
$H_2C{=}CH{-}CH_2{-}CH_3$	1-butene
$H_2C{=}CH{-}CH{=}CH_2$	1,3-butadiene
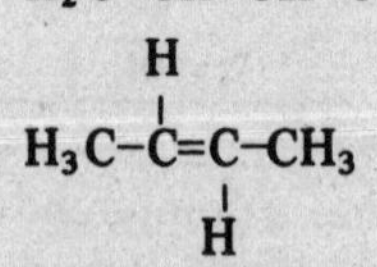	*trans*-2-butene
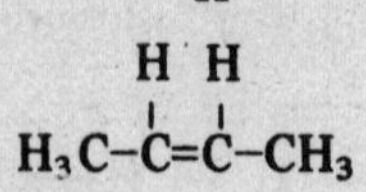	*cis*-2-butene

1. Synthesis:

a. *Dehydrohalogenation*

$$H_3C{-}CH_2Br + \text{alcoholic KOH} \longrightarrow H_2C{=}CH_2$$

b. *Dehydration*

$$H_3C{-}CH_2OH + H_2SO_4 \xrightarrow{\text{heat}} H_2C{=}CH_2$$

c. *Dehalogenation*

$$Br{-}CH_2{-}CH_2{-}Br + Zn \longrightarrow H_2C{=}CH_2 + ZnBr_2$$

d. *Cracking* (relatively nonspecific decomposition reactions)

$$H_3C{-}(CH_2)_4{-}CH_3 \xrightarrow[\text{cracking}]{\text{heat}} H_2C{=}CH_2 + H_3C{-}CH_2{-}CH_2{-}CH_3$$

2. Reactions:

a. *Addition of HX to the double bond*

$$H_3C{-}CH{=}CH_2 + HBr \longrightarrow H_3C{-}\overset{\displaystyle H}{\underset{\displaystyle Br}{C}}{-}CH_3$$

The Markownikoff Rule says that in the addition of an acid across a double bond, the double-bonded carbon having the most hydrogen will receive the H of HX. The above is true for ionic addition, but in the presence of peroxides we see a free radical anti-Markownikoff addition:

$$H_3C{-}CH{=}CH_2 + HBr \xrightarrow{\text{peroxide}} H_3C{-}CH_2{-}CH_2Br$$

b. *Hydrogenation* (catalyst such as Pt, Pd, or Ni)

$$H_2C{=}CH_2 + H_2 \xrightarrow{\text{Pt}} H_3C{-}CH_3$$

$$H_2C{=}CH{-}CH{=}CH_2 + H_2 \xrightarrow{\text{Pt}} H_3C{-}CH{=}CH{-}CH_3$$
$$+ H_2C{=}CH{-}CH_2{-}CH_3$$
$$+ H_3C{-}CH_2{-}CH_2{-}CH_3$$

c. $H_2C{=}CH_2 + Br_2 \longrightarrow BrCH_2{-}CH_2Br$

d. $H_2C{=}CH_2 \xrightarrow{\text{catalyst}}$ polymer (polyethylene in this case)

The Alkynes (derivatives of acetylene)

$HC{\equiv}CH$ acetylene or ethyne

1. Synthesis:

a. $CaC_2 + H_2O \longrightarrow C_2H_2 + CaO$

b. *Dehydrohalogenation*

$$H_3C{-}CHBr_2 + \text{alcoholic KOH} \longrightarrow HC{\equiv}CH$$

c. *Dehalogenation*

$$HCBr_2{-}CBr_2H + Zn \longrightarrow HC{\equiv}CH$$

2. Reactions:

a. *Hydrogenation*

$$HC{\equiv}CH + H_2 \xrightarrow{\text{Pt}} H_2C{=}CH_2 + H_2 \xrightarrow{\text{Pt}} CH_3{-}CH_3$$

b. *Hydrohalogenation*—see reactions of alkenes

c. *Halogenation*—see reactions of alkenes

d. *Reaction of active hydrogen*

$$H_3C{-}C{\equiv}CH + Ag^+ \longrightarrow H_3C{-}C{\equiv}CAg + H^+$$

$$H_3C{-}C{\equiv}CH + NaNH_2 \longrightarrow H_3C{-}C{\equiv}CNa + CH_3Br \longrightarrow H_3C{-}C{\equiv}C{-}CH_3$$

Aromatic Compounds

Aromatic compounds consist of benzene and compounds whose chemical reactions are similar to those of benzene. Almost all aromatic compounds that you would be expected to recognize as such are derivatives of benzene; there are other unrelated aromatic compounds.

1. Nature of Benzene: Although benzene is drawn as a conjugated cyclohexatriene, there are no discrete double or single bonds in the molecule. It is said to be a rêsonating structure.

2. Synthesis of the Aromatic Ring: This is unusual; in general one will only be interested in reactions of compounds containing the benzene ring rather than in the synthesis of the aromatic ring.

3. Reactions: (ϕ is sometimes used as a shorthand designation for the phenyl group. Thus, benzene would be indicated as ϕ-H.)

a. *Monosubstitution*

$$\phi + HNO_3 \longrightarrow \phi{-}NO_2 + H_2O$$

$$\phi + H_2SO_4 \longrightarrow \phi{-}SO_3H + H_2O$$

$$\phi + Br_2 \xrightarrow{Fe} \phi{-}Br + HBr$$

b. *Friedel-Crafts reaction*

$$\phi + RCl \xrightarrow{AlCl_3} \phi{-}R$$

$$\phi + R{-}\overset{\overset{\large O}{\|}}{C}{-}Cl \xrightarrow{AlCl_3} \phi{-}\overset{\overset{\large O}{\|}}{C}{-}R$$

c. *Substitution in a benzene ring that already has one substituent*

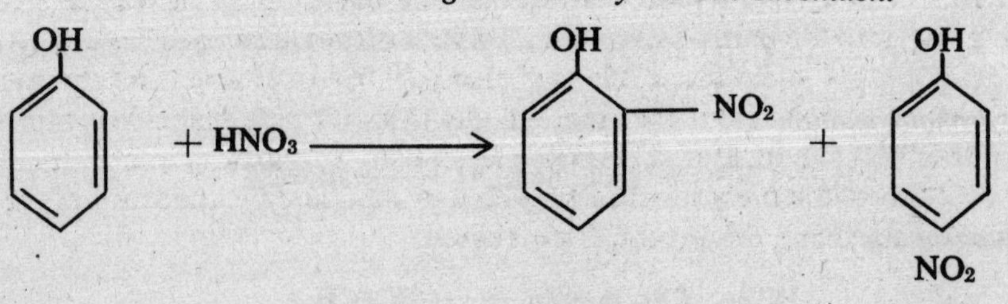

ortho isomer

para isomer

The placement of the second substituent is ordained by the first substituent. The OH substituent, as shown above, is an ortho, para-directing group. Other ortho, para-directing substituents include the CH_3 group and the halogens. The halogens deactivate the ring and also direct ortho, para. Many electrophilic substituents are said to be meta-directing: NO_2, CN, SO_3H, COOH, and so forth.

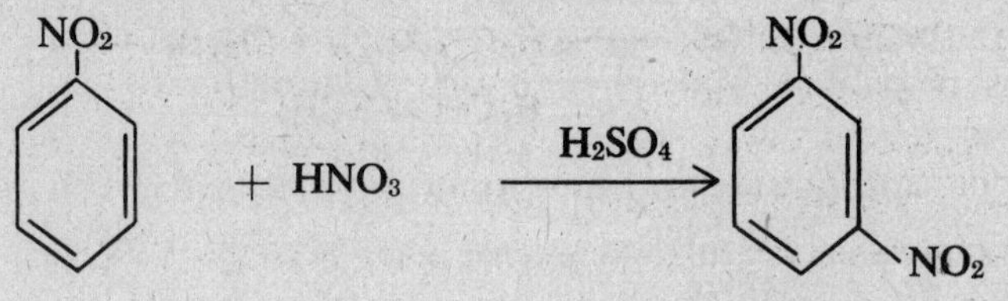

meta
isomer

The above meta-directing substituents also deactivate the ring.

d. *Diazotization of amines*

$$\phi\text{-}NH_2 + HNO_2 \longrightarrow \phi\text{-}N_2^+$$

e. *Reactions of diazonium salts* (see above)

$$\phi\text{-}N_2^+ + CuBr \longrightarrow \phi\text{-}Br$$

$$\phi\text{-}N_2^+ + CuCN \longrightarrow \phi\text{-}CN$$

$$\phi\text{-}N_2^+ + H_2O \xrightarrow{H^+} \phi\text{-}OH$$

$$\phi\text{-}N_2^+ + \phi\text{-}OH \longrightarrow \phi\text{-}N{=}N\text{-}\phi\text{-}OH \text{ (Coupling)}$$

$$\phi\text{-}N_2^+ + H_2 \xrightarrow{Pt} \phi\overset{H}{N}\text{-}NH_2$$

4. Acidity and Basicity:

a. *Acidity.* Phenol will ionize as an acid with a K_a of about 1×10^{-10}. A methyl substituent in the ortho position will lower the K_a (and the acidity) to about 6×10^{-11}. The electron-releasing methyl substituent contributes electrons to the ring and depresses release of H^+. A nitro substituent in the ortho position, conversely, increases the acidity (K_a about 7×10^{-8}) by withdrawing electrons from the ring.

b. *Basicity.* Aniline (aminobenzene or phenylamine) has a K_b of about 4×10^{-10}. The introduction of an electron-releasing methyl group in the para position (i.e., *p*-methylaniline) increases basicity (K_b about 1×10^{-9}). The introduction of the electron-withdrawing nitro group into the para position (i.e., *p*-nitroaniline) decreases basicity (K_b about 1×10^{-13}). The methyl substituent releases electrons into the ring, and the nitro substituent withdraws electrons from the ring. An electron-rich ring coincides with an electron-rich N in the NH_2 substituent. This will add stability to the NH_3^+ substituent which is formed by reaction of the NH_2 substituent with a proton, and the tendency of the NH_3^+ group to ionize by releasing the proton is decreased.

The Grignard Reagent

The Grignard reagent is one of the most important and versatile in organic chemistry. We will try to outline only a few of its reactions.

1. Synthesis: The Grignard reagent is synthesized by the reaction of an alkyl halide with elemental magnesium in the presence of anhydrous ether.

Example:

$$H_3C-CH_2Br + Mg \xrightarrow[\text{ether}]{\text{anhydrous}} H_3C-CH_2MgBr$$

or

$$RBr + Mg \xrightarrow[\text{ether}]{\text{anhydrous}} RMgBr$$

2. Reactions:

a. Reaction with active hydrogen. A Grignard reagent will react with any compound having active hydrogen (e.g., H_2O, an alcohol, an acid, or a 1-alkyne) to form a hydrocarbon.

$$RMgBr + H_2O \longrightarrow RH + MgBrOH$$

b. *Reaction with aldehydes and ketones*

$$RMgBr + HCHO \xrightarrow[\text{ether}]{\text{anhydrous}} R-CH_2OMgBr \xrightarrow{H^+} RCH_2OH \text{ (primary alcohol)}$$

$$RMgBr + R'\,CHO \xrightarrow[\text{ether}]{\text{anhydrous}} R\underset{\substack{|\\ H}}{\overset{\substack{R'\\ |}}{C}}-OMgBr \xrightarrow{H^+} R\underset{\substack{|\\ H}}{\overset{\substack{R'\\ |}}{C}}-OH \text{ (secondary alcohol)}$$

$$RMgBr + R'-\overset{\substack{R''\\ |}}{C}=O \xrightarrow[\text{ether}]{\text{anhydrous}} R'-\underset{\substack{|\\ R}}{\overset{\substack{R''\\ |}}{C}}-OMgBr \xrightarrow{H^+} R'-\underset{\substack{|\\ R}}{\overset{\substack{R''\\ |}}{C}}-OH \text{ (tertiary alcohol)}$$

c. *Reaction with CO_2*

$$RMgBr + CO_2 \xrightarrow[\text{ether}]{\text{anhydrous}} R-\overset{\substack{O\\ \|}}{C}-OMgBr \xrightarrow{H^+} RCOOH$$

d. *Reaction with an ester or an acyl halide*

$$RMgBr + R'\,COOR'' \xrightarrow[\text{ether}]{\text{anhydrous}} R'-\overset{\substack{O\\ \|}}{C}-R$$

$$RMgBr + R'\,COBr \xrightarrow[\text{ether}]{\text{anhydrous}} R'-\overset{\substack{O\\ \|}}{C}-R$$

Alcohols

Alcohols may be designated as ROH. The simplest alcohol is CH_3OH and is named methanol (i.e., methan-ol) as a derivative of the one-carbon hydrocarbon, methane. Other alcohols are similarly named as derivatives of hydrocarbons. The compound below is named 2-pentanol or 2-hydroxypentane.

$$H_3C{-}CH_2{-}CH_2{-}\underset{\underset{OH}{|}}{CH}{-}CH_3$$

The alcohols are very weak acids, even weaker than water. Polarity and hydrogen bonding cause short chain alcohols to be soluble in water.

1. **Synthesis:**
   a. *Hydration of alkenes*

$$H_2C{=}CH_2 + H_2O \xrightleftharpoons{H^+} H_3C{-}CH_2OH$$

   b. *Using Grignard reagents—discussed elsewhere*
   c. *Hydrolysis of alkyl halides*

$$R{-}I + H_2O \xrightleftharpoons{KOH} ROH + I^-$$

   d. *Reduction of aldehydes and ketones*

$$R{-}CHO + NaBH_4 \xrightarrow{H_2O} R{-}CH_2OH$$

2. **Reactions:**
   a. *Oxidation to form aldehydes or ketones*

$$R{-}CH_2OH + K_2Cr_2O_7 \xrightarrow{H^+} R{-}CHO$$

This is useful only if the aldehyde may be removed (sometimes by distillation) before further oxidation to the carboxylic acid. A ketone may not be easily oxidized further, but chain rupture is possible.
   b. *Dehydration to form alkenes—discussed elsewhere*
   c. *Formation of esters*

$$R{-}COOH + R{-}CH_2OH \xrightleftharpoons{H^+} R{-}COOCH_2{-}R$$

   d. *Conversion to halides*

$$ROH + HI \rightleftharpoons RI + H_2O$$

Amines

Amines have the structure $R{-}NH_2$. The simplest example is methylamine (or aminomethane):

$$H_3CNH_2$$

1. **Synthesis**
   a. $RX + NH_3 \longrightarrow R{-}NH_2$
   b. $RCN + LiAlH_4 \longrightarrow R{-}CH_2{-}NH_2$
   c. *Hofmann degradation*

$$R{-}CONH_2 \xrightarrow{Br_2,\ NaOH} RNH_2$$

2. Reactions

a. $R{-}NH_2 + HONO \xrightarrow{H_2O} ROH + N_2$

(This is the reaction for a primary alkyl amine)

b. $R{-}NH_2 + HONO \longrightarrow RN_2^+$

(This is the reaction for a primary aromatic amine. The diazonium salt is stable at the temperatures of ice water. It is capable of numerous further reactions under appropriate conditions.)

c. $R{-}NH_2 + R{-}COOH \longrightarrow R{-}NH{-}COOR$ (an amide)

Aldehydes and Ketones

1. Synthesis:

a. *Reaction of a Grignard reagent with a carboxylic ester or an acyl halide to form a ketone* (outlined above under "Grignard Reagent"—Section 2;d)

b. *Mild oxidation of an alcohol* (often feasible in the synthesis of ketones and sometimes in the synthesis of aldehydes)

$$RCH_2OH \xrightarrow{Cu,\ \Delta} R{-}CHO \text{ (aldehyde)}$$

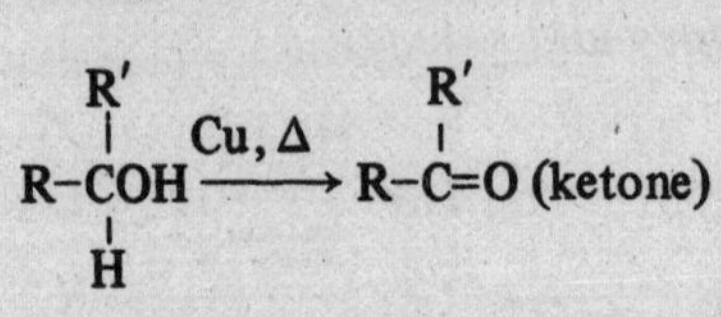

c. *Friedel-Crafts acylation to produce aromatic ketones* (see "Aromatic Compounds"—Section 3;b)

d. *Decarboxylation of acids to produce ketones*

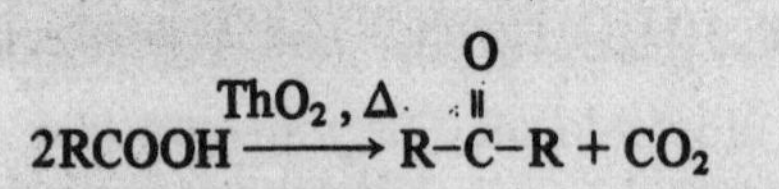

e. *Oxidation of diols to form aldehydes*

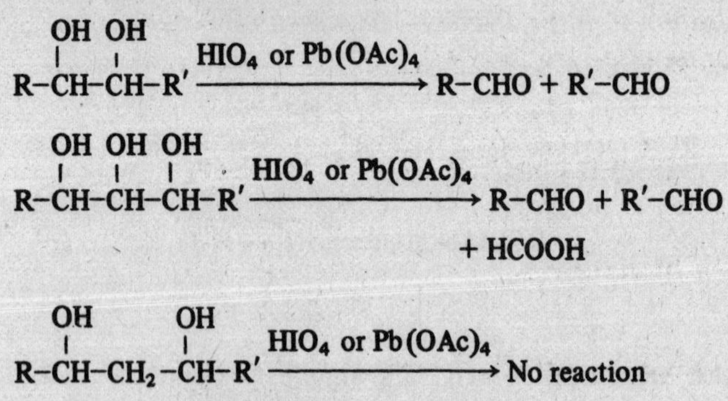

2. Reactions:

a. *Reaction with Grignard reagents*

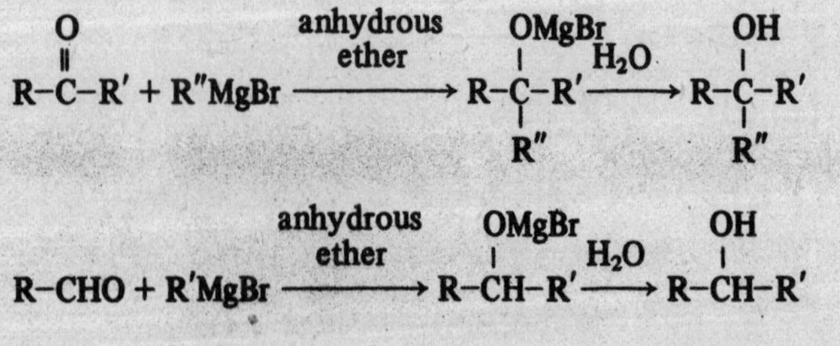

$$\mathrm{HCHO + RMgBr \xrightarrow[\text{ether}]{\text{anhydrous}} R{-}CH_2{-}OMgBr \xrightarrow{H_2O} R{-}CH_2OH}$$

b. *Reaction of aldehydes or ketones with HCN*

$$\mathrm{R{-}CHO + HCN \longrightarrow R{-}\overset{\overset{OH}{|}}{\underset{\underset{H}{|}}{C}}{-}CN \xrightarrow{H_2O,\ H^+} R{-}\overset{\overset{OH}{|}}{\underset{\underset{H}{|}}{C}}{-}COOH}$$

c. *Reaction of aldehydes or methyl ketones with* $NaHSO_3$

$$\mathrm{R{-}CHO + NaHSO_3 \longrightarrow R{-}\overset{\overset{OH}{|}}{\underset{\underset{H}{|}}{C}}{-}SO_3^-Na^+}$$

d. *Reaction with alcohols*

$$\mathrm{R{-}CHO + R'{-}OH \xrightarrow{H^+} R{-}\overset{\overset{OH}{|}}{\underset{\underset{H}{|}}{C}}{-}OR \xrightarrow{R'OH,\ H^+} R{-}\overset{\overset{OR'}{|}}{\underset{\underset{H}{|}}{C}}{-}OR'}$$

(a hemiacetal) (an acetal)

$$\mathrm{R{-}\overset{\overset{O}{\|}}{C}{-}R' + R''OH \xrightarrow{H^+} R{-}\overset{\overset{OH}{|}}{\underset{\underset{OR''}{|}}{C}}{-}R' \xrightarrow{R''OH,\ H^+} R{-}\overset{\overset{OR''}{|}}{\underset{\underset{OR''}{|}}{C}}{-}R'}$$

(a hemiketal) (a ketal)

e. *Reaction of ketones and aldehydes with hydroxylamine*

$$\mathrm{R{-}CHO + NH_2OH \xrightarrow{H^+} R{-}\overset{\overset{H}{|}}{C}{=}NOH}$$

(an oxime)

f. *Reaction of ketones and aldehydes with hydrazine or hydrazine derivatives*

$$\mathrm{R{-}CHO + NH_2NH_2 \xrightarrow{H^+} R{-}\overset{\overset{H}{|}}{C}{=}N{-}NH_2}$$

(a hydrazone)

g. *Oxidation of aldehydes*

$$\mathrm{R{-}CHO + Ag(NH_3)_2^+ \xrightarrow{OH^-} R{-}\overset{\overset{O}{\|}}{C}{-}O^- + Ag}$$

(Tollens' reagent) (silver mirror)

$$\mathrm{R{-}CHO + Cu^{++} \xrightarrow{OH^-,\ citrate} R{-}\overset{\overset{O}{\|}}{C}{-}O^- + Cu_2O}$$

(Benedict's reagent) (red ppt.)

h. *Haloform reaction with acetaldehyde or methyl ketones*

$$\mathrm{R{-}\overset{\overset{O}{\|}}{C}{-}CH_3 \xrightarrow{IO^-} R\overset{\overset{O}{\|}}{C}O^- + CHI_3}$$

i. *Aldol condensation* (requires alpha-hydrogen). Further reaction can also lead to polymers.

$$2CH_3-CHO \xrightarrow{OH^-} H_3C-C(OH)(H)-CH_2-CHO$$

j. *Cannizzaro reaction* (for aldehydes having no alpha-hydrogen)

$$2\ \phi-CHO \xrightarrow{OH^-} \phi-CH_2OH + \phi-\overset{O}{\overset{\|}{C}}-O^-$$

Carboxylic Acids

The carboxylic acids are organic compounds that ionize to produce free protons and carboxylate anions. The simplest example is formic acid, $H-\overset{O}{\overset{\|}{C}}-OH$

1. **Synthesis:**

   a. *Addition of carbon dioxide to a Grignard reagent*

$$R\,MgBr + CO_2 \rightarrow R-\overset{O}{\overset{\|}{C}}-OMgBr \xrightarrow{H^+} R-\overset{O}{\overset{\|}{C}}-OH$$

   b. *Oxidation of alkene*

$$R-C(H)=C(H)-R' + KMnO_4 \rightarrow R-C(H)(OH)-C(H)(OH)-R'$$

$$R-C(H)(OH)-C(H)(OH)-R' + KMnO_4 \rightarrow RCOOH + R'COOH$$

   c. *Oxidation of primary alcohol*

$$R-CH_2OH + KMnO_4 \rightarrow RCOOH$$

   d. *Hydrolysis of nitrile*

$$RCN \xrightarrow{H_2O,\ H^+} RCOOH$$

   e. *Hydrolysis of esters*

$$R-\overset{O}{\overset{\|}{C}}-O-R' + H_2O \overset{H^+}{\rightleftharpoons} R-COOH + R'OH$$

   f. *Saponification of esters*

$$R-\overset{O}{\overset{\|}{C}}-O-R' + NaOH \rightleftharpoons R'OH + R-\overset{O}{\overset{\|}{C}}-ONa \xrightarrow{H^+} R-COOH$$

2. **Reactions:**

   a. *Neutralization of base*

$$RCOOH + NaOH \rightarrow R\overset{O}{\overset{\|}{C}}-O-Na^+ + H_2O$$

b. *Esterification*

$$RCOOH + R'OH \overset{H^+}{\rightleftharpoons} R-\overset{\overset{O}{\|}}{C}-OR' + H_2O$$

c. *Formation of acylhalide*

$$RCOOH \xrightarrow{PBr_3} R\overset{\overset{O}{\|}}{C}-Br$$

d. *Formation of anhydride*

$$2RCOOH + H_3C-\overset{\overset{O}{\|}}{C}-O-\overset{\overset{O}{\|}}{C}-CH_3 \rightleftharpoons R-\overset{\overset{O}{\|}}{C}-O-\overset{\overset{O}{\|}}{C}-R + 2H_3C-\overset{\overset{O}{\|}}{C}-OH$$

e. *High temperature decomposition*

$$2RCOOH \xrightarrow{ThO_2,\,\Delta} R-\overset{\overset{O}{\|}}{C}-R + CO_2 + H_2O$$

Ethers

1. Synthesis:

a. *Dehydration. (Remember that the choice of conditions determines whether the ether or the unsaturated hydrocarbon, in this case ethylene, is the major product.)*

$$2CH_3-CH_2OH \xrightarrow{H_2SO_4\ \Delta} CH_3-CH_2-O-CH_2-CH_3$$

b. *Williamson synthesis*. Much more useful than the dehydration method if an unsymmetrical ether is desired.

$$RONa + R'Br \longrightarrow ROR'$$

2. Reactions: Ethers are generally unreactive compounds. They are often useful as solvents in organic reactions because of their unreactive nature. They may be cleaved by heated halogen acids:

$$ROR + HI \xrightarrow{heat} RI + ROH$$

The ROH which is formed may react with HI to form an additional RI.

Final remarks

As stated earlier, you cannot learn organic chemistry from a brief presentation such as this. We recognize that we have been able to present only some of the more important points. It is our intent that you use this material (and the questions and answers in the practice tests) to review the organic chemistry you have learned in your coursework. If you find areas of weakness in your preparation, we would recommend that you study those areas in your organic chemistry textbook.

Biochemistry

Some of you may have little or no background in biochemistry; in this section we will endeavor to introduce you to some of the terms and give you a better understanding of the importance of the various biochemical compounds. For those of you with more extensive backgrounds in biochemistry, perhaps this section will allow you to reorient your present biochemical information. Because of the brevity of presentation some statements may be noted that are generally but not universally true. Remember that dealing with the exceptions would have greatly lengthened the presentation and complicated your study at this time.

Definition

Biochemistry may be briefly stated to be the chemistry of living systems. This may be studied in a variety of ways, depending upon the goal.

Areas of Biochemistry

A. Proteins

1. **Structure:** polymers of L-α-amino acids (may contain other materials). The naturally occurring amino acids in higher animals are almost exclusively L-α-amino acids. Glycine is the simplest amino acid, of course, and it has no optical activity. D-Amino acids are more common in some bacteria. The peptide bond of peptides and proteins is formed by the removal of the elements of water between the amino group of one amino acid and the carboxyl of another amino acid (simply an amide linkage).

   The naturally occurring sugars in higher animals are D-isomers. The monomers (e.g., D-glucose) usually contain an internal ring; one monomer is attached to the next by a glycosidic linkage. The linkage between monomers in amylose (a simple starch) is α-1,4. In glycogen and in the more complex starch, amylopectin, there are also α-1,6 linkages in addition to the α-1,4. In cellulose there are β-1,4 linkages that are not susceptible to attack by mammalian hydrolytic enzymes. In animals that are able to utilize cellulose (e.g., cattle) the breakdown is accomplished by bacteria.

2. **Function:**
   a. *Structural proteins*—important components of structures such as biological membranes.
   b. *Enzymes*—serve as biological catalysts. They do not change the equilibrium quantities of reactants and products in an equilibrium reaction but do change the rate at which equilibrium is reached.
   c. *Amino acids*—Amino acids that cannot be synthesized in sufficient quantities by a particular organism are referred to as essential amino acids. Amino acids that can be synthesized in sufficient quantities by that organism are referred to as nonessential amino acids.

B. Carbohydrates

1. **Structure:** a group of polyhydroxy aldehydes, polyhydroxy ketones, and closely related compounds. They may occur as monomers (monosaccharides—e.g., glucose or fructose), dimers (disaccharides—e.g., sucrose or lactose), oligomers (few common other than disaccharides), or higher polymers (polysaccharides—e.g., starch and glycogen).
2. **Function:**
   a. *Metabolism for the production of energy*
   b. *Metabolism for the production of other required compounds*
   c. *Component of nucleic acids*
   d. *Structure—present in animal cell membranes as well as the cellulose of plants and the cell walls of bacteria*
   e. *Component of the lubricant of bone joints*
   f. *Blood cell antigen*
   g. *Heparin*

C. Lipids

1. **Definition:** material from organisms that may be extracted into nonpolar solvents such as chloroform or diethyl ether. The lipids are soluble in the latter solvents and virtually insoluble in water.
2. **Structure:** since the lipids are defined according to solubility rather than structure, the group is structurally heterogeneous.
3. **Function:**
   a. *Metabolism for the production of energy (important for food storage). The lipid utilized for storage is the triglyceride molecule. It is a 1,2,3-trihydroxy-propane (glycerol) that has been esterified in all three positions. The acid component of the ester is a carboxylic acid, usually containing a long straight alkyl chain. During metabolism 9 calories/gram are produced from triglyceride as compared to 4 calories/gram for carbohydrate or protein.*
   b. *Component of cell membranes*
   c. *Lipid hormones—steroid hormones and prostaglandins*
   d. *Fat-soluble vitamins—A, D, E, and K*

D. Nucleic acids

1. **Structure:**
   a. *Deoxyribonucleic acid*—contains the sugar deoxyribose
   b. *Ribonucleic acid*—contains the sugar ribose
2. **Function:**
   a. *Storage of genetic information*
   b. *Transmission of information by direction of the synthesis of proteins (including enzymes)*

E. Water-soluble vitamins

1. **Structure:** water solubility is main similarity—little structural similarity
2. **Function:** many serve as coenzymes in enzymatic reactions

PHYSICS—FREQUENTLY ENCOUNTERED PHYSICS PROBLEMS AND THEIR ANSWERS

I. Accelerated Motion

Example: A boat accelerates at a rate from 15 mi./hr. to 45 mi./hr. in 10 sec.

1. Calculate acceleration.

$$a = \frac{v_2 - v_1}{t}$$

a = acceleration
v_1 = initial speed *or* velocity
v_2 = final speed *or* velocity
t = time

$$a = \frac{45 \text{ mi./hr.} - 15 \text{ mi./hr.}}{10 \text{ sec.}} = \frac{30}{10} = 3 \text{ mi./hr./sec.}$$

2. Calculate average speed.

$$v = \frac{v_1 + v_2}{2} \qquad v = \text{average velocity}$$

$$v = \frac{15 \text{ mi./hr.} + 45 \text{ mi./hr.}}{2} = 30 \text{ mi./hr.}$$

3. Distance covered?

$$v = at \qquad v = \text{distance covered}$$

Recall: There are 5280 ft./mi. and 3600 sec./hr. In 30 mi., 158,400 ft. are covered. So,

$$\frac{158{,}400 \text{ ft.}}{3600 \text{ sec.}} = 44 \text{ ft./sec.}$$

Since the boat was in motion for 10 sec.,

$$\text{distance covered} = 44 \text{ ft./sec.} \times 10 \text{ sec.} = 440 \text{ ft.}$$

Example: An object is accelerated from rest to 600 mi./hr. in 30 sec.; the object has been subjected to an acceleration of 72,000 mi./hr.^{2}.

In any problem, it is best to convert the units to agree. Here, seconds were converted to hours.

$$\text{Velocity} = \text{Acceleration} \times \text{Time}$$

$$v = at$$

$$t = 30 \text{ sec.} = \frac{30}{3600} \text{ hr.}$$

$$600 = a\frac{30}{3600} = \frac{a}{120}$$

$$a = 72{,}000 \text{ mi./hr.}^2$$

Another way of expressing this type of phenomenon is to solve a problem as follows:

Example: A car is traveling at a speed of 31 mi./hr. and accelerates for 8 sec. to reach a speed of 55 mi./hr. Its rate of acceleration was 3 mi./hr./sec. Mathematically expressed:

$$a = \frac{\text{Final Velocity} - \text{Initial Velocity}}{\text{time}}$$

$$a = \frac{55 \text{ mi./hr.} - 31 \text{ mi./hr.}}{8 \text{ sec.}}$$

$$a = \frac{24 \text{ mi./hr.}}{8 \text{ sec.}} = 3 \text{ mi./hr./sec.}$$

Falling Objects—Gravity Acceleration

Recall: $g = 32 \text{ ft./sec.}^2$ or 980 cm/sec.^2

Example: An object in free fall travels for 1 sec.

1. Calculate speed (velocity) obtained.

$$v_2 = v_1 + at$$
$$v_2 = 0 + (32 \text{ ft./sec.}^2)(1 \text{ sec.})$$
$$v_2 = 32 \text{ ft./sec.}$$

v_1 = initial speed
v_2 = final speed
a = acceleration
t = time

2. The above body started from rest; the distance covered in the time was?

$$s = v_1 t + \frac{1}{2} at^2$$
$$s = 0 + \frac{1}{2}(32 \text{ ft./sec.}^2)(1 \text{ sec.})^2$$
$$s = 16 \text{ ft.}$$

v_1 = initial speed = 0
t = time
s = distance traversed
a = acceleration

Example: A rocket travels with an initial speed of 400 ft./sec. after its fuel has been used.

1. The distance covered after 1 sec. is?

$$s = v_1 t + \frac{1}{2} at^2$$

v_1 = 400 ft./sec.
a = 32 ft./sec.^{2}
t = 1 sec.

$$s = (400 \text{ ft./sec.})(1 \text{ sec.}) + \frac{1}{2}(-32 \text{ ft./sec.}^2)(1 \text{ sec.})^2$$
$$s = 240 \text{ ft.}$$

2. Calculate the speed obtained after 1 sec.

$$v_2 = v_1 + at$$
$$v_2 = 400 \text{ ft./sec.} + (-32 \text{ ft./sec.}^2)(1 \text{ sec.})$$
$$v_2 = 368 \text{ ft./sec.}$$

v_1 = initial velocity
v_2 = final velocity
a = acceleration
t = time

Example: a. At the end of 1 sec. a falling object will attain a velocity of 32 ft./sec.

$$v_f = at = 32 \text{ ft./sec.} \times 1 \text{ sec.} = 32 \text{ ft./sec.}$$

v_f = final velocity

b. During this 1 sec. of falling, however, an object previously at rest will have covered a distance of 16 ft.

$$s = v_0t + \frac{at^2}{2} \text{ or } s = v_1t + \frac{1}{2}at^2$$

$$s = (0 \text{ ft.})(1 \text{ sec.}) + \frac{(32 \text{ ft./sec.}^2)(1 \text{ sec.})^2}{2} = 16 \text{ ft.}$$

s = distance traversed
v_0 = velocity at rest
t = time

Uniform Velocity

Example: A car travels with a constant velocity of 30 mi./hr. for 40 mi. What time is needed to travel this distance?

$$t = \frac{x}{v}$$

$$t = \frac{40 \text{ mi.}}{30 \text{ mi./hr.}}$$

$$t = 1.33 \text{ hr.}$$

v = velocity = 30 mi./hr.
x = distance traversed = 40 mi.
t = time

Nonuniform Motion

Example: A rocket with an initial velocity of 25 m/sec. is accelerated at 75 m/sec.^{2} for 10 sec.

1. The rocket covers a distance of how many meters during the period of acceleration?

$$x = v_0t + \frac{1}{2}at^2$$

x = distance traversed

$$x = (25 \text{ m/sec.})(10 \text{ sec.}) + \frac{1}{2}(75 \text{ m/sec.}^2)(10 \text{ sec.})^2$$

$$x = 250 \text{ m} + \frac{7500 \text{ m}}{2}$$

$$x = 250 \text{ m} + 3750 \text{ m}$$

$$x = 4000 \text{ m}$$

2. How far would the rocket travel if it started from rest?

$$x = \frac{1}{2}(75 \text{ m/sec.}^2)(10 \text{ sec.})^2$$

$$x = 3750 \text{ m}$$

Uniform Deceleration

Example: A train travels at 60 mi./hr. (88 ft./sec.); the brakes are applied for 2 sec., and it decelerates at a rate of 22 ft./sec^2. Calculate its final velocity.

$$v = v_0 - at$$

$$v = 88 \text{ ft./sec.} - (22 \text{ ft./sec.}^2)(2 \text{ sec.})$$

$$v = 44 \text{ ft./sec. (or 30 mi./sec.)}$$

v_0 = initial velocity
a = acceleration or deceleration
t = time

Free Fall

Example: A construction worker drops a brick while working at a height of 900 ft.

$$v_0 = 0$$

$$g = 32 \text{ ft./sec.}$$

$$t = 3 \text{ sec.}$$

$$y = \text{distance traversed}$$

1. What distance does the brick cover in 3 sec.?

$$y = v_0 t + \frac{1}{2} g t^2$$

$$y = \frac{1}{2} g t^2$$

$$y = \frac{1}{2} (32 \text{ ft./sec.})(3 \text{ sec.}^2)$$

$$y = 144 \text{ ft.}$$

2. How long does it take for the brick to land on the ground?

$$y = \frac{1}{2} g t^2$$

$$t = \left(\frac{2y}{g}\right)^{1/2}$$

$$t = \left(\frac{(2)(900 \text{ ft.})}{32 \text{ ft./sec.}}\right)^{1/2}$$

$$t = (56 \text{ sec.})^{1/2}$$

$$t = 7.5 \text{ sec.}$$

3. What is the velocity of the brick at 2 sec. of travel?

$$v = gt$$

$$v = (32 \text{ ft./sec.})(2 \text{ sec.})$$

$$v = 74 \text{ ft./sec.}$$

II. Forces and Motion

Forces and Acceleration

Newton's Second Law: Force = Mass × Acceleration OR $f = ma$
Newton's Third Law: For every acting force there exists a reacting force of equal magnitude but in the opposite direction, that is, $F(\text{action}) = -F(\text{reaction})$.

$$f = \text{force}$$

$$m = \text{mass}$$

$$a = \text{acceleration}$$

Recall: The unit of force applied is the *dyne*; 1 dyne is the force that will impart a 1-gram mass an acceleration of 1 cm/sec.^{2}, that is, 1 dyne $= 1 \dfrac{\text{gm cm}}{\text{sec}^2}$.

Example: A force of 2000 dynes is applied to a mass of 250 gm. Calculate the acceleration obtained.

$$a = \frac{f}{m}$$

$$a = \frac{2000 \text{ dynes}}{250 \text{ gm}}$$

$$a = \frac{2000 \text{ gm cm/sec.}^2}{250 \text{ gm}}$$

$$a = 8 \text{ cm/sec.}^2.$$

Example: What is the force exerted on the surface of an asteroid by a man of 70-kg mass if the gravity of the asteroid is 2.5 m/sec.^{2}?

$$F = ma \text{ (gravity being one type of acceleration)}$$

$$F = 70 \text{ kg} \times 2.5 \text{ m/sec.}^2 = 175 \text{ N}$$

(A newton, abbreviated as N, is a unit of acceleration expressed in meter/second^2.)

Weight and Acceleration

$$F = \frac{W}{g} a \text{ OR } f = ma \qquad F \text{ or } f = \text{force}$$

$$W = mg \qquad a = \text{acceleration}$$

$$w = \text{weight}$$

$$m = \text{mass}$$

$$g = \text{gravity}$$

Example: A force of 30 lb. is applied to a weight or mass of 30 lb. Calculate the acceleration produced.

$$F = \frac{W}{g} a; \; a = \frac{Fg}{W}$$

$$a = \frac{30 \text{ lb.} \times 32 \text{ ft./sec.}^2}{30 \text{ lb.}}$$

$$a = 32 \text{ ft./sec.}^2$$

Example: A 180-lb. astronaut is accelerated upward by his rocket at 80 ft./sec.^{2}. Calculate the force that the seat exerts on him.

$$F = \frac{W}{g} a$$

$$F = \frac{(180 \text{ lb.})(80 \text{ ft./sec.}^2)}{32 \text{ ft./sec.}^2}$$

$$F = 450 \text{ lb.}$$

Example: A 20-kg mass located on a frictionless table is acted upon by a force of 250 N.

1. Calculate the acceleration of the object.

$$F = ma$$

$$a = \frac{F}{m}$$

$$a = \frac{240 \text{ N}}{20 \text{ kg}}$$

$$a = 12 \text{ m/sec.}^2$$

2. Calculate the distance the mass will travel in 10 sec.

$$x = v_0 t + \frac{1}{2} at^2$$

$$x = 0 + \frac{1}{2} (12 \text{ m/sec.}^2)(10 \text{ sec.})^2$$

$$x = \frac{1200 \text{ m}}{2}$$

$$x = 600 \text{ m}$$

Negative Acceleration

Example: A test vehicle weighing 3000 lb. travels at 60 mi./hr. (88 ft./sec.). Its stopping distance is 300 ft.

1. Calculate the braking force (negative acceleration).

$$v^2 = v_0 + 2ax$$

$$a = \frac{v^2 - v_0{}^2}{2x}$$

$$a = 0 - \frac{(88 \text{ ft./sec.})^2}{2(300 \text{ ft.})}$$

$$a = -12.90 \text{ ft./sec.}^2$$

2. What is the mass?

$$m = \frac{W}{g}$$

$$m = \frac{3000 \text{ lb.}}{32 \text{ ft./sec.}}$$

$$m = 93.75 \text{ lb.}$$

3. The relationship between mass and weight in the direction opposite the original motion is?

$$F = ma$$

$$F = (93.75 \text{ lb.}) - (-12.90 \text{ ft./sec.}^2)$$

$$F = -1209 \text{ lb.}$$

Example: A crane is lowering an air conditioning unit weighing 5000 kg onto the roof of a building. Its cable can support 15,000 kg. The speed of descent is 2 ft./sec.

1. The acceleration is?

The net force acting on the unit must be obtained: 15,000 kg − 5000 kg = 10,000 kg.

$$a = \frac{Fg}{W}$$

$$a = \frac{(10{,}000 \text{ kg})(-32 \text{ ft./sec.}^2)}{5000 \text{ kg}}$$

$$a = 64 \text{ ft./sec.}^2$$

2. The time necessary to stop the descent is?

$$t = \frac{v_2 - v_1}{a}$$

t = time
v_1 = initial velocity
v_2 = final velocity
a = acceleration

$$t = \frac{0 - 2 \text{ ft./sec.}}{-64 \text{ ft./sec.}^2}$$

$$t = 0.03 \text{ sec.}$$

3. The distance covered during this time is?

$$s = vt$$

$$s = \frac{2 \text{ ft./sec.} + 0}{2} (0.03 \text{ sec.})$$

$$s = 0.03 \text{ ft.}$$

Resultant Forces

a. Forces Acting Upon Each Other at Right Angles.

Example: If a force of 12 lb. and a force of 16 lb. acted upon each other at right angles, the resultant would be 20 lb. The answer is obtained by utilizing the formula:

$$R = \sqrt{(\text{Force } 1)^2 + (\text{Force } 2)^2}$$

Thus,

$$R = \sqrt{(12 \text{ lb.})^2 + (16 \text{ lb.})^2}$$

$$R = \sqrt{144 \text{ lb.} + 256 \text{ lb.}}$$

$$R = \sqrt{400 \text{ lb.}}$$

$$R = 20 \text{ lb.}$$

b. Forces Acting in the Same Direction.

Example: The resultant of two forces of 3 dynes and 10 dynes acting in the same direction is 13 dynes. Any combination of forces acting upon the same object in the same direction will result in an addition of the forces and the result will be equal to the sum of the forces.

III. Projectile Motion

v = initial velocity

v_h = horizontal component of path = $v \cos \theta$

v_v = vertical component of path = $v \sin \theta$

Example: A canonball travels with a speed of 200 ft./sec. with a 30° horizontal projection.

1. Determine the height the ball reaches. Look up the sine and cosine in a standard table.

$$\sin 30° = 0.5;\ v_v = \sin \theta = (200 \text{ ft./sec.})(\sin 30°) = 100 \text{ ft./sec.}$$

$$\cos 30° = 0.86;\ v_h = v \cos \theta = (200 \text{ ft./sec.})(\cos 30°) = 172 \text{ ft./sec.}$$

Utilize the equation:

$$v_2^2 - v_1^2 = 2as \qquad v_1 = 100 \text{ ft./sec.}$$

$$v_2 = 0$$

$$a = -32 \text{ ft./sec.}^2$$

Thus we have:

$$0 - (100 \text{ ft./sec.})^2 = 2(-32 \text{ ft./sec.}^2)s$$

$$s = \frac{10{,}000 \text{ ft.}^2/\text{sec.}^2}{64 \text{ ft./sec.}^2}$$

$$s = 156 \text{ ft.}$$

2. Calculate the time necessary to reach optimum height.

$$v_2 - v_1 = at$$

$$0 - 100 \text{ ft./sec.} = (-32 \text{ ft./sec.}^2)t$$

$$t = \frac{100 \text{ ft./sec.}}{32 \text{ ft./sec.}^2}$$

$$t = 3.12 \text{ sec.}$$

3. The ball will return to the earth in what time? If 3.12 sec. are used for ascending, $2t$ should be required. The answer is 6.24 sec.

4. Determine the range (R) of the ball.

$$R = v_h t$$

$$R = (172 \text{ ft./sec.})(6.24 \text{ sec.})$$

$$R = 1073 \text{ ft.}$$

IV. Friction

Formula $\mu = \dfrac{F}{N}$ $\qquad \mu$ = coefficient of friction

F = frictional force

N = normal or perpendicular force

Example: A 2500-lb. force draws a 30,000-lb. railroad car on level terrain.
1. Determine the coefficient of friction.

$$\mu = \frac{F}{N}$$

$$\mu = \frac{2500 \text{ lb.}}{30{,}000 \text{ lb.}} = 0.08$$

(The coefficient of friction is the ratio of the frictional force to the perpendicular force pressing the two surfaces together.)

2. The railroad car is pulled by a steel cable that makes a 30° angle above the horizontal. The tension in the cable is 300 lb. Determine the coefficient of friction.

$$F(\text{parallel frictional force}) = F = 300 \text{ lb.} \times \cos 30°$$
$$= 300 \text{ lb.} \times 0.866$$
$$= 259.8 \text{ lb.}$$

The normal force N—which is the weight of the car—is 30,000 lb. However, the vertical component of tension must be subtracted from it.

$$N = 30{,}000 \text{ lb.} - 300 \text{ lb.} \times \sin 30°$$
$$= 27{,}000 \text{ lb.} \times 0.5$$
$$= 13{,}500 \text{ lb.}$$
$$\mu = \frac{F}{N}$$
$$\mu = \frac{259.8 \text{ lb.}}{13{,}500 \text{ lb.}}$$
$$\mu = 0.01$$

V. Work and Power

Work (W) equals the force (F) times the displacement (d) in the direction of the force, that is, $W = Fd$.

Example: A machine is pushed 50 ft. on a level floor. The frictional force is determined as 300 lb. Calculate the work performed.

$$W = Fd$$
$$W = (300 \text{ lb.})(50 \text{ ft.})$$
$$W = 15{,}000 \text{ ft.-lb.}$$

Example: Instead of being pushed, the above machine is dragged via a steel cable at an angle of 30° and a force on the cable of 600 lb. The work performed is?

$$W = (F \cos 30°)d$$
$$W = 300 \text{ lb.} \times 0.866 \times 50 \text{ ft.}$$
$$W = 12{,}990 \text{ ft.-lb.}$$

Work and Energy

Example: A man pushes his snowblower with a constant force of 50 lb. The angles on the handle are 45° in both directions. The work done by the man after 150 ft. is?

$$W = Fd \cos 45°$$

$$W = (50 \text{ lb.})(150 \text{ ft.})(0.707)$$

$$W = 5302 \text{ ft.-lb.}$$

Power and Power Units

$$\text{Power} = \frac{\text{Work}}{\text{Time}} \text{ or } P = \frac{W}{t}$$

Units: 1 watt = 10^7 ergs/sec. = 1 joule/sec.
1 horsepower (hp.) = 550 ft.-lb./sec. = 746 watts
1 kilowatt = 1000 watts = 1.34 hp.

Example: By means of its steel pulleys, a crane raises a machine weighing 500 lb. to a height of 100 ft. in 200 sec. The average horsepower necessary is?

$$P = \frac{W}{t}$$

$$P = \frac{\text{Force} \times \text{Distance}}{\text{Time}}$$

$$P = \frac{(500 \text{ lb.})(100 \text{ ft.})}{200 \text{ sec.}}$$

$$P = 250 \text{ ft.-lb./sec.}$$

$$P = \frac{250 \text{ ft.-lb./sec.}}{550 \dfrac{\text{ft.-lb./sec.}}{1 \text{ hp.}}}$$

$$P = 0.45 \text{ hp.}$$

Example: A man weighing 180 lb. is taking a stress test. The test equals the activity of climbing a 30-ft. set of stairs in 5 sec. Calculate the horsepower he develops.

$$P = \frac{W}{t}$$

$$P = \frac{180 \text{ lb.} \times 30 \text{ ft.}}{5 \text{ sec.}}$$

$$P = \frac{5400 \text{ ft.-lb.}}{5 \text{ sec.}}$$

$$P = 1080 \text{ ft.-lb./sec.}$$

$$P = \frac{1080 \text{ ft.-lb./sec.}}{550 \dfrac{\text{ft.-lb./sec.}}{1 \text{ hp.}}}$$

$$P = 1.96 \text{ hp.}$$

Example: To take the MCAT examination you must climb 60 ft. of stairs, and you weigh 180 lb. The work you do against the force of gravity is 10,800 ft.-lb.

$$W = F \times D$$

$$W = 180 \text{ lb.} \times 60 \text{ ft.} = 10{,}800 \text{ ft.-lb.}$$

VI. Energy

Potential Energy

Potential energy (*PE*)—or stable energy, energy of position—is the product of the weight (w) of an object and the height (h) to which the object is elevated, or the work done in elevating it: $PE = wh$.

Example: A machine weighing 5000 lb. is raised onto the roof of a building 150 ft. high. Calculate the increase in potential energy or the work done in lifting the machine.

$$PE = wh$$

$$PE = (5000 \text{ lb.})(150 \text{ ft.})$$

$$PE = 750{,}000 \text{ ft.-lb.}$$

Kinetic Energy

Kinetic energy = energy of motion.

Formulas: 1. $KE = \frac{1}{2}\frac{w}{g}v^2$ w = weight in lb.

2. $KE = \frac{1}{2}mv^2$ g = ft./sec./sec.

v = ft./sec.

KE = ft.-lb.

Example: Determine the kinetic energy of a locomotive weighing 250,000 lb. and traveling at a speed of 30 mi./hr. (44 ft./sec.).

$$KE = \frac{1}{2}\frac{w}{g}v^2$$

$$KE = \frac{1}{2}\frac{(250{,}000 \text{ lb.})(44 \text{ ft./sec.})^2}{32 \text{ ft./sec.}^2}$$

$$KE = 7{,}562{,}500 \text{ ft.-lb.}$$

Recall: The joule (J) is a unit of energy. It is the heat produced by an ampere flowing against an ohm for one second. One joule is equal to 10^7 ergs and to a newton-meter, and 4.187 J are equal to one calorie.

Example: A rocket weighing 2000 kg is fired vertically upward with an initial velocity of 100 m/sec.

1. Calculate the change in kinetic energy at maximum height reached.

$$\Delta K = K - K_0$$

$$-K_0 = -\frac{1}{2} m v_0^2$$

$$-K_0 = -\frac{1}{2} (2000 \text{ kg})(100 \text{ m/sec.})^2$$

$$-K_0 = -10{,}000{,}000 \text{ J}$$

K = kinetic energy at maximum height

K_0 = initial kinetic energy

V_0 = initial velocity

Answer: At maximum height reached, the rocket has lost 10,000,000 J of kinetic energy.

2. Calculate the potential energy at maximum height, and the change in kinetic energy upon return to lift-off point.

a. $v^2 = v_0^2 - 2gy$

$$y = \frac{v_0^2}{2g}$$

$$y = \frac{(100 \text{ m/sec.})^2}{2(100 \text{ m/sec.})}$$

$$y = \frac{10{,}000 \text{ m/sec.}}{200 \text{ m/sec.}}$$

$$y = 50 \text{ m/sec.}$$

v_0 = initial velocity

y = maximum height

g = gravitational acceleration

b. $PE = mgh$

$$PE = (2000 \text{ kg})(100 \text{ m/sec.})(50 \text{ m/sec.})$$

$$PE = 10{,}000{,}000 \text{ J}$$

The increase in potential energy, then, is 10,000,000 J, and one can deduce that the rocket returns to its lift-off point with the same velocity it had at the beginning. The rocket had gained 10,000,000 J of kinetic energy on the original flight, but lost this amount in potential energy and, therefore, the total change in potential energy was zero. The *KE* and *PE* balance each other and are constant; the principle of conservation of energy is demonstrated.

VII. Momentum

Momentum is the product of the mass and velocity of an object:

$$p = mv$$

p = momentum

m = mass

v = velocity

You may use $\frac{W}{g}$ in place of m(mass), since $m = \frac{W}{g}$ (see p. 56).

Example: A 180-lb. man is shot out of a cannon at the speed of 30 ft./sec. What is his momentum?

$$p = \frac{W}{g} v$$

$$p = \frac{180 \text{ lb.}}{32 \text{ ft./sec.}} (30 \text{ ft./sec.})$$

$$p = 169 \text{ lb.-sec.}$$

Example: On landing, a plane is traveling at 60 mi./hr. Brakes are applied, and the plane comes to a stop in 10 sec. Assuming the average weight to be 160 lb., what is the force of the seat belts on the passengers?

Step 1 Calculate the change in momentum (momentum lost = momentum gained).

$$p = -mv_0$$

$$p = -(160 \text{ lb.})(88 \text{ ft./sec.})$$

$$p = -14{,}080 \text{ ft.-lb./sec.}$$

Step 2 Now calculate the force applied by the seat belts.

$$F = \frac{p}{t}$$

$$F = \frac{-14{,}080 \text{ ft.-lb./sec.}}{10 \text{ sec.}}$$

$$F = -1408 \text{ ft.-lb.}$$

VIII. Uniform Circular Motion

Centripetal Acceleration

Example: A subway car traveling at a speed of 30 mi./hr. (44 ft./sec.) negotiates a curve whose radius is 600 ft. What is its acceleration?

$$a = \frac{v^2}{r}$$

a = acceleration
v = velocity
r = radius

$$a = \frac{(44 \text{ ft./sec.})^2}{600 \text{ ft.}}$$

$$a = \frac{1936 \text{ ft.}^2/\text{sec.}^2}{600 \text{ ft.}}$$

$$a = 3.22 \text{ ft./sec.}^2$$

Circular Motion

Recall: $\theta = \frac{360°}{2\pi} = 1 \text{ rad} = 57.3°$

$$360° = 2\pi \text{ rad} = 180° = \pi \text{ rad}; \; 90° = \frac{\pi}{2 \text{ rad}}$$

The radian is a unit of measurement equal to the angle obtained at the center of a circle making an arch equal to the length of the radius.

Example: An airplane has its automatic pilot fly a circular route at a constant speed of 60 mi./hr. The route has a diameter of 10,000 ft.

1. Calculate the plane's angular speed.

w = angular speed

$$w = \frac{v}{r}$$

v = velocity = 60 mi./hr. = 88 ft./sec.

$$w = \frac{88 \text{ ft./sec.}}{5000 \text{ ft.}}$$

d = diameter = 10,000 ft.

$$w = 0.0176 \text{ rad/sec.}$$

r = radius $= \frac{d}{2}$ = 5,000 ft.

2. Calculate the angular distance and the arc length flown in 45 sec.

$$\text{Angular distance } \theta = wt$$

$$\theta = (0.0176 \text{ rad/sec.})\ (45 \text{ sec.})$$

$$\theta = 0.792 \text{ rad}$$

$$\text{Arc length } s = r\theta$$

$$s = (5000 \text{ ft.})\ (0.792 \text{ rad})$$

$$s = 3960 \text{ ft.}$$

OR

$$s = vt$$

$$s = (88 \text{ ft./sec.})\ (45 \text{ sec.})$$

$$s = 3960 \text{ ft.}$$

Centripetal Force or Newton's Second Law

Centripetal force may be expressed as mass times velocity squared divided by the radius, that is, $F_c = \frac{mv^2}{r}$ or $F_c = \frac{W}{g} \times \frac{v^2}{r}$.

Example: The previously cited subway car weighs 300,000 lb., travels at 30 mi./hr., and rounds the above radius of 600 ft. Its centripetal force is?

$$F_c = \frac{W}{g} \times \frac{v^2}{r}$$

W = 300,000 lb.
g = 32 ft./sec.^{2}
v = 30 mi./hr. (44 ft./sec.)
r = 600 ft.

$$F_c = \frac{300{,}000 \text{ lb.}}{32 \text{ ft./sec.}^2} \times \frac{(44 \text{ ft./sec.})^2}{600 \text{ ft.}}$$

$$F_c = 9375 \times 3.22$$

$$F_c = 30187.5 \text{ lb.}$$

Example: A satellite is in circular orbit at an altitude of 5.0×10^2 km. One complete revolution takes 90 min.

1. Calculate the tangential velocity.

$h = 5.0 \times 10^2 = 5.0 \times 10^5 \text{ m} = 500{,}000 \text{ m}$

$t = 90 \text{ min.} = 5.4 \times 10^3 \text{ sec.} = 5400 \text{ sec. for } \theta = 2\pi \text{ rad}$

$r =$ the radius of the earth, about $6.4 \times 10^6 \text{ m} = 6{,}400{,}000$ m. Hence,

$r = (6.4 \times 10^6 \text{ m}) + (5.0 \times 10^5 \text{ m})$

$r = (6.4 \times 10^6 \text{ m}) + (0.5 \times 10^6 \text{ m})$

$r = 6.9 \times 10^6 \text{ m}$

2. Calculate the angular speed.

$$w = \frac{\theta}{t}$$

$$w = \frac{2\pi}{5.4 \times 10^3}$$

$$w = 1.2 \times 10^{-3} \text{ rad/sec.}$$

Next:

$$v = rw$$

$$v = (6.9 \times 10^6 \text{ m})(1.2 \times 10^{-3} \text{ rad/sec.})$$

$v = 8.28 \times 10^3$ m/sec., tangent to the orbit in the direction of the motion.

3. Calculate the centripetal acceleration.

$$a_c = \frac{v^2}{r}$$

$$a_c = \frac{(8.28 \times 10^3 \text{ m/sec.})^2}{6.9 \times 10^6 \text{ m}}$$

$$a_c = 9.94 \text{ m/sec.}^2$$

Centrifugal Force

$$F_r = \frac{mv^2}{r} \quad \text{or} \quad F_r = \frac{W}{g} \times \frac{v^2}{r}$$

Example: An astronaut weighing 160 lb. is being spun in a centrifuge with a radius of 120 ft. at a speed of 60 mi./hr. What is the centripetal force on the astronaut?

$$F_r = \frac{mv^2}{r} \qquad w = mg$$

$$m = \frac{160 \text{ lb.}}{32 \text{ ft./sec.}^2} = 5 \text{ slugs}$$

$$F = \frac{5 \text{ slugs } (88 \text{ ft./sec.})^2}{120 \text{ ft.}}$$

$$F = 32{,}316 \text{ lb.}$$

Example: A 0.5-kg. object is traveling in a circular orbit 20 m in diameter at a speed of 2 m/sec.; the cord is subjected to a force of 0.2 N.

$$F = \frac{mv^2}{r} = \frac{(0.5 \text{ kg})(2 \text{ m/sec.})^2}{10 \text{ m}} = 0.2 \text{ N}$$

Since the mass is expressed in kilograms, velocity in meters per second, and distance in meters, the unit of force will be the newton. Note that the diameter of the circle was given, but the radius is required in the equation.

IX. Fluids at Rest

Pressure

$$P = \frac{F}{A}$$

P = Pressure

F = Force

A = Area

Example: The end of a pillar of a building has an area of 400 in.^{2}. The air hammer applies a force of 600 lb. as the pillar is driven into the ground. What is the pressure under the pillar?

$$P = \frac{F}{A}$$

$$P = \frac{600 \text{ lb.}}{400 \text{ in.}}$$

$$P = 1.5 \text{ lb./in.}^2$$

Example: A man weighs 185 lb.; his shoes have a surface area of 13 in.^{2}, and therefore, the pressure exerted because of his weight is 14.23 lb./in.^{2}. The formula to be employed is:

$$P = \frac{F}{A}$$

$$P = \frac{185 \text{ lb.}}{13 \text{ in.}^2} = 14.23 \text{ lb./in.}^2$$

Density

Density is the mass per unit volume of a substance.

$$P = hdg$$

P = pressure

h = height

d = density

g = gravity

Example: A tank 10 × 10 × 10 ft. is filled with gasoline (weight-density 42 lb./ft.^{3}).

1. Calculate the pressure at the bottom of the tank in lb./ft.^{2} and lb./in.^{2}.

$$P = hd$$

$$P = 10 \times 42 \text{ lb./ft.}^3$$

$$P = 420 \text{ lb./ft.}^2$$

$$P = \frac{420 \text{ lb./ft.}^2}{144 \text{ in.}^2/\text{ft.}^2}$$

$$P = 2.92 \text{ lb./in.}^2$$

2. Calculate the force at the bottom of the tank.

$$P = \frac{F}{A}$$

$$F = PA$$

$$F = (420 \text{ lb./ft.}^2)(100 \text{ ft.}^2)$$

$$F = 42{,}000 \text{ lb.}$$

Example: Find the pressure due to a column of mercury 100 cm high.

$$P = hdg \qquad h = 100 \text{ cm}$$

$$P = (100 \text{ cm})(13.6 \text{ gm/cm}^3)(980 \text{ cm/sec.}^2) \qquad d = 13.6 \text{ gm/cm}^3\text{(given)}$$

$$P = 1{,}332{,}800 \text{ dynes/cm}^2 \qquad g = 980 \text{ cm/sec}^2$$

Specific Gravity

$$\text{Specific Gravity} = \frac{d}{d_?} \qquad d = \text{density of a substance}$$

$d_?$ = density of a standard substance, usually water (d_w)

Example: A metal bar weighs 300 oz. in air and 200 oz. when submerged in water.

1. Calculate the specific gravity.

$$\text{Specific Gravity} = \frac{\text{Weight in Air}}{\text{Weight Lost in Water}}$$

$$\text{Specific Gravity} = \frac{300 \text{ oz.}}{100 \text{ oz.}}$$

$$\text{Specific Gravity} = 3$$

2. Calculate the weight-density of the metal.

$$d_w = 62.4 \text{ lb./ft.}^3$$

$$d = \text{Specific Density} \times d_w$$

$$d = (3)(62.4 \text{ lb./ft.}^3)$$

$$d = 187.2 \text{ lb./ft.}^3$$

X. Gases

Buoyancy

Example: A balloon on a transatlantic flight is operating where the weight-density of air is 0.050 lb./ft.^{3}. It weighs 300 lb., has a volume of 8000 ft.^{3}, and is filled with helium, with a d of 0.011 lb./ft.^{3}. What load can it support?

Step 1. $W = Vd$ W = weight
V = volume
d = density

Weight of Air Displaced = 8000 ft.^{3} × 0.050 lb./ft.^{3} = 400 lb.
Weight of Helium = 8000 ft. × 0.01 lb./ft.^{3} = 88 lb.
Weight of Balloon = 300 lb.

Step 2. $L = W_a - W_h - W_b$ L = load balloon can support

L = 400 lb. − 88 lb. − 300 lb. W_a = weight of air displaced

L = 12 lb. W_h = weight of helium

W_b = weight of balloon

The load the balloon can support is 12 lb.

Pressure and Volume of Gas or Boyle's Law

$$P_1V_1 = P_2V_2$$

(Note that the product of pressure and volume is constant if there is no change in temperature.)

Example: A gas exhibits a volume of 500 in.^{3} under standard atm. pressure (760 mm of mercury). If the temperature remains the same but the pressure is raised to 100 cm, what is its new volume?

$$P_1V_1 = P_2V_2$$

$$76 \text{ cm} \times 500 \text{ in.}^3 = 100 \text{ cm} \times V_2$$

$$V_2 = \frac{76 \text{ cm}}{100 \text{ cm}} \times 500 \text{ in.}^3$$

$$V_2 = 380 \text{ in.}^3$$

Example: A tractor-trailer tire has a volume of 3000 in.^{3} at a pressure of 60 lb./in.^{2}. How much air (at standard pressure) must be added to elevate the pressure to 90 lb./in.^{2}?

$P_1V_1 = P_2V_2$

P_1 = 60 lb./in.^{2} + 14.7 lb./in.^{2} (14.7 lb./in.^{2} = 760 mm Hg)

P_1 = 74.7 lb./in.^{2}

P_2 = 90 lb./in.^{2} + 14.7 lb./in.^{2}

P_2 = 104.7 lb./in.^{2}

(74.7 lb./in.^{2})(3000 in.^{3}) = (104.7 lb./in.^{2})(V_2)

V_2 = 2140.4 in.^{3}

The volume of air that must be added to elevate the pressure to 90 lb./in.^{2} is:

$$3000 \text{ in.}^3 - 2140.4 \text{ in.}^3 = 859.6 \text{ in.}^3$$

XI. Temperature Calculations and Measurement

Recall:

	Freezing Point	Boiling Point of Water
Centigrade	0°	100°
Fahrenheit	32°	212°
Kelvin	273°	373°
Rankine	492°	672°

Formulas: $C = \frac{5}{9} \times (F - 32°)$

$$F = \frac{9}{5}C + 32°$$

Example: A centigrade thermometer records a temperature in a patient of 37°C. What is the temperature on the Fahrenheit scale?

$$F = \frac{9}{5} \times 37° + 32°$$

$$F = 66.6° + 32°$$

$$F = 98.6°\text{F}$$

Example: An indoor arena is kept at a temperature of 72°F. What is the corresponding reading on the centigrade scale?

$$C = \frac{5}{9} \times (72° - 32°)$$

$$C = \frac{5}{9} \times 40°$$

$$C = 22°\text{C}$$

Absolute Scales: Fahrenheit absolute is expressed on the Rankine scale ($R = 460° + F$) while centigrade absolute is expressed on the Kelvin scale ($K = 273° + C$).

Example: 40°C and −40°C can be expressed on the Kelvin scale as follows:

a. $K = 273° + 40°$

$K = 313°\text{K}$

b. $K = 273° + (-40°)$

$K = 233°\text{K}$

Example: 80°F and −20°F can be expressed on the Rankine scale as follows:

a. $R = 460° + 80°$

$R = 540°R$

b. $R = 460° + (-20°)$

$R = 420°R$

XII. The General Gas Law

Formula(s): $\frac{P_1V_1}{t_1} = \frac{P_2V_2}{t_2}$

or $\frac{P_1V_1}{m_1t_1} = \frac{P_2V_2}{m_2t_2}$

or $\frac{P_1}{d_1t_1} = \frac{P_2}{d_2t_2}$

P = pressure

V = volume

m = mass

t = temperature

Example: A 10,000-cm³ steel container holds 10 gm of a gas. The pressure of mercury is 85 cm, and the temperature reads 60°C. Calculate the pressure if 12 gm of this gas are placed in a 5000-cm³ steel container at a temperature of 10°C.

$$\frac{P_1V_1}{m_1t_1} = \frac{P_2V_2}{m_2t_2}$$

$$\frac{P_1 \times 5000 \text{ cm}^3}{12 \text{ gm} \times 283°\text{K}} = \frac{85 \text{ cm Hg} \times 10{,}000 \text{ cm}^3}{10 \text{ gm} \times 333°\text{K}}$$

$$\frac{5000P_1}{3396} = \frac{850{,}000}{3330}$$

$$16{,}650{,}000P_1 = 2{,}886{,}600{,}000$$

$$P_1 = 173 \text{ cm Hg}$$

Example: The weight-density of carbon dioxide at 32°F and 30 in. of mercury pressure is 0.123 lb./ft.³. Calculate the weight-density at an altitude where a pressure of 15 in. of mercury and a temperature of 16°F are recorded.

$$\frac{P_1}{d_1t_1} = \frac{P_2}{d_2t_2}$$

$$\frac{30 \text{ in.}}{0.123 \text{ lb./ft.}^3 \times 492°\text{R}} = \frac{15 \text{ in.}}{d_2 \times 460°\text{R}}$$

$t_1 = 32° + 460° = 492°R$
$t_2 = 16° + 460° = 476°R$

$$\frac{30 \text{ in.}}{60.5} = \frac{15 \text{ in.}}{460d_2}$$

$$13{,}800d_2 = 907.5$$

$$d_2 = 0.066 \text{ lb./ft.}^3$$

Example: Gasoline is pumped at a pressure of 20 lb./in.² into a storage tank with a volume of 200 ft.³. What volume of gasoline must be pumped to raise the pressure to 60 lb./in.² if concomitantly the temperature is raised from 50°F to 70°F?

$$P_1 = 20 \text{ lb./in.}^2$$

$$P_2 = 20 \text{ lb./in.}^2 + 60 \text{ lb./in.}^2 = 80 \text{ lb./in.}^2$$

$$t_1 = 50° + 460° = 510°\text{R}$$

$$t_2 = 70° + 460° = 530°\text{R}$$

$$\frac{P_1V_1}{t_1} = \frac{P_2V_2}{t_2}$$

$$\frac{20 \text{ lb./in.}^2 \times V_1}{510°\text{R}} = \frac{80 \text{ lb./in.}^2 \times 200 \text{ ft.}^3}{530°\text{R}}$$

$$\frac{20V_1}{510} = \frac{16{,}000}{530}$$

$$V_1 = 769.8 \text{ ft.}^3$$

The volume present at the beginning was 200 ft.^{3}. The volume added is calculated in the following manner:

$$V = 770 \text{ ft.}^3 - 200 \text{ ft.}^3$$

$$V = 570 \text{ ft.}^3$$

XIII. Heat

Heat is expressed in British thermal units or in calories. One British thermal unit (Btu) is the amount of heat required to raise the temperature of one pound of water one Fahrenheit degree, and one calorie (cal.) is the amount of heat necessary to raise the temperature of one gram of water one centigrade degree. One British thermal unit equals about 250 calories.

Specific Heat

Example: How much heat is required to raise the temperature of 10 lb. of ethylene glycol (0.528 cal./gm°C or Btu/lb.°F) from 70°F to 140°F?

$$H = (10 \text{ lb.})(0.528 \text{ Btu/lb.°F})(140° - 70°\text{F})$$

$$H = (10 \text{ lb.})(0.528 \text{ Btu/lb.°F})(70°\text{F})$$

$$H = 370 \text{ Btu}$$

Heat Lost = Heat Gained

Example: Five hundred lb. of steel at 300°F are cooled in 5000 lb. of water at 100°F. The temperature obtained in the water is 150°F. Calculate the specific heat of the steel. Remember that the heat lost by the steel equals the heat gained by the water.

M_B = weight of first object (steel)

S_B = specific heat of first object

Δt_B = initial temperature of first object − final temperature of first object

M_w = weight of second object (water)

S_w = unit of heat (1 Btu/lb.°F)

Δt_w = final temperature of second object − initial temperature of second object

$$M_B S_B \,\Delta t_B = M_w S_w \,\Delta t_w$$

$$(500 \text{ lb.})S_B(300°\text{F} - 150°\text{F}) = (5000 \text{ lb.})(1.00 \text{ Btu/lb.°F})(150°\text{F} - 100°\text{F})$$

$$S_B = \frac{(5000 \text{ lb.})(1.00 \text{ Btu/lb.°F})(50°\text{F})}{(500 \text{ lb.})(150°\text{F})}$$

$$S_B = 3.33 \text{ Btu/lb.°F}$$

Heat of Vaporization

Example: How much heat is necessary to change 100 lb. of ice at 10°F to steam at 212°F? Ice, 0.51 Btu/lb.°F; heat of fusion of ice, 144 Btu/lb.; water, 1.00 Btu/lb.°F; vaporized water, 970 Btu/lb.

Step 1. Heat required to raise the temperature of ice to melting point

$$= M_i S_i(32°\text{F} - 10°\text{F})$$
$$= (100 \text{ lb.})(0.51 \text{ Btu/lb.°F})(22°\text{F})$$
$$= 1122 \text{ Btu}$$

Step 2. Heat required to melt ice

$$= (100 \text{ lb.})(144 \text{ Btu/lb.})$$
$$= 14{,}400 \text{ Btu}$$

Step 3. Heat required to bring water to its boiling point

$$= (100 \text{ lb.})(1 \text{ Btu/lb.°F})(212° - 32°\text{F})$$
$$= 18{,}000 \text{ Btu}$$

Step 4. Heat required to vaporize water

$$= (100 \text{ lb.})(970 \text{ Btu/lb.})$$
$$= 97{,}000 \text{ Btu}$$

Step 5. Total heat required:

$$\begin{array}{r} 1{,}122 \text{ Btu} \\ 14{,}400 \text{ Btu} \\ 18{,}000 \text{ Btu} \\ \underline{97{,}000 \text{ Btu}} \\ 130{,}522 \text{ Btu} \end{array}$$

XIV. Thermodynamics

Work and Heat

The following conversion values of mechanical energy to heat should be utilized:

4.18×10^7 ergs equals 1 cal.
4.18 J equals 1 cal.
1 J equals 0.239 cal.
778 ft.-lb. equals 1 Btu
1055 J equals 1 Btu

$W = J \text{ (constant) } H$ $\qquad W$ = work
J = constant
H = heat

Example: Water drops 300 ft. over the horseshoe falls at Niagara. Calculate the rise in temperature of the water if its potential energy were converted into heat.

Step 1. Energy transformed per pound of water

$$= (1.00 \text{ lb.})(300 \text{ ft.})$$

$$= 300 \text{ ft.-lb.}$$

Step 2. Heat produced

$$= \frac{300 \text{ ft.-lb.}}{778 \text{ ft.-lb./Btu}}$$
$$= 0.39 \text{ Btu}$$

Step 3. Rise in temperature:

Δt = rise (change) in temperature

H = heat change in material

M = mass (1 lb. of water)

S = energy or units of work (Btu), or the specific heat of a substance (heat/unit mass/degree change in temperature)

$$\Delta t = \frac{H}{MS}$$

$$\Delta t = \frac{0.39 \text{ Btu}}{(1.00 \text{ lb.})(1.00 \text{ Btu/lb.°F})}$$

$$\Delta t = 0.39\text{°F}$$

Specific Heat of a Gas

Example: A compressed gas at a constant pressure of 75 lb./in.^{2} enters a cylinder 5 in. in diameter and pushes a piston 5 in. The work done by the gas is?

$W = P \Delta V$ $\qquad P = 75 \text{ lb./in.}^2$

$W = (75 \text{ lb./in.}^2)(5\pi \text{ in.}^3)$ $\qquad \Delta V = \pi r^2 s$

$W = 1200 \text{ in.-lb.}$ $\qquad = \pi(1.0 \text{ in.})^2 \times 5 \text{ in.}$

$W = 100 \text{ ft.-lb.}$ $\qquad = 5\pi \text{ in.}^3$

Efficiency of a Boiler

Recall: The maximum efficiency of a heat engine supplied with heat at temperature T_1 and delivering heat to a reservoir at temperature T_2 can be calculated as follows:

$$E = \frac{T_1 - T_2}{T_1} = 1 - \frac{T_2}{T_1}$$

Example: An engine driven by a boiler receives steam at 300°C. Its exhaust temperature is 100°C. Its efficiency is?

$$E = \frac{T_1 - T_2}{T_1}$$

$$E = \frac{(300 + 273)°K - (100 + 273)°K}{(300 + 273)°K}$$

$$E = \frac{573°K - 173°K}{573°K}$$

$$E = 0.6980$$

$$E = 69.8\%$$

Example: A heat engine removes 6000 J per cycle of heat energy from the heat chamber and exhausts 1000 J to a cold chamber.

1. What is the thermal efficiency of the engine?

$$E = 1 - \frac{T_{cold}}{T_{hot}}$$

$$E = 1 - \frac{1000 \text{ J}}{6000 \text{ J}}$$

$$E = 1 - 0.17$$

$$E = 83\%$$

2. What is the work done by the engine?

$$W = Q_{hot} - Q_{cold}$$

$$W = 6000 \text{ J} - 1000 \text{ J}$$

$$W = 5000 \text{ J}$$

XV. Magnetism

Recall: A unit pole is the force of one dyne exerted by an object when placed at a distance of one centimeter from another object that has a unit pole (magnet) in a medium of unit permeability (vacuum or air).

Example: A magnetic pole with a strength of 600 u.p. (unit pole) exerts a force of 200 dynes upon a second pole located 10 cm away. Calculate the strength of the second pole.

F = force between poles

m = magnetic pole strength of one pole

m' = magnetic pole strength of second pole

S = distance between the two points

μ = a quantity called permeability (for air it is 1)

$$F = \frac{mm'}{\mu s^2} \text{ OR } \textit{Coulomb's Law}$$

$$200 \text{ dynes} = \frac{600 \text{ u.p.} \times m'}{1 \times (10 \text{ cm})^2}$$

$$200 \text{ dynes} = \frac{600 \text{ u.p.} \times m'}{100 \text{ cm}}$$

$$600 \text{ u.p.} \times m' = 20{,}000 \text{ dynes/cm}$$

$$m' = 33.33 \text{ u.p.}$$

Example: A force of 15,000 dynes is exerted upon the above magnetic pole. Calculate the strength of the magnetic field.

$$H = \frac{F}{m}$$

$$H = \frac{15{,}000 \text{ dynes}}{600 \text{ u.p.}}$$

$$H = 2.5 \text{ oersteds}$$

Example: What is the force exerted upon the above magnetic pole of 600 u.p. when it is placed in a magnetic field with a strength of 10 oersteds?

$$F = Hm$$

$$F = 10 \text{ oersteds} \times 600 \text{ u.p.}$$

$$F = 6000 \text{ dynes}$$

Example: Calculate the magnetic field strength 25 cm, in air, under the influence of a pole strength of 600 u.p.

$$H = \frac{m}{\mu s^2}$$

$$H = \frac{600 \text{ u.p.}}{1.0 \times (25 \text{ cm})^2}$$

$$H = \frac{600 \text{ u.p.}}{625 \text{ cm}}$$

$$H = 0.96 \text{ oersted}$$

XVI. Electricity

Ohm's Law: The ratio of the voltage to the current is a constant, that is,

$$R \text{ (a constant)} = \frac{V}{P}$$

Ohm's Law: The value in volts is equal to the amount of current in amperes times the distance in ohms, that is,

$$\text{Volts} = \text{Amperes} \times \text{Ohms}$$

$$\text{Amperes} = \frac{\text{Volts}}{\text{Ohms}}$$

$$\text{Ohms} = \frac{\text{Volts}}{\text{Amperes}}$$

Example: The difference in potential between two terminals is 10 volts. A current of 5 A passes; calculate the resistance.

$$R = \frac{V}{I}$$

$$R = \frac{10 \text{ volts}}{5 \text{ A}}$$

$$R = 2 \text{ ohms}$$

Example: Increase the difference of the above potential to 20 volts. Calculate the current that passes. Remember that according to Ohm's law, the resistance (R) will remain the same when the voltage is increased—it is constant.

$$I = \frac{V}{R}$$

$$I = \frac{20 \text{ volts}}{2 \text{ ohms}}$$

$$I = 10 \text{ A}$$

Example: A waffle iron needs a current of 8 A and has a resistance of 40 ohms. What voltage is necessary for the operation?

$$V = IR$$

$$V = 8 \text{ A} \times 40 \text{ ohms}$$

$$V = 320 \text{ volts}$$

Example: A 150-watt bulb draws 110 volts.

1. Calculate the current drawn.

$$P = IV$$

$$I = \frac{P}{V}$$

$$I = \frac{150 \text{ watts}}{110 \text{ volts}}$$

$$I = 1.36 \text{ A}$$

2. Calculate the resistance.

$$V = IR$$

$$R = \frac{V}{I}$$

$$R = \frac{110 \text{ volts}}{1.36 \text{ A}}$$

$$R = 80.88 \text{ ohms}$$

Example: A current of 10 A flows through a wire for 45 min. The charge that passes through a cross section of the wire may be calculated as follows:

$$I = \frac{q}{t}$$

$$q = It$$

$$q = (10 \text{ A})(2700 \text{ sec.})$$

$$q = 27{,}000 \text{ A}$$

XVII. Electric Circuits

Emf and Internal Resistance

$$V = E - Ir$$

V = terminal potential difference
E = potential difference
r = internal resistance
I = current

Example: A battery powering a portable television has an emf of 10 volts and an internal resistance of 0.20 ohm. It supplies a current of 6 A. Calculate the voltage.

$$V = E - IR$$

$$V = 10 \text{ volts} - (6 \text{ A} \times 0.20 \text{ ohm})$$

$$V = 10 \text{ volts} - 1.2 \text{ volts}$$

$$V = 8.8 \text{ volts}$$

Resistors in Series

Example: A direct-current circuit is wired with resistances of 3 ohms, 6 ohms, and 2 ohms in series. These resistances could be replaced by one resistor of 11 ohms to produce equivalent resistance.

Example: Three lamps are connected in series and exhibit a resistance of 15, 10, and 5 ohms, respectively. The current feeding them produces a potential difference of 100 volts across its terminals.

1. Determine the current in the lamp.

$$R = (15 + 10 + 5) \text{ ohms}$$

$$R = 30 \text{ ohms}$$

$$I = \frac{V}{R}$$

$$I = \frac{100 \text{ volts}}{30 \text{ ohms}}$$

$$I = 3.33 \text{ A}$$

2. Determine the voltage across each lamp; it is the product of its resistance and the current.

$$v_1 = (3.33 \text{ A})(15 \text{ ohms}) = 49.95 \text{ volts}$$

$$v_2 = (3.33 \text{ A})(10 \text{ ohms}) = 33.33 \text{ volts}$$

$$v_3 = (3.33 \text{ A})(5 \text{ ohms}) = 16.65 \text{ volts}$$

Resistors in Parallel

$$\frac{1}{R} = \frac{1}{R_1} + \frac{1}{R_2} + \frac{1}{R_3}$$

Recall that addition to a circuit of resistors in series increases the resistance while addition to a circuit of resistors in parallel decreases the resistance.

Example: Using the example of 3, 6, and 2 ohms, the equivalent resistance can be calculated as follows:

$$\frac{1}{R_{eq}} = \frac{1}{R_1} + \frac{1}{R_2} + \frac{1}{R_3}$$

$$\frac{1}{R_{eq}} = \frac{1}{3 \text{ ohms}} + \frac{1}{6 \text{ ohms}} + \frac{1}{2 \text{ ohms}}$$

$$= \frac{2}{6 \text{ ohms}} + \frac{1}{6 \text{ ohms}} + \frac{3}{6 \text{ ohms}} = \frac{6}{6 \text{ ohms}}$$

$$\frac{1}{R_{eq}} = 1 \text{ ohm, OR, } R_{eq} = 1 \text{ ohm}$$

Example: A circuit has resistances of 15, 10, and 5 ohms. If these are wired in parallel what is their combined resistance?

$$\frac{1}{R} = \frac{1}{R_1} + \frac{1}{R_2} + \frac{1}{R_3}$$

$$\frac{1}{R} = \frac{1}{15 \text{ ohms}} + \frac{1}{10 \text{ ohms}} + \frac{1}{5 \text{ ohms}}$$

$$\frac{1}{R} = (0.07 + 0.1 + 0.2) \text{ ohm}$$

$$\frac{1}{R} = 0.37 \text{ ohm}$$

$$R = \frac{1}{0.37} \text{ ohm}$$

$$R = 2.7 \text{ ohms}$$

Example: Find the current in a circuit with two energy sources (E_1 = 12 volts, E_2 = −4 volt) and two resistors (R_1 = 15 ohms, R_2 = 10 ohms).

$$E_1 + E_2 = I_1(R_1 + R_2)$$

$$I_1 = \frac{E_1 + E_2}{R_1 + R_2}$$

$$I_1 = \frac{(12 - 4) \text{ volts}}{(15 + 10) \text{ ohms}}$$

$$I_1 = \frac{8 \text{ volts}}{25 \text{ ohms}} = 0.32 \text{ A}$$

Example: A circuit has three resistors—of 2 ohms, 4 ohms, and 8 ohms.

1. What is the resistance of these three resistors when connected in series?

$$R_s = R_1 + R_2 + R_3$$

$$R_s = (2 + 4 + 8) \text{ ohms}$$

$$R_s = 14 \text{ ohms}$$

2. What is their resistance when connected in parallel?

$$\frac{1}{R_p} = \frac{1}{R_1} + \frac{1}{R_2} + \frac{1}{R_3}$$

$$\frac{1}{R_p} = \frac{1}{2 \text{ ohms}} + \frac{1}{4 \text{ ohms}} + \frac{1}{8 \text{ ohms}}$$

$$\frac{1}{R_p} = \frac{4}{8 \text{ ohms}} + \frac{2}{8 \text{ ohms}} + \frac{1}{8 \text{ ohms}}$$

$$\frac{1}{R_p} = \frac{7}{8 \text{ ohms}}$$

$$R_p = \frac{8}{7} \text{ ohms}$$

3. A 12-volt battery would draw what current?

SERIES

$$I = \frac{V}{R_s} = \frac{12 \text{ volts}}{14 \text{ ohms}} = 0.857 \text{ A}$$

Potential drop in each resistor:

$$V_1 = IR_1 = (0.857 \text{ A})(2 \text{ ohms}) = 1.7 \text{ volts}$$

$$V_2 = IR_2 = (0.857 \text{ A})(4 \text{ ohms}) = 3.4 \text{ volts}$$

$$V_3 = IR_3 = (0.857 \text{ A})(8 \text{ ohms}) = 6.9 \text{ volts}$$

The drop equals the voltage rise in the battery:

$$V_i = V_1 + V_2 + V_3$$

$$V_i = 12 \text{ volts}$$

PARALLEL

$$I = \frac{V}{R_p} = \frac{12 \text{ ohms}}{8/7 \text{ ohms}} = 10.5 \text{ A}$$

Current in each resistor:

$$I_1 = \frac{V}{R_1} = \frac{12 \text{ volts}}{2 \text{ ohms}} = 6 \text{ A}$$

$$I_2 = \frac{V}{R_2} = \frac{12 \text{ volts}}{4 \text{ ohms}} = 3 \text{ A}$$

$$I_3 = \frac{V}{R_3} = \frac{12 \text{ volts}}{8 \text{ ohms}} = 1.5 \text{ A}$$

$$I_i = I_1 + I_2 + I_3 = 10.5 \text{ A}$$

Cells in Series

Example: Three cells are connected in series; each has an emf of 10 volts and a resistance of 2 ohms. Calculate the current in the middle cell after it is connected to an external resistance of 20 ohms.

$$\text{Total emf} = 10 \text{ volts} + 10 \text{ volts} + 10 \text{ volts} = 30 \text{ volts}$$

$$\text{Total Resistance } (R) = 2 \text{ ohms} + 2 \text{ ohms} + 2 \text{ ohms} = 6 \text{ ohms}$$

$$\text{Total Current} = \frac{\text{Total emf}}{\text{Total Resistance}}$$

$$\text{Total Current} = \frac{30 \text{ volts}}{(20 + 6) \text{ ohms}}$$

$$\text{Total Current} = 1.15 \text{ A}$$

Cells in Parallel

Example: Consider the following three arrangements:

a. A single cell
b. Two cells in series
c. Two cells in parallel

Compare the currents maintained in a 5-ohm resistor under each condition. Each cell has an emf of 3 volts. The emf of (a) is 3 volts, of (b) 6 volts, and of (c) 3 volts.

$$I_{total} = \frac{E_{total}}{R_{total}}$$

$$I_a = \frac{3 \text{ volts}}{5 \text{ ohms}}$$

$$I_a = 0.6 \text{ A}$$

$$I_b = \frac{6 \text{ volts}}{5 \text{ ohms}}$$

$$I_b = 1.2 \text{ A}$$

$$I_c = \frac{3 \text{ volts}}{5 \text{ ohms}}$$

$$I_c = 0.6 \text{ A}$$

In each cell, however, the current is 0.3 A.

XVIII. Electric Energy

$$\text{Voltage} = \frac{\text{Work}}{\text{Charge}} \qquad V = \text{volts}$$

$$V = \frac{W}{Q} \qquad W = \text{usually in joules}$$

$$\text{OR } VIt = I^2Rt \qquad Q = \text{usually in coulombs}$$

Rewriting $W = VQ$, we can make the substitutions $Q = It$ and $V = IR$. Then, the basic equation for electric energy may be $W = VQ = VIt = I^2Rt$. This equation indicates that one joule must be expanded in maintaining for one second a current of one ampere in a circuit of a one-ohm resistance.

Example: A motor is used for 45 min. to drive a conveyor belt. It uses 35 A at 110 volts. Calculate the energy supplied.

$$W = VIt$$

$$W = (110 \text{ volts})(35 \text{ A})(2700 \text{ sec.})$$

$$W = 10{,}395{,}000 \text{ J}$$

$$W = 10.4 \times 10^6 \text{ J}$$

Example: How many calories are produced in a central electric resistance heating system in 5 min. as it draws 30 A connected to a 220-volt line?

Recall: 1 cal = 4.18 J

$$H = \frac{VIt}{J} \text{ or } H = \frac{W}{J}$$

$$H = \frac{(220 \text{ volts})(30 \text{ A})(300 \text{ sec.})}{4.18 \text{ J/cal.}}$$

$$H = \frac{1{,}980{,}000}{4.18 \text{ J/cal.}}$$

$$H = 473{,}684 \text{ cal.}$$

Power and Resistance

Example: The above furnace operating at 220 volts requires 2 hp. What are the current and the resistance of the unit?

1. Current

$$P = 2 \text{ hp.} \times 746 \frac{\text{watts}}{\text{hp.}}$$

$$P = 1492 \text{ watts}$$

2. Resistance

$$P = VI$$

$$1492 \text{ watts} = 220 \text{ volts} \times I$$

$$I = 6.78 \text{ A}$$

$$R = \frac{V}{I}$$

$$R = \frac{220 \text{ volts}}{6.78 \text{ A}}$$

$$R = 32.45 \text{ ohms}$$

XIX. Machines and Mechanical Advantage

Actual Mechanical Advantage (AMA) $= \frac{F_o}{F_i}$,

where F_o = output force and F_i = input force.

Theoretical Mechanical Advantage (TMA) $= \frac{d_i}{d_o}$

$$Efficiency\ (E) = \frac{F_o/F_i}{d_i/d_o} = \frac{\text{AMA}}{\text{TMA}} = \frac{\text{Output Work}}{\text{Input Work}}$$

Example: A man pushing down with a force of 50 lb. lifts a 200-lb. crate by utilizing a lever system. The lever arms are 6 and 1.2 ft., respectively.

1. Calculate the AMA.

$$\text{AMA} = \frac{F_o}{F_i}$$

$$\text{AMA} = \frac{200 \text{ lb.}}{50 \text{ lb.}}$$

$$\text{AMA} = 4 \text{ lb.}$$

2. Calculate the TMA.

$$\text{TMA} = \frac{d_i}{d_o}$$

$$\text{TMA} = \frac{6 \text{ ft.}}{1.2 \text{ ft.}}$$

$$\text{TMA} = 5 \text{ ft.}$$

3. What is the efficiency?

$$E = \frac{\text{AMA}}{\text{TMA}}$$

$$E = \frac{4}{5}(100\%)$$

$$E = 80\%$$

Example: A car weighing 1500 lb. is pushed up a 50-ft. ramp exhibiting an incline of 30°. A parallel force of 1000 lb. is used to accomplish this task.

1. What is the AMA?

$$\text{AMA} = \frac{F_0}{F_i} = \frac{1500\text{ lb.}}{1000\text{ lb.}} = 1.5\text{ lb.}$$

2. What is the efficiency of the system?

$$E = \frac{1}{\sin\theta}$$

$$E = \frac{1.5\text{ lb.}}{2}$$

$$E = 75\%$$

XX. Wavelength

Example: What is the wavelength of a beam of monochromatic light that passes through two slits 0.50 mm apart? The third-order bright fringe of the interference patterns observed on a screen 1.5 m from the slits is 5 mm from the center of central maximum.

$$\gamma = \frac{yd}{nL} \qquad \begin{aligned} d &= 0.50\text{ mm} \\ L &= 1500\text{ mm} \\ y &= 5\text{ mm} \\ n &= 3 \end{aligned}$$

$$\gamma = \frac{(5\text{ mm})(0.50\text{ mm})}{(3)(1500\text{ mm})}$$

$$\gamma = 0.0005555\text{ mm}$$

$$\gamma = 5.5 \times 10^{-4}\text{ mm}$$

Answer Sheet—Model Test A

SCIENCE KNOWLEDGE

Biology

1. (A) (B) (C) (D) (E)
2. (A) (B) (C) (D) (E)
3. (A) (B) (C) (D) (E)
4. (A) (B) (C) (D) (E)
5. (A) (B) (C) (D) (E)
6. (A) (B) (C) (D) (E)
7. (A) (B) (C) (D) (E)
8. (A) (B) (C) (D) (E)
9. (A) (B) (C) (D) (E)
10. (A) (B) (C) (D) (E)
11. (A) (B) (C) (D) (E)
12. (A) (B) (C) (D) (E)
13. (A) (B) (C) (D) (E)
14. (A) (B) (C) (D) (E)
15. (A) (B) (C) (D) (E)
16. (A) (B) (C) (D) (E)
17. (A) (B) (C) (D) (E)
18. (A) (B) (C) (D) (E)
19. (A) (B) (C) (D) (E)
20. (A) (B) (C) (D) (E)
21. (A) (B) (C) (D) (E)
22. (A) (B) (C) (D) (E)
23. (A) (B) (C) (D) (E)
24. (A) (B) (C) (D) (E)
25. (A) (B) (C) (D) (E)
26. (A) (B) (C) (D) (E)
27. (A) (B) (C) (D) (E)
28. (A) (B) (C) (D) (E)
29. (A) (B) (C) (D) (E)
30. (A) (B) (C) (D) (E)
31. (A) (B) (C) (D) (E)
32. (A) (B) (C) (D) (E)
33. (A) (B) (C) (D) (E)
34. (A) (B) (C) (D) (E)
35. (A) (B) (C) (D) (E)
36. (A) (B) (C) (D) (E)
37. (A) (B) (C) (D) (E)
38. (A) (B) (C) (D) (E)

Chemistry

1. (A) (B) (C) (D) (E)
2. (A) (B) (C) (D) (E)
3. (A) (B) (C) (D) (E)
4. (A) (B) (C) (D) (E)
5. (A) (B) (C) (D) (E)
6. (A) (B) (C) (D) (E)
7. (A) (B) (C) (D) (E)
8. (A) (B) (C) (D) (E)
9. (A) (B) (C) (D) (E)
10. (A) (B) (C) (D) (E)
11. (A) (B) (C) (D) (E)
12. (A) (B) (C) (D) (E)
13. (A) (B) (C) (D) (E)
14. (A) (B) (C) (D) (E)
15. (A) (B) (C) (D) (E)
16. (A) (B) (C) (D) (E)
17. (A) (B) (C) (D) (E)
18. (A) (B) (C) (D) (E)
19. (A) (B) (C) (D) (E)
20. (A) (B) (C) (D) (E)
21. (A) (B) (C) (D) (E)
22. (A) (B) (C) (D) (E)
23. (A) (B) (C) (D) (E)
24. (A) (B) (C) (D) (E)
25. (A) (B) (C) (D) (E)
26. (A) (B) (C) (D) (E)
27. (A) (B) (C) (D) (E)
28. (A) (B) (C) (D) (E)
29. (A) (B) (C) (D) (E)
30. (A) (B) (C) (D) (E)
31. (A) (B) (C) (D) (E)
32. (A) (B) (C) (D) (E)
33. (A) (B) (C) (D) (E)
34. (A) (B) (C) (D) (E)
35. (A) (B) (C) (D) (E)
36. (A) (B) (C) (D) (E)
37. (A) (B) (C) (D) (E)
38. (A) (B) (C) (D) (E)
39. (A) (B) (C) (D) (E)
40. (A) (B) (C) (D) (E)
41. (A) (B) (C) (D) (E)
42. (A) (B) (C) (D) (E)
43. (A) (B) (C) (D) (E)
44. (A) (B) (C) (D) (E)
45. (A) (B) (C) (D) (E)
46. (A) (B) (C) (D) (E)
47. (A) (B) (C) (D) (E)
48. (A) (B) (C) (D) (E)
49. (A) (B) (C) (D) (E)

Physics

1. Ⓐ Ⓑ Ⓒ Ⓓ Ⓔ
2. Ⓐ Ⓑ Ⓒ Ⓓ Ⓔ
3. Ⓐ Ⓑ Ⓒ Ⓓ Ⓔ
4. Ⓐ Ⓑ Ⓒ Ⓓ Ⓔ
5. Ⓐ Ⓑ Ⓒ Ⓓ Ⓔ
6. Ⓐ Ⓑ Ⓒ Ⓓ Ⓔ
7. Ⓐ Ⓑ Ⓒ Ⓓ Ⓔ
8. Ⓐ Ⓑ Ⓒ Ⓓ Ⓔ
9. Ⓐ Ⓑ Ⓒ Ⓓ Ⓔ
10. Ⓐ Ⓑ Ⓒ Ⓓ Ⓔ
11. Ⓐ Ⓑ Ⓒ Ⓓ Ⓔ
12. Ⓐ Ⓑ Ⓒ Ⓓ Ⓔ
13. Ⓐ Ⓑ Ⓒ Ⓓ Ⓔ
14. Ⓐ Ⓑ Ⓒ Ⓓ Ⓔ
15. Ⓐ Ⓑ Ⓒ Ⓓ Ⓔ
16. Ⓐ Ⓑ Ⓒ Ⓓ Ⓔ
17. Ⓐ Ⓑ Ⓒ Ⓓ Ⓔ
18. Ⓐ Ⓑ Ⓒ Ⓓ Ⓔ
19. Ⓐ Ⓑ Ⓒ Ⓓ Ⓔ
20. Ⓐ Ⓑ Ⓒ Ⓓ Ⓔ
21. Ⓐ Ⓑ Ⓒ Ⓓ Ⓔ
22. Ⓐ Ⓑ Ⓒ Ⓓ Ⓔ
23. Ⓐ Ⓑ Ⓒ Ⓓ Ⓔ
24. Ⓐ Ⓑ Ⓒ Ⓓ Ⓔ
25. Ⓐ Ⓑ Ⓒ Ⓓ Ⓔ
26. Ⓐ Ⓑ Ⓒ Ⓓ Ⓔ
27. Ⓐ Ⓑ Ⓒ Ⓓ Ⓔ
28. Ⓐ Ⓑ Ⓒ Ⓓ Ⓔ
29. Ⓐ Ⓑ Ⓒ Ⓓ Ⓔ
30. Ⓐ Ⓑ Ⓒ Ⓓ Ⓔ
31. Ⓐ Ⓑ Ⓒ Ⓓ Ⓔ
32. Ⓐ Ⓑ Ⓒ Ⓓ Ⓔ
33. Ⓐ Ⓑ Ⓒ Ⓓ Ⓔ
34. Ⓐ Ⓑ Ⓒ Ⓓ Ⓔ
35. Ⓐ Ⓑ Ⓒ Ⓓ Ⓔ
36. Ⓐ Ⓑ Ⓒ Ⓓ Ⓔ
37. Ⓐ Ⓑ Ⓒ Ⓓ Ⓔ
38. Ⓐ Ⓑ Ⓒ Ⓓ Ⓔ

SCIENCE PROBLEMS

1. Ⓐ Ⓑ Ⓒ Ⓓ Ⓔ
2. Ⓐ Ⓑ Ⓒ Ⓓ Ⓔ
3. Ⓐ Ⓑ Ⓒ Ⓓ Ⓔ
4. Ⓐ Ⓑ Ⓒ Ⓓ Ⓔ
5. Ⓐ Ⓑ Ⓒ Ⓓ Ⓔ
6. Ⓐ Ⓑ Ⓒ Ⓓ Ⓔ
7. Ⓐ Ⓑ Ⓒ Ⓓ Ⓔ
8. Ⓐ Ⓑ Ⓒ Ⓓ Ⓔ
9. Ⓐ Ⓑ Ⓒ Ⓓ Ⓔ
10. Ⓐ Ⓑ Ⓒ Ⓓ Ⓔ
11. Ⓐ Ⓑ Ⓒ Ⓓ Ⓔ
12. Ⓐ Ⓑ Ⓒ Ⓓ Ⓔ
13. Ⓐ Ⓑ Ⓒ Ⓓ Ⓔ
14. Ⓐ Ⓑ Ⓒ Ⓓ Ⓔ
15. Ⓐ Ⓑ Ⓒ Ⓓ Ⓔ
16. Ⓐ Ⓑ Ⓒ Ⓓ Ⓔ
17. Ⓐ Ⓑ Ⓒ Ⓓ Ⓔ
18. Ⓐ Ⓑ Ⓒ Ⓓ Ⓔ
19. Ⓐ Ⓑ Ⓒ Ⓓ Ⓔ
20. Ⓐ Ⓑ Ⓒ Ⓓ Ⓔ
21. Ⓐ Ⓑ Ⓒ Ⓓ Ⓔ
22. Ⓐ Ⓑ Ⓒ Ⓓ Ⓔ
23. Ⓐ Ⓑ Ⓒ Ⓓ Ⓔ
24. Ⓐ Ⓑ Ⓒ Ⓓ
25. Ⓐ Ⓑ Ⓒ Ⓓ Ⓔ
26. Ⓐ Ⓑ Ⓒ Ⓓ Ⓔ
27. Ⓐ Ⓑ Ⓒ Ⓓ Ⓔ
28. Ⓐ Ⓑ Ⓒ Ⓓ Ⓔ
29. Ⓐ Ⓑ Ⓒ Ⓓ Ⓔ
30. Ⓐ Ⓑ Ⓒ Ⓓ Ⓔ
31. Ⓐ Ⓑ Ⓒ Ⓓ Ⓔ
32. Ⓐ Ⓑ Ⓒ Ⓓ Ⓔ
33. Ⓐ Ⓑ Ⓒ Ⓓ Ⓔ
34. Ⓐ Ⓑ Ⓒ Ⓓ Ⓔ
35. Ⓐ Ⓑ Ⓒ Ⓓ Ⓔ
36. Ⓐ Ⓑ Ⓒ Ⓓ Ⓔ
37. Ⓐ Ⓑ Ⓒ Ⓓ Ⓔ
38. Ⓐ Ⓑ Ⓒ Ⓓ Ⓔ
39. Ⓐ Ⓑ Ⓒ Ⓓ Ⓔ
40. Ⓐ Ⓑ Ⓒ Ⓓ Ⓔ
41. Ⓐ Ⓑ Ⓒ Ⓓ Ⓔ
42. Ⓐ Ⓑ Ⓒ Ⓓ Ⓔ
43. Ⓐ Ⓑ Ⓒ Ⓓ Ⓔ
44. Ⓐ Ⓑ Ⓒ Ⓓ Ⓔ
45. Ⓐ Ⓑ Ⓒ Ⓓ Ⓔ
46. Ⓐ Ⓑ Ⓒ Ⓓ Ⓔ
47. Ⓐ Ⓑ Ⓒ Ⓓ Ⓔ
48. Ⓐ Ⓑ Ⓒ Ⓓ Ⓔ
49. Ⓐ Ⓑ Ⓒ Ⓓ Ⓔ
50. Ⓐ Ⓑ Ⓒ Ⓓ Ⓔ
51. Ⓐ Ⓑ Ⓒ Ⓓ Ⓔ
52. Ⓐ Ⓑ Ⓒ Ⓓ Ⓔ
53. Ⓐ Ⓑ Ⓒ Ⓓ Ⓔ
54. Ⓐ Ⓑ Ⓒ Ⓓ Ⓔ
55. Ⓐ Ⓑ Ⓒ Ⓓ Ⓔ
56. Ⓐ Ⓑ Ⓒ Ⓓ Ⓔ
57. Ⓐ Ⓑ Ⓒ Ⓓ Ⓔ
58. Ⓐ Ⓑ Ⓒ Ⓓ Ⓔ
59. Ⓐ Ⓑ Ⓒ Ⓓ Ⓔ
60. Ⓐ Ⓑ Ⓒ Ⓓ Ⓔ
61. Ⓐ Ⓑ Ⓒ Ⓓ Ⓔ
62. Ⓐ Ⓑ Ⓒ Ⓓ Ⓔ
63. Ⓐ Ⓑ Ⓒ Ⓓ Ⓔ
64. Ⓐ Ⓑ Ⓒ Ⓓ Ⓔ
65. Ⓐ Ⓑ Ⓒ Ⓓ Ⓔ
66. Ⓐ Ⓑ Ⓒ Ⓓ Ⓔ

SKILLS ANALYSIS: READING

1. Ⓐ Ⓑ Ⓒ
2. Ⓐ Ⓑ Ⓒ
3. Ⓐ Ⓑ Ⓒ
4. Ⓐ Ⓑ Ⓒ
5. Ⓐ Ⓑ Ⓒ
6. Ⓐ Ⓑ Ⓒ
7. Ⓐ Ⓑ Ⓒ
8. Ⓐ Ⓑ Ⓒ
9. Ⓐ Ⓑ Ⓒ
10. Ⓐ Ⓑ Ⓒ
11. Ⓐ Ⓑ Ⓒ
12. Ⓐ Ⓑ Ⓒ
13. Ⓐ Ⓑ Ⓒ
14. Ⓐ Ⓑ Ⓒ Ⓓ Ⓔ
15. Ⓐ Ⓑ Ⓒ Ⓓ Ⓔ
16. Ⓐ Ⓑ Ⓒ Ⓓ Ⓔ
17. Ⓐ Ⓑ Ⓒ Ⓓ Ⓔ
18. Ⓐ Ⓑ Ⓒ Ⓓ Ⓔ
19. Ⓐ Ⓑ Ⓒ Ⓓ Ⓔ
20. Ⓐ Ⓑ Ⓒ Ⓓ Ⓔ
21. Ⓐ Ⓑ Ⓒ Ⓓ Ⓔ
22. Ⓐ Ⓑ Ⓒ Ⓓ Ⓔ
23. Ⓐ Ⓑ Ⓒ Ⓓ Ⓔ
24. Ⓐ Ⓑ Ⓒ
25. Ⓐ Ⓑ Ⓒ
26. Ⓐ Ⓑ Ⓒ
27. Ⓐ Ⓑ Ⓒ
28. Ⓐ Ⓑ Ⓒ
29. Ⓐ Ⓑ Ⓒ
30. Ⓐ Ⓑ Ⓒ
31. Ⓐ Ⓑ Ⓒ
32. Ⓐ Ⓑ Ⓒ Ⓓ Ⓔ
33. Ⓐ Ⓑ Ⓒ Ⓓ Ⓔ
34. Ⓐ Ⓑ Ⓒ Ⓓ Ⓔ
35. Ⓐ Ⓑ Ⓒ Ⓓ Ⓔ
36. Ⓐ Ⓑ Ⓒ Ⓓ Ⓔ
37. Ⓐ Ⓑ Ⓒ
38. Ⓐ Ⓑ Ⓒ
39. Ⓐ Ⓑ Ⓒ
40. Ⓐ Ⓑ Ⓒ
41. Ⓐ Ⓑ Ⓒ
42. Ⓐ Ⓑ Ⓒ
43. Ⓐ Ⓑ Ⓒ
44. Ⓐ Ⓑ Ⓒ
45. Ⓐ Ⓑ Ⓒ
46. Ⓐ Ⓑ Ⓒ
47. Ⓐ Ⓑ Ⓒ
48. Ⓐ Ⓑ Ⓒ
49. Ⓐ Ⓑ Ⓒ Ⓓ Ⓔ
50. Ⓐ Ⓑ Ⓒ Ⓓ Ⓔ
51. Ⓐ Ⓑ Ⓒ Ⓓ Ⓔ
52. Ⓐ Ⓑ Ⓒ Ⓓ Ⓔ
53. Ⓐ Ⓑ Ⓒ Ⓓ Ⓔ
54. Ⓐ Ⓑ Ⓒ
55. Ⓐ Ⓑ Ⓒ
56. Ⓐ Ⓑ Ⓒ
57. Ⓐ Ⓑ Ⓒ
58. Ⓐ Ⓑ Ⓒ
59. Ⓐ Ⓑ Ⓒ
60. Ⓐ Ⓑ Ⓒ
61. Ⓐ Ⓑ Ⓒ
62. Ⓐ Ⓑ Ⓒ Ⓓ
63. Ⓐ Ⓑ Ⓒ Ⓓ
64. Ⓐ Ⓑ Ⓒ Ⓓ
65. Ⓐ Ⓑ Ⓒ Ⓓ
66. Ⓐ Ⓑ Ⓒ Ⓓ
67. Ⓐ Ⓑ Ⓒ Ⓓ
68. Ⓐ Ⓑ Ⓒ Ⓓ

SKILLS ANALYSIS: QUANTITATIVE

1. Ⓐ Ⓑ Ⓒ
2. Ⓐ Ⓑ Ⓒ
3. Ⓐ Ⓑ Ⓒ
4. Ⓐ Ⓑ Ⓒ
5. Ⓐ Ⓑ Ⓒ
6. Ⓐ Ⓑ Ⓒ
7. Ⓐ Ⓑ Ⓒ
8. Ⓐ Ⓑ Ⓒ
9. Ⓐ Ⓑ Ⓒ
10. Ⓐ Ⓑ Ⓒ
11. Ⓐ Ⓑ Ⓒ
12. Ⓐ Ⓑ Ⓒ
13. Ⓐ Ⓑ Ⓒ
14. Ⓐ Ⓑ Ⓒ
15. Ⓐ Ⓑ Ⓒ
16. Ⓐ Ⓑ Ⓒ
17. Ⓐ Ⓑ Ⓒ
18. Ⓐ Ⓑ Ⓒ
19. Ⓐ Ⓑ Ⓒ Ⓓ Ⓔ
20. Ⓐ Ⓑ Ⓒ Ⓓ Ⓔ
21. Ⓐ Ⓑ Ⓒ Ⓓ Ⓔ
22. Ⓐ Ⓑ Ⓒ Ⓓ
23. Ⓐ Ⓑ Ⓒ Ⓓ
24. Ⓐ Ⓑ Ⓒ Ⓓ
25. Ⓐ Ⓑ Ⓒ Ⓓ
26. Ⓐ Ⓑ Ⓒ Ⓓ
27. Ⓐ Ⓑ Ⓒ Ⓓ
28. Ⓐ Ⓑ Ⓒ Ⓓ
29. Ⓐ Ⓑ Ⓒ Ⓓ
30. Ⓐ Ⓑ Ⓒ Ⓓ
31. Ⓐ Ⓑ Ⓒ Ⓓ
32. Ⓐ Ⓑ Ⓒ
33. Ⓐ Ⓑ Ⓒ
34. Ⓐ Ⓑ Ⓒ
35. Ⓐ Ⓑ Ⓒ
36. Ⓐ Ⓑ Ⓒ
37. Ⓐ Ⓑ Ⓒ
38. Ⓐ Ⓑ Ⓒ
39. Ⓐ Ⓑ Ⓒ
40. Ⓐ Ⓑ Ⓒ
41. Ⓐ Ⓑ Ⓒ
42. Ⓐ Ⓑ Ⓒ
43. Ⓐ Ⓑ Ⓒ
44. Ⓐ Ⓑ Ⓒ
45. Ⓐ Ⓑ Ⓒ Ⓓ
46. Ⓐ Ⓑ Ⓒ Ⓓ
47. Ⓐ Ⓑ Ⓒ Ⓓ
48. Ⓐ Ⓑ Ⓒ
49. Ⓐ Ⓑ Ⓒ
50. Ⓐ Ⓑ Ⓒ
51. Ⓐ Ⓑ Ⓒ
52. Ⓐ Ⓑ Ⓒ
53. Ⓐ Ⓑ Ⓒ
54. Ⓐ Ⓑ Ⓒ
55. Ⓐ Ⓑ Ⓒ
56. Ⓐ Ⓑ Ⓒ
57. Ⓐ Ⓑ Ⓒ
58. Ⓐ Ⓑ Ⓒ Ⓓ
59. Ⓐ Ⓑ Ⓒ Ⓓ
60. Ⓐ Ⓑ Ⓒ Ⓓ
61. Ⓐ Ⓑ Ⓒ Ⓓ
62. Ⓐ Ⓑ Ⓒ Ⓓ
63. Ⓐ Ⓑ Ⓒ Ⓓ
64. Ⓐ Ⓑ Ⓒ
65. Ⓐ Ⓑ Ⓒ
66. Ⓐ Ⓑ Ⓒ
67. Ⓐ Ⓑ Ⓒ
68. Ⓐ Ⓑ Ⓒ

The New MCAT Model Examination A*

SCIENCE KNOWLEDGE

135 MINUTES
125 QUESTIONS

The following questions are based on your knowledge of science. The questions are varied; therefore, you are advised to pay careful attention to the instructions for each portion.

Biology

DIRECTIONS: In the following questions, five words or phrases are presented that have been labeled A-E. For each question, choose the word or phrase that is most closely associated with the given item. You may use a choice more than once, or not at all. Eliminate those choices that you think to be incorrect and mark the letter of your choice on the answer sheet.

Questions 1-6:

(A) Placenta
(B) Hypothalamus
(C) Adrenal cortex
(D) Saliva
(E) Pancreas

1. Chorionic gonadotropin
2. Relaxin
3. Cortisol
4. Ptyalin
5. Vasopressin
6. Maltase

DIRECTIONS: Each of the statements or questions is followed by five suggested completions or answers. Choose the one that best completes the statement or answers the question, and mark the letter of your choice on the answer sheet.

7. Epithelial cells cover and protect the body. Which of the following is a secretion of this tissue?
(A) chitin
(B) mucus
(C) keratin
(D) none of the above
(E) all of the above

*Explanations for science answers can be found on p. 133.

8. A fiber of striated (skeletal) muscle
   (A) possesses only one nucleus.
   (B) possesses no clear Z bands.
   (C) possesses more than one nucleus.
   (D) has the same characteristics as smooth muscle.
   (E) possesses few mitochondria.

9. The insect vector for African sleeping sickness is the
   (A) ant lion.
   (B) anopheles mosquito.
   (C) tsetse fly.
   (D) fruit fly.
   (E) fire ant.

10. Metamorphosis follows an orderly sequence. Which is the proper one?
   (A) egg → spore → adult
   (B) egg → larva → pupa → adult
   (C) egg → nymph → adult
   (D) egg → larva → pupa → nymph → adult
   (E) egg → pupa → larva → adult

11. All chordates are said to possess
   (A) a dorsal tubular nerve cord.
   (B) a vertebral column.
   (C) jaws.
   (D) appendages.
   (E) a maxilla.

12. The smallest unit possessing the capability to maintain life and to reproduce is
   (A) an organ.
   (B) a cell.
   (C) DNA.
   (D) RNA.
   (E) a nucleus.

13. Of the following, which is not considered a membranous organelle?
   (A) ribosome
   (B) endoplasmic reticulum
   (C) Golgi body
   (D) mitochondrion
   (E) lysosome

14. Cellular "digestive" or "suicide" packages is a common description or name for
   (A) mitochondria.
   (B) Golgi zones or Golgi bodies.
   (C) lysosomes.
   (D) centrosomes.
   (E) multivesicular bodies.

15. Housed in the sella tursica is the
   (A) pineal organ.
   (B) pituitary gland.
   (C) olfactory bulb.
   (D) optic chiasm.
   (E) hypothalamus.

16. ____________ gives origin to the nervous system.
   (A) Ectoderm
   (B) Mesoderm
   (C) Endoderm
   (D) Ectoderm and endoderm
   (E) Endoderm and mesoderm

17. Social stress will affect most severely the
   (A) pancreas.
   (B) pineal.
   (C) adrenal.
   (D) parathyroid.
   (E) thyroid.

18. ____________ gives origin to the skeletal system.
   (A) Ectoderm
   (B) Mesoderm
   (C) Endoderm
   (D) Ectoderm and endoderm
   (E) Ectoderm and mesoderm

19. One of the outstanding features of connective tissue may be listed as
(A) an orderly arrangement of cells into sheets.
(B) possessing a fairly large amount of intercellular material.
(C) making up the majority of the ducts of secretory organs.
(D) all of the above.
(E) none of the above.

20. Human sperm and ova are similar in the respect that they
(A) are haploid.
(B) both possess flagella which give them good mobility.
(C) are approximately the same in size.
(D) both carry the identical genetic information.
(E) are diploid.

21. We speak in terms of an aggregation of nerve cell bodies in the central nervous system as the site of a (an)
(A) ganglion.
(B) nucleus.
(C) cranial nerve.
(D) association area.
(E) decussation.

22. The neurolemma of an axon is part of the
(A) nerve cell body.
(B) Schwann cell.
(C) node of Ranvier.
(D) axoplasm.
(E) axon hillock.

23. Exchange in the lung of CO_2 and O_2 takes place in the
(A) bronchi.
(B) bronchioles.
(C) alveoli.
(D) broncho-pulmonary segment.
(E) dust cells.

24. A common feature of sweat glands, salivary glands, and sebaceous glands is that they are
(A) endocrine in nature.
(B) exocrine in nature.
(C) apocrine in nature.
(D) merocrine in nature.
(E) none of the above.

25. The appendix can be found by the surgeon by locating the
(A) jejunum.
(B) cecum.
(C) colon (transverse).
(D) duodenum.
(E) right iliac fossa.

26. The process by which a cell can move a substance from a point of lower concentration to a point of higher concentration (against the diffusion gradient) is called
(A) osmosis.
(B) plasmolysis.
(C) turgor pressure.
(D) diffusion.
(E) active transport.

27. The internal structure of a cilium or flagellum, no matter what organism, has the same arrangement. The fibrillar arrangement is
(A) 7 outer, 2 inner.
(B) 9 outer, 2 inner.
(C) 11 outer, 2 inner.
(D) 9 outer, 1 inner.
(E) 9 outer, 3 inner.

28. The most elaborate, active, and functional system in the tapeworm is the
(A) digestive system.
(B) reproductive system.
(C) sensory system.
(D) muscular system.
(E) cardiovascular system.

29. Treatment of drinking water with ____________ is thought to lower the incidence of tooth decay.
(A) fluorine
(B) chlorine
(C) sodium chloride
(D) potassium fluoride
(E) sodium fluoride

30. Municipal water supplies in this country are commonly treated with ____________ to kill harmful organisms.
(A) fluorine
(B) sodium fluoride
(C) chlorine
(D) calcium chloride
(E) bromine

31. During metaphase of mitosis
(A) there is a dissolution of the chromosomal material.
(B) the centrioles with asters are at the opposite poles.
(C) the cell membrane starts to reappear.
(D) the nuclear membrane disappears.
(E) there is a slowdown in metabolic activity.

32. Locomotion of planaria is accomplished by
(A) cilia.
(B) cauda equina.
(C) flagella.
(D) microvilli.
(E) pseudopodia.

33. Two types of circulatory systems are utilized by organisms: a closed and an open one. An open one as found in the crayfish denotes that
(A) the heart has a patent foramen ovale.
(B) the auricles receive mixed and unmixed blood.
(C) the blood is not always encased in defined blood vessels.
(D) blood can flow in either direction within the vessels depending on need.
(E) none of the above.

34. The two cerebral hemispheres of the mammalian brain are connected via the
(A) corpus callosum.
(B) posterior commissure.
(C) anterior commissure.
(D) anterior peduncle.
(E) third ventricle.

35. Man is considered a (an)
(A) heterotroph.
(B) autotroph.
(C) geotroph.
(D) phototroph.
(E) chemotroph.

36. In order for speciation to occur the following factor(s) must have been met:
(A) adequate time elapsed
(B) genetic isolation occurred
(C) mutations are essential
(D) A and C
(E) A and B

37. Filtration in the kidneys results mainly from
(A) blood flow (m/sec.).
(B) reabsorption.
(C) blood pressure.
(D) secretion.
(E) osmotic phenomenon.

38. Blood-sucking insects usually carry parasites in their
(A) salivary glands.
(B) blood.
(C) lungs.
(D) colon.
(E) tentacles.

Chemistry

DIRECTIONS: In the following questions, five choices are presented and have been labeled A-E. For each question, choose the alternative that is most closely associated with the given item. You may use a choice more than once, or not at all. Eliminate those choices that you think to be incorrect, and mark the letter of your choice on the answer sheet.

Questions 1-5:

(A) Synthesis reaction
(B) Decomposition reaction
(C) Single replacement reaction
(D) Double replacement reaction
(E) None of the above

1. $NaCl + AgNO_3 \rightarrow NaNO_3 + AgCl$
2. $HCl + NaOH \rightarrow NaCl + H_2O$
3. $Fe + S \xrightarrow{\Delta} FeS$
4. $Fe + CuSO_4 \rightarrow FeSO_4 + Cu$
5. $2KClO_3 \rightarrow 2KCl + 3O_2$

Questions 6-8:

(A) $C_m(H_2O)_n$
(B) $C_nH_{2n}O_2$
(C) C_nH_{2n+2}
(D) C_nH_{2n}
(E) C_nH_{n+2}

6. A saturated fatty acid
7. A carbohydrate
8. A saturated hydrocarbon

DIRECTIONS: Each of the statements is followed by five suggested answers or completions. Choose the one that best completes each of the statements, and mark the letter of your choice on the answer sheet.

9. A reaction that needs energy is an _____________ reaction.
   (A) endergonic
   (B) exergonic
   (C) exopthalmus
   (D) equilibrium
   (E) insipid

10. Of the functional groups listed below which is incorrectly identified?
   (A) $-NH_2$ amino group
   (B) $-C(=O)-CH_3$ acetyl group
   (C) $-C(=O)-NH_2$ amide group
   (D) $-C(=O)-OH$ hydroxyl group
   (E) $-O-P(=O)(OH)-OH$ phosphate group

11. The positively charged electrode is the
(A) cathode.
(B) anode.
(C) filament.
(D) nematode.
(E) positron.

12. If 1-butene is reacted with HBr in the presence of peroxides, the major product is
(A) butane.
(B) 1-bromobutane.
(C) 2-bromobutane.
(D) 1,2-dibromobutane.
(E) 2-butene.

13. A gain of electrons is known as
(A) oxidation.
(B) valence.
(C) reduction.
(D) electrolysis.
(E) hydrolysis.

14. The eutectic temperature is the
(A) lowest melting temperature of any alloy produced by varying the percentages of its two components.
(B) temperature at which all motion ceases; i.e., –273°C.
(C) highest temperature at which a gas may be liquefied, no matter how high the applied pressure.
(D) most efficient temperature for electrolytic production of metals such as aluminum.
(E) none of the above.

15. The common zinc-cased dry cell used in flashlights uses a carbon rod as the positive terminal and the zinc case as the negative terminal. One half-cell reaction during discharge is

$$2NH_4^+ + 2e^- \rightarrow 2NH_3 + H_2$$

and the other half-cell reaction (with electrons not indicated) is
(A) $C + O_2 \rightarrow CO_2$
(B) $Zn \rightarrow Zn^{++}$
(C) $Zn^{++} \rightarrow Zn$
(D) $CO_2 \rightarrow C + O_2$
(E) $Pb^{++} \rightarrow Pb$

16. To a solution of $AgNO_3$ is added Na_2CO_3 until no more precipitation occurs. If we know that the K_{sp} for Ag_2CO_3 is 6.2×10^{-12}, and if we find that the $(CO_3^=)$ in the supernatant is 6.2×10^{-6} moles/liter, then the (Ag^+) in the supernatant will be
(A) 1×10^{-3} moles/liter.
(B) 1×10^{-6} moles/liter.
(C) 1×10^{-9} moles/liter.
(D) 38×10^{-18} moles/liter.
(E) 6.2×10^{-6} moles/liter.

17. The solubility product constant (K_{sp}) of NiS is given as 1×10^{-26}. In an experiment $Ni(NO_3)_2$ solution is treated with H_2S and a precipitate forms. If the (Ni^{++}) in the supernatant is found to be 1×10^{-20} moles/liter, the $(S^=)$ in the supernatant will be
(A) $1 \times 10^{-1.4}$ moles/liter.
(B) 1×10^{-6} moles/liter.
(C) 1×10^{-20} moles/liter.
(D) 1×10^{-26} moles/liter.
(E) 1×10^{-46} moles/liter.

18. An alloy of mercury with another metal is called
(A) a metalloid.
(B) pollution.
(C) an eluent.
(D) ecology.
(E) an amalgam.

19. Acetone may be produced by pyrolysis of ____________ acid in the presence of ThO_2.
(A) acetic
(B) propionic
(C) butyric
(D) oleic
(E) pyruvic

20. D-glucose is an aldohexose. Not considering ring structures, how many isomeric aldohexoses are there?
(A) 6
(B) 8
(C) 10
(D) 13
(E) 17

21. The compound ______________ reacts with glass; this allows use of the compound in the etching of glass.
(A) hydrofluoric acid
(B) carbolic acid
(C) boric acid
(D) ammonium nitrate
(E) nitric acid

22. Oxidation of coal that contains sulfur often produces ______________, the anhydride of sulfuric acid.
(A) SO_3
(B) SO_2
(C) SO_4
(D) H_2S
(E) CS_2

Questions 23 and 24:

In the uncharged atom, the atomic number equals the sum of all the ___(23)___ in the shells surrounding the nucleus; an atom that has lost two orbital electrons has a charge of ___(24)___.

23. (A) protons
(B) neutrons
(C) electrons
(D) positrons
(E) mesons

24. (A) +1
(B) +2
(C) −1
(D) −2
(E) −3

25. A.I. Oparin suggested that in order for the complex molecules (organic molecules) to have originated and have given rise to life, the early atmosphere of the earth was probably deficient in free
(A) xenon.
(B) oxygen.
(C) hydrogen.
(D) methane.
(E) nitrogen.

26. Addition of sodium to bromobenzene in dry ether will produce
(A) naphthalene.
(B) cyclohexane.
(C) benzene.
(D) biphenyl.
(E) no reaction.

27. An individual has at his disposal benzyl chloride, benzene, aluminum chloride, and sodium, and he wishes to synthesize diphenylmethane. He should react
(A) all four compounds.
(B) benzyl chloride and sodium.
(C) benzyl chloride, benzene, and aluminum chloride.
(D) benzyl chloride, benzene, and sodium.
(E) benzyl chloride and aluminum chloride.

28. Among the properties ordinarily possessed by organic compounds can be listed those that
(A) possess mainly covalent bonds.
(B) are insoluble in water but soluble in nonpolar solvents.
(C) are generally nonconducting.
(D) all of the above.
(E) none of the above.

29. You have at your disposal benzene, bromine, nitric acid, and sulfuric acid. If you wish to produce m-bromonitrobenzene, you should
(A) nitrate the benzene and then brominate.
(B) brominate the benzene and then nitrate.
(C) either (A) or (B). They work equally well.
(D) forget it. You cannot obtain the desired product with these materials.
(E) mix all except sulfuric acid.

30. The conversion of 1,2-dichloropropane to propene may be achieved by heating with
(A) alcoholic KOH.
(B) aqueous KOH.
(C) sulfuric acid.
(D) zinc duct in alcohol.
(E) sodium in dry ether.

31. In the usual commercial vulcanization process crosslinking is introduced by addition of
(A) ethylene.
(B) propylene.
(C) silicon.
(D) sulfur.
(E) toluene.

32. Ethylene will react with 1,3-butadiene to produce
(A) cyclohexene.
(B) cyclohexane.
(C) benzene.
(D) toluene.
(E) octadiene.

33. An uncharged atom of a particular element has an electron distribution of $1s^2$, $2s^2$, $2p^5$. You would expect this to be a (an)
(A) metal.
(B) nonmetal.
(C) metalloid.
(D) amalgam.
(E) can't tell from the information given.

34. The element above would most often be expected to gain or lose electrons and thus exhibit a valence of
(A) +1
(B) +3
(C) −1
(D) −2
(E) −3

35. Which of the following will react with water to form an acidic solution?
(A) Na_2O
(B) K_2O
(C) CaO
(D) BaO
(E) P_2O_3

36. In the nucleotides of nucleic acids are found what sugars?
(A) D-galactose and D-ribose
(B) L-ribose and D-glucose
(C) L-ribose and D-ribose
(D) L-deoxyribose and D-ribose
(E) D-deoxyribose and D-ribose

37. Which of the following is NOT an anhydride?
(A) 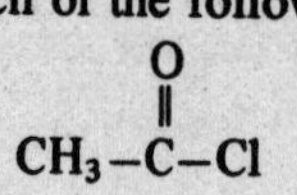
(B) 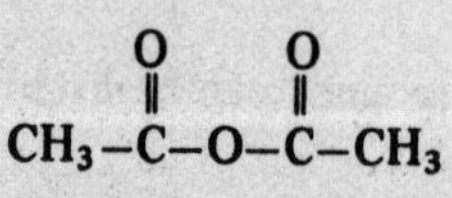
(C) P_2O_5
(D) 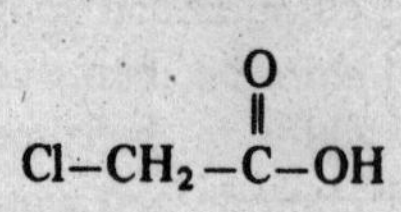
(E) SO_3

38. Ionic bonding is seen in
(A) O_2
(B) H_2
(C) ClF
(D) HCl
(E) N_2

39. Which scientist is NOT matched to his specific accomplishment?
(A) Lavoisier — identified O_2 as a component of air
(B) Rubner — devised the calorimeter
(C) Wohler — synthesized urea
(D) Coulomb — synthesized insulin
(E) Buchner — disproved the belief that fermentation requires whole live cells

40. One crystal of sodium chloride is added to a sodium chloride supersaturated solution. We would expect to see
(A) the added crystal dissolve.
(B) nothing other than the added crystal falling into the bottom of the container.
(C) precipitation begin.
(D) the volume decrease.
(E) the formation of ice crystals on the surface.

41. A polymer of tetrafluoroethylene is useful because of its
(A) flexibility.
(B) chemical inertness.
(C) high water solubility.
(D) high chemical reactivity.
(E) release of fluoride for water treatment.

42. Enzymes act in a reaction such as $A + B \rightarrow C + D$
(A) changing the equilibrium constant.
(B) increasing the rate of the forward reaction without changing the rate of the reverse reaction.
(C) decreasing the rate of the reverse reaction without changing the rate of the forward reaction.
(D) decreasing the activation energy.
(E) increasing the rate of the reverse reaction and decreasing the rate of the forward reaction.

43. In comparison to β-D-glucose acid-catalyzed mutarotation, the mutarotation of the β-methyl glucoside of D-glucose will occur
(A) more slowly.
(B) more rapidly.
(C) only in the presence of CaO.
(D) only in the presence of KOH.
(E) not at all.

44. The Lobry de Bruyn-van Ekenstein Transformation utilizes the treatment of an aldose or kétose with very dilute aqueous alkali (e.g., $Ba\ (OH)_2$) at room temperature to produce various products. If D-glucose is treated in this manner, we may produce
(A) D-gluconic acid.
(B) D-glucuronic acid.
(C) D-fructose.
(D) L-glucose.
(E) a saccharic acid.

45. The iron in hemoglobin is said to be held in place by
(A) hydrogen bonds.
(B) chelation.
(C) ionic bonds.
(D) covalent bonds.
(E) surface tension.

46. The nitration of toluene produces a compond that is most useful as a (an)
(A) lubricant.
(B) explosive.
(C) fertilizer.
(D) dye.
(E) dry cleaning agent.

47. Phenolphthalein is an organic compound that is quite useful as a result of
(A) its high glucose content.
(B) a change in color at a pH of about 8 to 10.

(C) a high content of polyunsaturated fatty acids.
(D) its flammability.
(E) all of the above.

48. Sodium bisulfite reacts with ____________ to yield a sparingly soluble bisulfite addition compound.
(A) any aldehyde or ketone
(B) aldehydes only
(C) aldehydes and unhindered methyl ketones
(D) ketones only
(E) none of the above

49. An aromatic aldehyde will react with primary amines to form
(A) amides.
(B) aromatic acids.
(C) nitriles.
(D) tertiary amines.
(E) none of the above.

Physics

DIRECTIONS: In the following questions, five words or phrases are presented that have been labeled A-E. For each question, choose the word or phrase that is most closely associated with the given item. You may use a choice more than once, or not at all. Eliminate those choices that you think to be incorrect and mark the letter of your choice on the answer sheet.

Questions 1-4:
(A) Graham's law of diffusion
(B) Charles' law
(C) Centripetal force
(D) Ohm's law
(E) Gresham's law

1. $I = E/R$
2. $V/V_1 = T/T_1$
3. $R_1/R_2 = \sqrt{M_2/M_1}$
4. $F = MV^2/R_2$

DIRECTIONS: Each of the statements is followed by five suggested answers or completions. Choose the one that best completes each of the statements, and mark the letter of your choice on the answer sheet.

5. What would be the resultant, if a force of 12 pounds and a force of 16 pounds act upon each other at right angles?
(A) 14 lbs.
(B) 18 lbs.
(C) 28 lbs.
(D) 20 lbs.
(E) 192 lbs.

6. The resultant of two forces of 96 dynes and 74 dynes acting in the same direction is equal to
(A) 170 dynes.
(B) 12 dynes.
(C) 85 dynes.
(D) 7104 dynes.
(E) none of the above.

7. A man weighing 185 pounds wears a pair of thick-soled boots having an area of 15 inch^2. The pressure exerted on each sole due only to his weight is
(A) 14.23 lb./in.^{2}
(B) 1423 lb./in.^{2}
(C) 1.423 lb./in.^{2}
(D) 142.3 lb./in.^{2}
(E) 71.15 lb./in.^{2}

8. A ball of steel weighs 720 grams in air; when submerged in water, its weight is recorded as 360 grams. What is the specific gravity of this ball?
(A) 360
(B) 7
(C) 2
(D) 1
(E) .05

9. A test animal is partially shielded from *X*-rays by a 1-cm thickness of a uniform metal. If this metal shield stops 50% of the radiation, a similar shield of 3-cm thickness would stop ____________ of the original radiation.
(A) 50%
(B) 75%
(C) 85%
(D) 98%
(E) 150%

10. A flywheel of 10-cm radius is operating at a speed of 1000 rev/min. If a particle breaks away from the circumference of the wheel, what will be its linear velocity?
(A) 10,000 cm/min.
(B) 60,000 cm/min.
(C) 110,000 cm/min.
(D) 110,000 km/sec.
(E) 10,000 rev./min.

11. In the northern hemisphere winds circulate about a ____________ in a clockwise direction.
(A) cold front
(B) warm front
(C) stationary front
(D) high pressure area
(E) low pressure area

12. The image in a plane mirror appears to be ____________ behind the mirror as (than) the object is in front of the mirror.
(A) the same size as the object and a greater distance
(B) a smaller size than the object and a lesser distance
(C) a larger size than the object and a lesser distance
(D) a larger size than the object and a greater distance
(E) none of the above

13. A 120-lb. boy scout climbed a flagpole 40 feet tall. How much work did he do against gravitational forces?
(A) 480 ft.-lb.
(B) 4800 ft.-lb.
(C) 160 ft.-lb.
(D) 4.8×10^5 ft.-lb.
(E) 220 ft.-lb.

14. A gas occupies a volume of 16 liters at STP. It is heated to 546°C and compressed to 4 atm. What volume does it now occupy?
(A) 12 liters
(B) 16 liters
(C) 8 liters
(D) 64 liters
(E) 566 liters

15. If the absolute pressure on a gas is doubled at constant temperature, the volume
(A) remains unchanged.
(B) doubles.
(C) quadruples.
(D) is halved.
(E) decreases by 25%.

16. An object is thrown upward with a vertical velocity of 128 ft./sec. It will return in
(A) 2 seconds.
(B) 4 seconds.
(C) 8 seconds.
(D) 16 seconds.
(E) 64 seconds.

17. The boiling point of any liquid at atmospheric pressure is
(A) 3 (273) ⅓ Fahrenheit molecular weight +212.
(B) a function of the shape and type of vessel holding the liquid.
(C) the temperature at which sublimation takes place.
(D) the temperature at which the vapor pressure is equal to atmospheric pressure.
(E) all of the above.

18. In order to determine the density of an alloy, small particles (50 g) of the alloy are added to a graduated cylinder containing 100 ml of water. After adding the particles the volume reads 125 ml. The density of the alloy is
(A) 2 g/ml.
(B) 2.5 g/ml.
(C) 25 g/ml.
(D) 12.5 g/ml.
(E) 6.8 g/ml.

19. To explain the properties of light, we must rely on the
(A) assimilation theory.
(B) propagation theory.
(C) dissolution theory.
(D) wave theory.
(E) wave and particle theories.

20. A parcel dropped from a low-flying helicopter hits the ground 8 seconds later. From what height was it dropped?
(A) 256 ft.
(B) 1024 ft.
(C) 512 ft.
(D) 64 ft.
(E) 128 ft.

21. An astronaut is accelerated in his spacecraft from rest to 800 mi./hr. in 60 sec. He was subjected to an acceleration of
(A) 4800 mi./hr.^{2}
(B) 1200 mi./hr.^{2}
(C) 4800 ft./sec./sec.
(D) 48,000 mi./hr.^{2}
(E) 48,000 ft./sec.^{2}

22. In a plane two forces of 60 newtons and 40 newtons are acting on an object to produce a resultant force of 20 newtons. The forces in question are oriented at ____________ with respect to each other.
(A) 45°
(B) 90°
(C) 60°
(D) 180°
(E) 360°

23. Which of the factors listed below is NOT a type of heat transfer?
(A) conduction
(B) convection
(C) consumption
(D) radiation and absorption
(E) evaporation

24. Which of the matched pairs is incorrect?
(A) Boyle's law — ($PV = k$)
(B) Torricelli's theorem — ($v = \sqrt{2gh}$)
(C) Avogadro's number — (6.023×10^{23})
(D) 1 liter — (1.057 liquid quarts)
(E) F — ($5/9C + 32°$)

25. A radioactive isotope has a half-life of 21 days; at the end of 42 days ____________ of the original radioactive isotope will be left.
(A) 100%
(B) 50%
(C) 25%
(D) 12.5%
(E) none

26. A pin may be floated on the surface of water; the fact may be explained by which of the following?
(A) Water is at a higher temperature than the pin.
(B) Water is at a lower temperature than the pin.
(C) Surface tension allows the pin to float.
(D) Water is rich in minerals.
(E) The temperature of the water is within 3° of 0°C.

27. Into about how many kilograms can 165 lb. be converted?
(A) 82
(B) 75
(C) 40
(D) 100
(E) 165

28. A locomotive accelerates at a constant rate from 10 mi./hr. to 50 mi./hr. in 20 seconds while traveling in a straight line. What is the locomotive's acceleration?
(A) 10 mi./hr. per sec.
(B) 2.5 mi./hr. per sec.
(C) 5 mi./hr.^{2}
(D) 2 mi./hr. per sec.
(E) 5 mi./hr. per sec.

29. A 200-lb. man uses an elevator that is accelerated upward 10 ft./sec^2. The total force exerted upon him by the floor of the elevator is
(A) 200 lb.
(B) 20 lb.
(C) 2000 lb.
(D) 65.2 lb.
(E) 265.2 lb.

30. Air resistance has an effect on projectiles. Which factor(s) does it influence?
(A) speed
(B) maximum height
(C) range
(D) all of the above
(E) none of the above

31. A 300-lb. horizontal force is able to draw a 20,000-lb. railroad car. What is the value of the coefficient of friction?
(A) 0.013
(B) 0.13
(C) 1.3
(D) 66
(E) 6.6

32. A 50-lb. sack of cement is carried to the 20th floor (160 ft) of a building. By how much did the potential energy of the sack of cement increase?
(A) 80 ft.-lb.
(B) 32 ft.-lb.
(C) 160 ft.-lb.
(D) 8000 ft.-lb.
(E) 5 ft.-lb.

33. A pillar that is being driven into the ground during the construction of a new building has an area of 144 in^2. What is the pressure under it when an air hammer force of 400 lbs. is applied to it during construction?
(A) 28 lb./in.^{2}
(B) 2.8 lb./in.^{2}
(C) 14 lb./in.^{2}
(D) 2.8 kg/cm^2
(E) 140 lb./in.^{2}

DIRECTIONS: Each of the statements or questions is followed by five suggested completions or answers. Choose the one that best completes the statement or answers the question, and mark the letter of your choice on the answer sheet.

34. What voltage is required to maintain a current of 15 amps in a wire that has resistance of 36 ohms?
(A) 54 volts
(B) 51 volts
(C) 22 volts
(D) 220 volts
(E) 540 volts

35. What is the energy used by a boiler during a period of 30 minutes using 5.0 amps at 110 volts?
(A) 5.0×10^6 joules
(B) 550 amp-volts
(C) 150 amps
(D) 50×10^5 joules
(E) 55 amps

36. A photoelectric cell consists of a cathode with a photosensitive surface and an anode. Common light-sensitive surfaces are
(A) potassium and cesium.
(B) sodium and barium.
(C) rubidium and certain oxides.
(D) all of the above.
(E) none of the above.

37. The range of distances on the near and far sides of a plane focused upon, within which the details can be imaged, is called
(A) hyperfocal distance.
(B) depth of field.
(C) infinity of the lens.
(D) parfocal distance.
(E) anastigmatic distance.

38. The basic constituent of all electricity is the
(A) ion.
(B) atom.
(C) positron.
(D) electron.
(E) molecule.

STOP. If you finish before the time limit is up, go over your work for this section. DO NOT look at any other sections of the model examination. When your time limit is up, go on to the next section.

SCIENCE PROBLEMS

85 MINUTES
66 QUESTIONS

The following questions require you to use your knowledge of science to solve problems.

DIRECTIONS: The following questions are in groups of three. Preceding each series of questions is a paragraph or a short explanatory statement, a formula or set of formulas, or a definition. Read the written material and then answer the questions. Eliminate those choices that you think to be incorrect and mark the letter of your choice on the answer sheet.

A patient is brought into the emergency room and, upon examination, a thyroid goiter is discovered. You suspect that he is suffering from a thyroid disorder. You ask the intern for a definition of *hypothyroidism* and he responds with:

1. *Hypothyroidism* is the general term for syndromes that reflect
   (A) increased secretion of thyroid hormones.
   (B) decreased secretion of thyroid hormones.
   (C) no change in secretion of thyroid hormones.
   (D) increased secretion of thyroid stimulating hormone releasing factor.
   (E) increased metabolism of iodine.

2. A basal metabolism rate test is ordered that measures the rate of oxidative metabolism. In hypothyroidism, this rate is
   (A) above normal.
   (B) normal.
   (C) below normal.
   (D) not significant in your diagnosis.
   (E) a sure diagnosis.

3. Because of the hypothyroidism that you suspect, you would also consider that this patient
   1. has gained weight
   2. converts less food into energy
   3. stores more food as fat
   4. has had no shift in weight
   (A) 1, 3, 4 above
   (B) 2, 3, 4 above
   (C) 1, 2, 3 above
   (D) all of the above
   (E) none of the above

Utilize the following formulas in answering the next three questions:

Equation 1: $6CO_2 + 6H_2O + \text{Energy} \rightarrow C_6H_{12}O_6 + 6O_2$
Equation 2: $C_6H_{12}O_6 + 6O_2 \rightarrow 6H_2O + 6CO_2 + \text{Energy}$
Equation 3: $C_6H_{12}O_6 \rightarrow 2C_2H_5OH + 2CO_2 + \text{Energy}$
Equation 4: $C_6H_{12}O_6 \rightarrow 2CH_3CHOHCOOH + \text{Energy}$

4. Which of the following combinations of the above equations listed below were exothermic reactions?
   (A) 1, 2, 3
   (B) 2, 3, 4
   (C) 1, 3, 4
   (D) 1, 2, 4
   (E) all of the above

5. Equation 1 essentially could be considered
   (A) aerobic respiration.
   (B) anaerobic respiration.
   (C) photosynthesis reaction.
   (D) butyric acid fermentation.
   (E) glycolysis.

6. Equation 2 demonstrates
   (A) aerobic respiration.
   (B) fermentation.
   (C) photosynthesis.
   (D) anaerobic respiration.
   (E) glycogenolysis.

Standard temperature and pressure (STP) is defined as 0°C (273°K) and 760 mm mercury. The specific gravity of mercury is about 14.

7. Standard pressure could also be stated as ____________ mm of water.
   (A) 1×10^4
   (B) 1400
   (C) 760
   (D) 54
   (E) 380

8. If 100 ml of air at standard pressure in a balloon is taken to a location where the pressure is lower, the balloon will ____________. (Assume no temperature change.)
   (A) burst
   (B) become smaller
   (C) exhibit no change in appearance
   (D) become larger
   (E) do nothing predictable

9. A tin can is equilibrated with the atmosphere at an altitude at which the pressure is 300 mm mercury and then sealed. If the can is taken to standard pressure (assuming no change in temperature), the can may
   (A) explode.
   (B) collapse.
   (C) rust.
   (D) be noted to condense the water vapor from the contained air.
   (E) show oxidation of the tin rather than the iron.

You have been given a sample of three anhydrides:

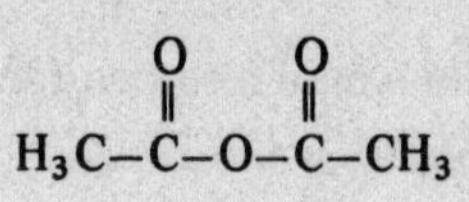

1.

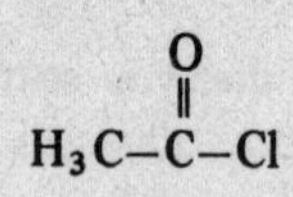

2.

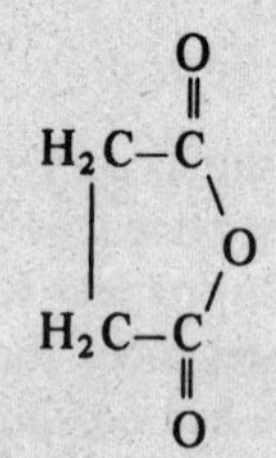

3.

10. When all three have been hydrolyzed in water, at least one of them gives two acid products. This would be which of the above formulas?
   (A) 1
   (B) 2
   (C) 3
   (D) 1 and 2
   (E) 1 and 3

11. A mole of which of the above will give only one mole of acid product after hydrolysis?
   (A) 1
   (B) 2
   (C) 3
   (D) 1 and 2
   (E) 2 and 3

12. A mole of at least one of the above will give two moles of acid on hydrolysis, but there is chemically only one acid product. The anhydride is which of the above?
   (A) 1
   (B) 2
   (C) 3
   (D) 1 and 2
   (E) 2 and 3

For osmotic pressure, $P = cRT$ where P is osmotic pressure, c is the number of particles in solution, R is the gas constant, and T is the absolute temperature.

13. A one-molar solution of which of the following would have the greatest osmotic pressure?
(A) NaCl
(B) glucose
(C) sucrose
(D) $Ba(NO_3)_2$
(E) HCl

14. A one-degree increase in temperature will induce the greatest percentage increase in osmotic pressure in the solution of
(A) NaCl.
(B) glucose.
(C) HCl.
(D) $Ba(NO_3)_2$.
(E) none of the above.

15. The difference in the osmotic pressures of one molar solutions of different compounds at a given temperature results from
(A) different values for R.
(B) different values for Avogadro's number.
(C) ionization to produce different numbers of particles per mole.
(D) all of the above.
(E) none of the above.

Black (B) is dominant over white (b); rough coat (R) is dominant over smooth (r).

16. A purebred white-rough coat male is mated to a purebred black-smooth female; their offspring are
(A) all white with rough coat.
(B) all white with smooth coat.
(C) all black with smooth coat.
(D) all agouti.
(E) all black with rough coat.

17. When these F_1 are mated, you expect how many types of offspring?
(A) 2
(B) 4
(C) 1
(D) 16
(E) 8

18. In what ratio will they appear?
(A) 1:2:1
(B) 3:1
(C) 9:3:3:1
(D) 2:4
(E) 12:3:3:1

The change in length of a bar of material is given by the formula $\Delta L = \alpha L_i \Delta t$ where ΔL is the change in length, α is coefficient of linear expansion, L_i is the initial length, and Δt is the change in temperature.

19. If the temperature increases from 27 to 30°C, then the bar will be
(A) three times as long as initially.
(B) one-third as long as initially.
(C) increased by 1/9.
(D) increased by $3\alpha L_i$.
(E) none of the above.

20. If length is given in centimeters and temperature in °C, the coefficient of expansion will be given in
(A) centimeters.
(B) cm/°C.
(C) cm^{-1}.
(D) $°C^{-1}$.
(E) °C/cm.

21. If thin strips of two metals are joined, an increase in temperature will cause the joined strip to
(A) curve toward the one with the greatest α.
(B) be longer than a similar strip of either metal alone.
(C) curve away from the metal with the greatest α.
(D) assume the shape of a sine wave.
(E) none of the above.

The solubility product constant, K_{sp}, of a slightly soluble salt is given as the product of the concentrations of its ions in solution raised to the exponential powers of their coefficients in ionization.

$$BaF_2 \rightleftharpoons Ba^{++} + 2F^- \qquad K_{sp} = [F^-]^2\,[Ba^{++}] = 2 \times 10^{-6}$$
$$BaCO_3 \rightleftharpoons Ba^{++} + CO_3^{=} \qquad K_{sp} = [Ba^{++}]\,[CO_3^{=}] = 7 \times 10^{-9}$$

22. In the precipitation of Ba^{++} from identical solutions in two beakers, beaker (1) contains $[F^-] = 1 \times 10^{-2}$ and beaker (2) contains $[CO_3^{=}] = 7 \times 10^{-5}$. The higher concentration of Ba^{++} in solution is
(A) in beaker (1).
(B) in beaker (2).
(C) in neither beaker (i.e., no difference).
(D) not possible to predict with the information given.
(E) directly related to the difference of atmospheric pressure over the two beakers.

23. To precipitate the Ba^{++} from a 5×10^{-4} molar solution we consider adding either F^- to produce a concentration of 0.1 molar or $CO_3^{=}$ to produce a concentration of 0.01 molar. The lesser concentration of Ba^{++} left in solution will be noted after addition of
(A) 0.1 molar F^-.
(B) 0.01 molar $CO_3^{=}$.
(C) 0.05 molar F^-.
(D) 0.003 molar $CO_3^{=}$.
(E) either of the above (i.e., no difference).

24. You wish to precipitate F^- from a 0.001 molar solution in beaker (5) or $CO_3^{=}$ from a 0.002 molar solution in beaker (7). The addition of 0.1 molar Ba^{++} will result in a lower concentration of the anion mentioned in _______________ as compared to the mentioned anion in the other beaker.
(A) beaker (5)
(B) beaker (7)
(C) neither of the above (i.e., no difference)
(D) one of the beakers but the information is insufficient to allow prediction

The iodine number of a fatty acid is defined as the number of grams of iodine that will react with the double bonds of 100 grams of the fatty acid.

$$R{-}CH{=}CH{-}R' + I_2 \rightarrow R{-}\underset{H}{\overset{I}{C}}{-}\underset{I}{\overset{H}{C}}{-}R'$$

$H_3C{-}(CH_2)_7{-}CH{=}CH{-}(CH_2)_5{-}\overset{O}{\overset{\|}{C}}{-}OH$ 1. molecular wt. 254

$H_3C{-}(CH_2)_6{-}CH{=}CH{-}(CH_2)_6{-}\overset{O}{\overset{\|}{C}}{-}OH$ 2. molecular wt. 254

$H_3C{-}(CH_2)_{14}{-}\overset{O}{\overset{\|}{C}}{-}OH$ 3. molecular wt. 256

$H_3C{-}(CH_2)_9{-}CH{=}CH{-}CH_2{-}CH{=}CH{-}(CH_2)_2$ 4. molecular wt. 280

$H_3C{-}(CH_2)_{16}{-}\overset{O}{\overset{|}{C}}{-}OH$ 5. molecular wt. 284

25. The highest iodine number in the group above would be shown by
(A) 1.
(B) 2.
(C) 3.
(D) 4.
(E) 5.

26. The lowest iodine number in the group above would be shown by
(A) 1.
(B) 2.
(C) 3.
(D) 4.
(E) more than one of the above.

27. Equal iodine numbers would be found for
(A) 1 and 3.
(B) 2 and 4.
(C) 3 and 5.
(D) 2 and 5.
(E) none of the above combinations.

The hematology laboratory reports to the surgeon that his patient's blood clumped with both anti A and anti B serum.

28. The patient's blood type is
(A) AB.
(B) A.
(C) B.
(D) O.
(E) Rh^+.

29. The test is based upon the presence or absence of
1. antigens (agglutinogens) in red blood cells
2. antibodies (agglutinins) in the serum
3. antigens in white blood cells
4. agglutinins in white blood cells
(A) 1 and 3 above
(B) 2 and 4 above
(C) 1 and 2 above
(D) 3 and 4 above
(E) none of the above

30. The surgeon in this case could expect approximately ____________ percent of the population to have the blood type of the patient.
(A) 47
(B) 41
(C) 9
(D) 15
(E) 3

Recall that force on any surface is the pressure on the surface times the area of the surface. The pressure exerted on a surface can be expressed as the height of an object times the specific density occupying a space. Use the diagram below in your calculations.

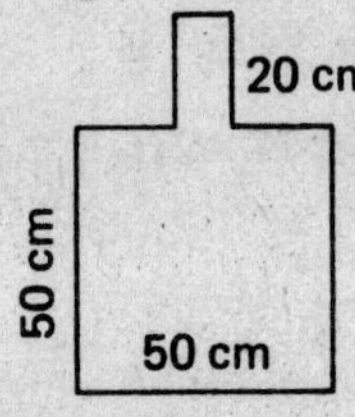

This cubical container is filled with hexabromoethane which has a specific gravity of 2.8. The cross-section of the elevated area is 15 cm².

31. The force exerted upon the bottom of this container is
(A) 40 kg.
(B) 4000 kg.
(C) 4000 gm.
(D) 500 gm.
(E) 500 kg.

32. The area of the top of the container that is exposed to hexabromoethane is
(A) 2485 cm^2.
(B) 500 cm^2.
(C) 980 cm^2.
(D) 1200 cm^2.
(E) more than 3000 cm^2.

33. The force exerted upon the top of this container is
(A) 1390 gm.
(B) 125 gm.
(C) 139 kg.
(D) 10 kg.
(E) 42 kg.

One mole of sodium, potassium, or lithium will react with an excess of ethanol to form one gram atomic weight of hydrogen. Hydrogen is also produced by the reaction of these metals with a number of alcohols, organic acids, and water.

34. The addition of 0.1 mole of lithium to excess ethanol will produce ____________ liter of hydrogen at standard temperature and pressure.
(A) 0.1
(B) 0.05
(C) 0.2
(D) 1.1
(E) 11.2

35. The addition of 0.001 mole of potassium to excess ethanol will produce enough hydrogen to react with ____________ of oxygen in the production of water.
(A) 5 ml
(B) 20 ml
(C) 100 ml
(D) 220 ml
(E) 11200 ml

36. If one is given a choice of adding 0.001 mole of potassium, lithium, or sodium to excess ethanol, the greatest amount of hydrogen will be produced after the addition of
(A) sodium.
(B) lithium.
(C) potassium.
(D) A or B (equal).
(E) A, B, or C (all equal).

Density is defined as the mass of a body divided by the volume of a body. The density of water is 1 g/cm^3 or 62.4 $lb./ft.^3$ Specific gravity usually is expressed as

$$\frac{\text{density or weight of a body}}{\text{density or weight of an equal volume of water}}$$

The specific gravity of water is 1. The specific gravity of a piece of steel is 8.0.

37. The density of this piece of steel in g/cm^3 is
(A) 6.15
(B) less than 0.6.
(C) 0.8
(D) 8.0.
(E) more than 10.

38. The density of this piece of steel in $lb./ft.^3$ is
(A) 499.
(B) 800.
(C) 61.5.
(D) less than 60.
(E) more than 825.

39. The weight of 35 $ft.^3$ of this steel is
(A) 2152 lb.
(B) 17,400 lb.
(C) 2.8×10^4 lb.
(D) 1.5×10^3 lb.
(E) less than 2000 lb.

It is known that periodate will oxidize OH groups or amines on adjacent carbon atoms to form aldehydes.

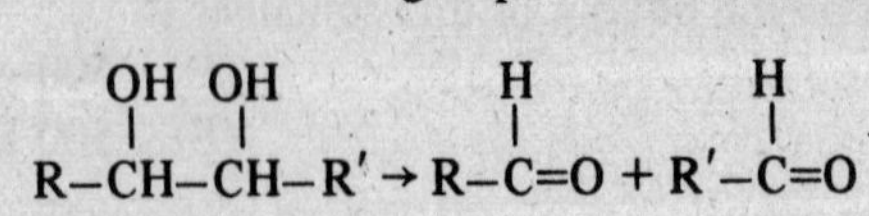

In the case of three adjacent alcohol or amino groups, there is oxidation to produce formic acid and two aldehydes.

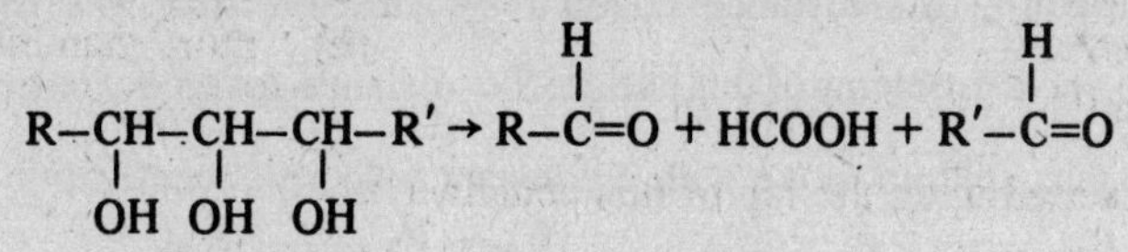

You have been given pure samples of three diol compounds, but you do not know the identity of any of them. The possible structures are

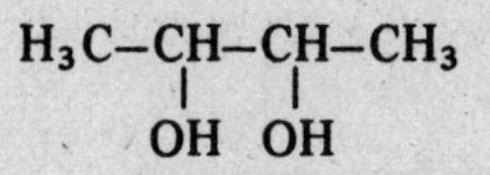

1.

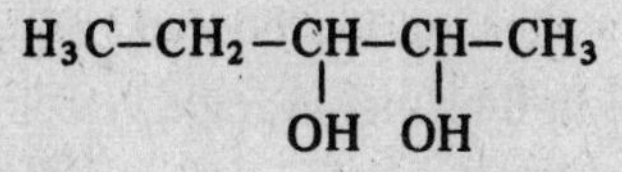

2.

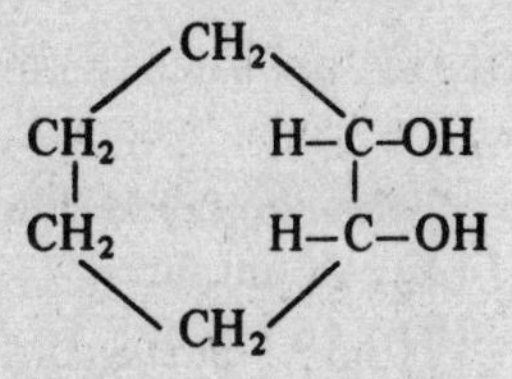

3.

Each of the unknown compounds is subjected to periodate oxidation and the products are examined.

40. One compound produces two different aldehydes. The structure of this compound must be
(A) 1.
(B) 2.
(C) 3.
(D) 1 or 2.
(E) 1 or 3.

41. Another compound produces one mole of aldehyde from one mole of the starting material. This compound must be
(A) 1.
(B) 2.
(C) 3.
(D) 1 or 2.
(E) 2 or 3.

42. The remaining compound yields only one aldehyde on oxidation by periodate. *Disregarding any data presented and conclusions you have reached in study of the other two compounds,* this compound must be
(A) 1.
(B) 2.
(C) 3.
(D) 1 or 2.
(E) 1 or 3.

A 10-kg piece of glass is weighed in air, and then while suspended in water. The density of the glass is 6.0 gm/cm^3.

43. If the piece of glass were suspended in air, it would weigh (the buoyancy of air is neglected)
(A) 10 newtons.
(B) 50 newtons.
(C) 100 newtons.
(D) 500 newtons.
(E) 600 newtons.

44. The volume of the piece of glass is
(A) 1.6 cm^3.
(B) 60 cm^3.
(C) 166 cm^3.
(D) 6 cm^3.
(E) 1666 cm^3.

45. If the buoyant force of the water is equal to the weight of the water displaced, then the piece of glass suspended in water weighs
(A) 83 N.
(B) 100 N.
(C) 16 N.
(D) 6 N.
(E) 50 N.

Velocity of a moving object is defined as the distance covered per unit of time; the average speed is calculated by dividing the distance covered by the time that was required. The equation $\overline{v} = \frac{S}{t}$ is utilized to solve problems of this nature; S = distance covered, t = time and $\overline{v}$ = the average velocity. Since objects seldom move with a constant velocity, acceleration defined as

$$a = \frac{V_2 - V_1}{t}$$

(where V_1 = initial velocity, V_2 = final velocity and t = time) must be taken into consideration.

46. A particle travels 336 mi. in 6 hr.; its average velocity is
(A) 56 mi./hr.
(B) 66 mi./hr.
(C) 33.6 mi./hr.
(D) 56 km/hr.
(E) 40 mi./km/hr.

47. The particle accelerated at a constant rate from 23 mi./hr. to 58 mi./hr. in 3.5 sec. Its acceleration was
(A) 23 mi./hr. per sec.
(B) 58 mi./hr. per sec.
(C) 10 mi./hr. per sec.
(D) 17 mi./hr. per sec.
(E) less than 10 mi./hr. per sec.

48. Since speed changed at a uniform rate and the average velocity is equal to the average of the initial and final speeds, how far has the particle traveled while it was accelerating?
(A) 210 ft.
(B) 600 ft.
(C) 51 ft.
(D) 21 mi.
(E) less than 20 mi.

The number of possible optical isomers of a particular organic compound is equal to 2^n (where n = the number of asymmetric carbon atoms) when no two of the asymmetric carbon atoms are attached to the same four kinds of groups.

49. Based on the above statement, 1,2-dibromobutane would have ______________ isomers.
(A) 1
(B) 2
(C) 4
(D) 8
(E) none of the above

50. The number of possible isomers of 1,3-dibromobutane is
(A) 1.
(B) 2.
(C) 4.
(D) 8.
(E) none of the above.

51. The number of possible isomers of 1,4-dibromobutane is
(A) 1.
(B) 2.
(C) 4.
(D) 8.
(E) 12.

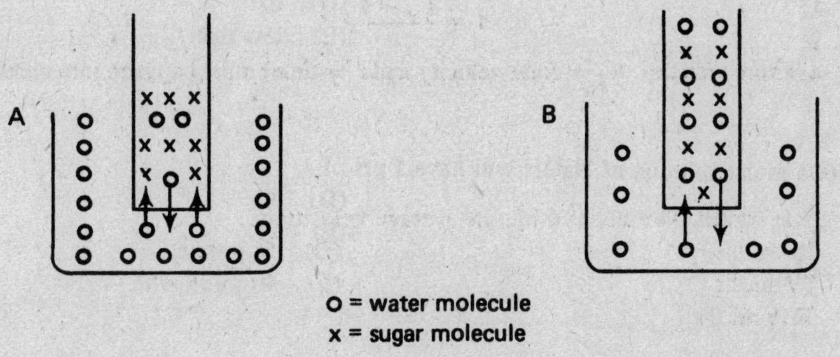

The diagrams demonstrate the principle of osmosis. As indicated, water molecules pass freely across the semipermeable membrane, while the starch molecules do not. In *A*, more water molecules move into the tube; the water level rises and the solution becomes more dilute. In *B*, osmotic equilibrium has been reached, and the same number of water molecules pass through the membrane in either direction.

52. If a cell were put into a solution of greater osmotic pressure than its protoplasm,
(A) water would pass out through the plasma membrane faster than in.
(B) water would pass in through the plasma membrane faster than out.
(C) the cell would swell.
(D) no unequal rates would be experienced.
(E) the result could not be predicted.

53. The principle of osmosis depends upon the concentration of:
1. diffusible particles
2. nondiffusible particles
3. protons
4. starch molecules

(A) 1 and 2 above
(B) 1 and 3 above
(C) 1 and 4 above
(D) 2 and 3 above
(E) 3 and 4 above

54. If a red blood cell is placed in a solution and hemolysis occurs due to the osmotic relationships, we can deduce that the cell was placed in a
(A) hypertonic solution.
(B) hypotonic solution.
(C) isotonic solution.
(D) none of the above.
(E) no conclusion — insufficient data.

The pH of a solution is equal to the negative $\log_{10}$ of $[H^+]$. In an aqueous solution $[H^+][OH^-] = 10^{-14}$.

55. A 0.01 molar solution of HCl will have a pH of
(A) 1.
(B) 2.
(C) 4.
(D) 6.
(E) less than 1.

56. A 0.001 molar solution of NaOH will have a pH of
(A) 3.
(B) 4.
(C) 13.
(D) 8.
(E) 11.

57. The above solution of NaOH will have a pOH of
(A) 3.
(B) 4.
(C) 8.
(D) 11.
(E) 13.

The schema of thyroxine formation is outlined below:

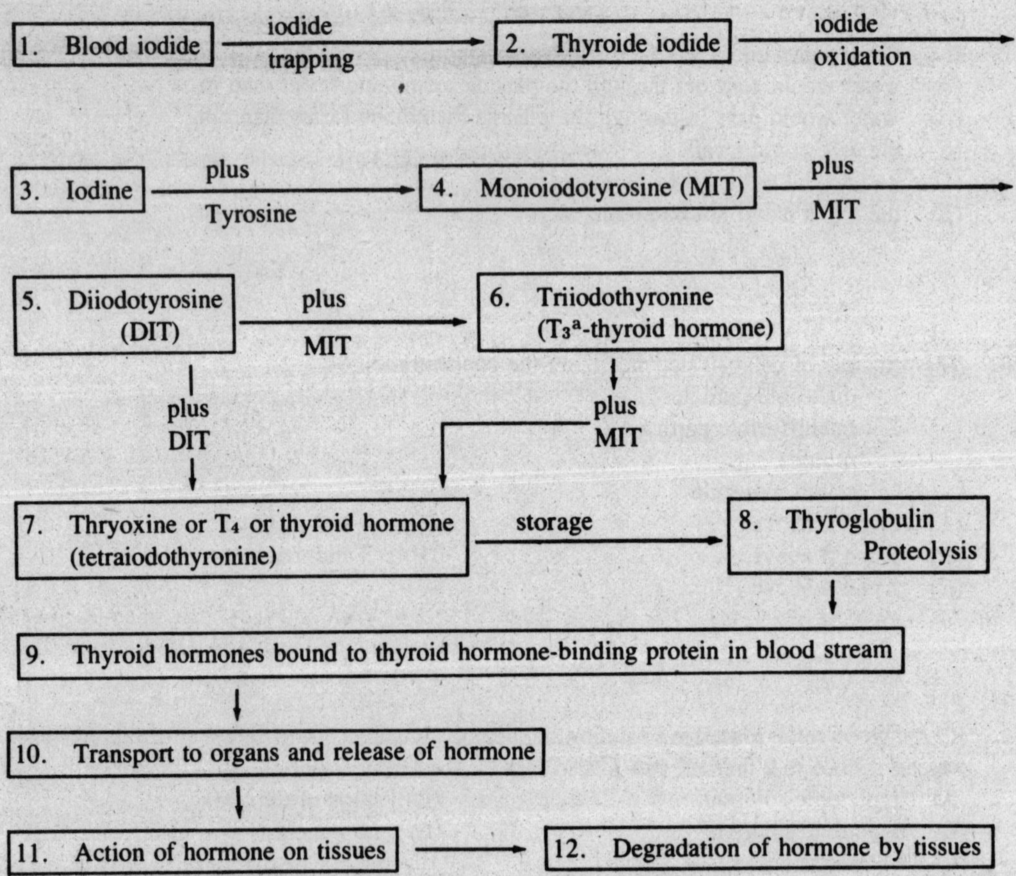

58. Chemically, thyroid hormones are
(A) iodotyrosines.
(B) iodothyronines.
(C) iodides.
(D) iodines.
(E) tyrosines.

59. In proceeding from compound 3 to compound 4, the amino acid tyrosine is
(A) oxidized.
(B) reduced.
(C) iodinated.
(D) synthesized.
(E) none of the above.

60. During transport thyroid hormones are inactive because they are
(A) in the form of thyroglobulin.
(B) free hormones.
(C) protein-bound.
(D) on red blood cells.
(E) deactivated.

Reduction of an alkyne by lithium in liquid ammonia produces a trans-alkene. Hydrogenation of an alkyne with hydrogen over palladium-calcium carbonate partially deactivated by lead salt produces a cis-alkene.

61. A sample of 2,3-dichlorobutane is reacted with alcoholic KOH to form an alkyne. This product is then treated with sodium in liquid ammonia to produce
(A) 1-butyne.
(B) 2-butyne.
(C) cis-2-butene.
(D) trans-2-butene.
(E) none of the above.

62. If the final product of the reaction sequence above is reacted with Cl_2, there will be production of
(A) 2,3-dichlorobutane.
(B) 2-butyne.
(C) 2,2,3,3-tetrachlorobutane.
(D) 2-butene.
(E) no reaction.

63. The final product of the previous step can be reacted with alcoholic KOH to produce
(A) 2-chloro-2-butene.
(B) 2-butyne.
(C) trans-2,3-dichlorobutene.
(D) 2-butene.
(E) none of the above.

The equivalent weight of an acid is equal to the molecular weight divided by the number of available protons. The equivalent weight of base is equal to the molecular weight divided by the number of available hydroxyls.

64. The equivalent weight of an acid, H_3Y, having a molecular weight of 270 would be
(A) 60.
(B) 90.
(C) 135.
(D) 180.
(E) 270.

65. The equivalent weight of a base, $Z_3(OH)_3$, having a molecular weight of 180 would be

(A) 60.
(B) 90.
(C) 120.
(D) 135.
(E) 250.

66. One mole each of the above acid and the above base mixed together would produce a solution that is

(A) weakly acidic.
(B) weakly alkaline.
(C) strongly acidic.
(D) strongly alkaline.
(E) neutral.

STOP. If you finish before the time limit is up, go over your work for this section. DO NOT look at any other sections of the model examination. When your time limit is up, go on to the next section.

SKILLS ANALYSIS: READING

85 MINUTES
68 QUESTIONS

The following questions are to be answered based on your careful reading of selections from scientific writings.

DIRECTIONS: Read each passage carefully, then answer the questions following it. Consider only the material within the passage in answering the questions. Eliminate those choices that you think to be incorrect and mark the letter of your choice on the answer sheet.

Cellular regeneration has attracted great interest among both the experimenter and the clinician interested in liver disease. The liver is the largest organ of the body and is the main processing, as well as detoxification, plant of the organism. Insult and injury are common. Many of the abnormalities of liver disease are attributed to regeneration phenomena. Its absence or deficiency is responsible for many of the hepatic failures observed. Cellular hypertrophy, arrangement and distortion of the normal morphological pattern may cause portal hypertension and lead to cirrhosis. Portal hypertension may result in severe esophageal varices and necessitate the surgical creation of a porta-caval shunt. Uncontrolled regenerative hyperplasia is the hallmark of hepatic carcinoma. To study liver regeneration investigators have untilized a good animal model; after partial hepatectomy (removal of about ⅔ of liver mass) regeneration is rapid and it regains its normal size within about 20 days. The study of the specific processes has been enhanced by the development of tools such as *in vivo* techniques to measure humoral factors, transmission and scanning electron microscopy, ultra-centrifugation and analysis of subcellular fractions and radioactive tracers. The needle biopsy now allows easy access to the liver of man for study.

After partial hepatectomy or carbon tetrachloride insult, mitotic activity reaches a peak around 35 hours. The new growth encompasses not only the liver parenchymal cells but also the elements of the biliary system, reticuloendothelial system, connective tissue system and the vascular system. Utilizing ultra-centrifugation the nuclear fraction (containing DNA and RNA), the mitochondrial fraction (containing the cytochrome oxidase enzymes) and microsomal fraction (containing RNA and phospholipids) have been investigated and have yielded data that allow for a meaningful comparison of the composition and chemical processes that are prominent in normal and regenerating liver. Despite the vast amount of knowledge concerning regeneration the clinical utilization of results of animal experimentation has been very difficult because of the lack of methodology for assessing regeneration in human beings.

The following statements are related to the passage above. Based on the information given, select:

(A) if the statement is *supported by* the information in the passage.
(B) if the statement is *contradicted by* the information in the passage.
(C) if the statement is *neither supported nor contradicted by* information in the passage.

1. The paragraph emphasizes liver degeneration.
2. In routine histological examinations most importance has been placed on the mitotic activity of the regenerating liver.
3. The liver is a very important functional organ.
4. Deficiency of the regenerative process may lead to liver failures.
5. A good animal model is in existence for investigators to utilize.
6. Results of animal experiments can directly be correlated with man.
7. Scanning and transmission electron microscopy are the most useful tools in the study of liver regeneration.
8. Several systems are involved in liver regeneration.
9. Mitotic activity ceases around 35 hours.

10. Partial hepatectomy and carbon tetrachloride poisoning are alike in their injury to the liver.

11. Only the nuclear fraction contains RNA.

12. Ultra-centrifugation is the most useful tool in regeneration studies.

13. Animal experimentation has yielded much information that is directly applied in clinical treatment in man.

Throughout the various phyla of the plant and animal kingdom numerous species have evolved. It is apparent that sexual reproduction plays an important role in the continuation of the species and in the expression of different phenotypes within the species. This mode of reproduction is accomplished by the fusion of two gametes which will give rise to a zygote. In order for future generations to maintain the same number of chromosomes as their parents the gametes must undergo a reduction in chromosome number. If the offspring express phenotypic traits that are different from those of their parents, there must be a rearrangement of the DNA within the chromosomes. The reduction of the number of chromosomes and mixing of the gene pool are accomplished by the process of meiosis.

The process of meiosis is characterized by a naturally occurring sequence of events which are usually artificially subdivided into ten different stages. The first five stages comprise the first or reductional division of meiosis. At the end of the reductional division the chromosomes are reduced to one-half their original number (haploid). The last five stages comprise the second or equatorial division of meiosis. Germ cells undergoing meiosis give rise to haploid gametes which contain one representative of each type of chromosome. The chromosomes of the gametes may also demonstrate variations in genetic composition due to crossing over which takes place during the first prophase.

Replication of DNA occurs during interphase before the process of meiosis begins. The condensation and coiling of chromotin to form chromosomes marks the beginning of prophase I, the first stage of meiosis. Homologous chromosomes pair with one another to form a structure called a bivalent. Next each chromosome splits lengthwise to form two chromatids. The homologous pairs of chromosomes are now composed of four chromatids which are referred to as a tetrad. The chromatids of tetrads become short and thick and breaks may occur in them. The breaks are eventually repaired but segments of different chromatids may be joined together. This process, referred to as crossing over, enables segments of two different chromatids to be joined together. This enables the gametes to receive chromosomes derived from segments of both homologous chromosomes. In the second stage of meiosis or metaphase I, the nuclear membrane disappears, a spindle apparatus forms, and the homologous pairs align along the equatorial plate of the cell. In anaphase I the homologous chromosomes migrate to opposite poles of the cell. Telophase I is characterized by the complete separation of the homologous pairs, and the spindle apparatus disappears. The nuclear membrane begins to reform and in many organisms a cytoplasmic division may occur at this stage.

After a brief interphase, prophase II begins. Prophase II is the first stage in the second or equatorial division of meiosis. It is characterized by the condensing of chromatin to form the chromosomes. During metaphase II the spindle apparatus forms and the chromosomes line up along the equatorial plate. In anaphase II the daughter chromosomes migrate to opposite poles of the cell. Anaphase II differs from the first anaphase in that the centromere divides and the two chromatids now become the daughter chromosomes. The daughter chromosomes separate completely and reach opposite poles of the cell in telophase II. Subsequent divisions of the cytoplasm result in the formation of two daughter cells which have a haploid number of chromosomes.

The two divisions of the germ cell during meiosis produce four gametes with one-half the original number of chromosomes.

14. According to this passage, at the end of the reductional division of meiosis
(A) four haploid sets of chromosomes are produced.
(B) the homologous pairs of chromosomes are completely separated.
(C) the chromatin duplicates and coils.
(D) the centromeres divide and daughter chromosomes move to opposite poles of the cell.
(E) the chromatids of the tetrads form breaks.

15. According to this passage, crossing over occurs
(A) during the equatorial division.
(B) before the tetrad separates.
(C) during anaphase I.
(D) during prophase II.
(E) just before the first prophase begins.

16. According to this passage, duplication of the chromatin occurs during
(A) metaphase I.
(B) anaphase II.
(C) telophase I.
(D) interphase.
(E) the reductional division.

17. According to this passage, variation in genetic composition is made possible by
(A) the formation of homologous pairs.
(B) mitotic division of germ cells.
(C) crossing over.
(D) random mutations.
(E) fusion of gametes to form a zygote.

18. It can be inferred from this passage that
(A) all species in both the plant and animal kingdom are capable of sexual reproduction.
(B) haploid cells are only found in animals.
(C) four functional gametes are always formed by the process of meiosis.
(D) zygote formation may produce an offspring which has the same number of chromosomes as its parents.
(E) fusion of gametes will produce offspring that have ½ the original number of chromosomes.

Unlike skeletal muscle, smooth muscle can be stretched without developing a lasting increase in tension. When stretched slowly, smooth muscle initially contracts to resist the stretching force. However, the tension then begins to decrease and the muscle fibers adjust to new lengths without contracting against the force which continues to stretch them. This property is very useful in the case of smooth muscle in the walls of hollow visceral organs. Such organs can serve as reservoirs because, as they become filled, the smooth muscle in their walls can adapt to new lengths without raising the internal pressure of the organ. For example, the urinary bladder can contain 100 or 1000 ml of urine with approximately the same internal or intraluminal pressure. There is a limit, however, to the amount of stretch that smooth muscle can sustain before an increase in tension occurs. When this limit is reached, continued stretching stimulates the muscle to contract forcefully and consequently causes expulsion of the contents of the organ. Smooth muscle can be over-stretched, and, as is the case with skeletal muscle, once the optimal length has been exceeded the amount of tension developed will be less.

19. The main topic of this passage is
(A) a comparison of the response of smooth and skeletal muscle to stretch.
(B) the plasticity of smooth muscle.
(C) the storage and release properties of hollow organs.
(D) the contraction of smooth muscle.
(E) the lengthening of smooth muscle.

20. By inference from this passage, skeletal muscle
(A) can be stretched and responds by developing a lasting increase in tension.
(B) does not develop a lasting increase in tension when stretched.
(C) plays no role in the emptying of hollow organs.
(D) continues to increase in tension as its optimal length is exceeded.
(E) contracts more rapidly than smooth muscle.

21. An increase in tension does *not* occur
(A) when skeletal muscle is stretched.
(B) when smooth muscle is over-stretched.
(C) as smooth muscle is initially stretched.
(D) when the limit of stretch of smooth muscle is exceeded.
(E) unless smooth muscle is over-stretched.

22. According to this passage, hollow visceral organs
(A) may have skeletal muscle in their walls.
(B) may have constant internal pressure over a wide range of internal volumes.
(C) cannot contract if their volume is rapidly increased.
(D) increase their internal pressure continuously as their volume increases.
(E) do not show an initial increase in wall-tension when initially stretched.

23. It can be concluded from the passage that
(A) skeletal muscle always responds to length increases differently than smooth muscle.
(B) the ability of smooth muscle to adjust to increased length without increased contraction is necessary to the reservoir function of certain hollow organs.
(C) smooth muscle does not increase the internal pressure of hollow organs.
(D) smooth muscle has no response to stretch.
(E) smooth muscle has a different morphology than skeletal muscle.

Migration of birds, butterflies, and fishes is still a subject of intrigue and study. Since recorded time the sounds and sights of the great migrations of birds have awed man, and we still marvel at the great distances that are covered and the accuracy of guidance that the animals possess. Migration routes of many species have been mapped as they travel south in the fall to feed and head north in the spring to breed. The fall migration seems to be triggered by the change in weather, but an endogenous factor, probably chemical in nature, is responsible for the spring migration. The question as to how the animals find their destinations with pin-point accuracy has received great attention. Experiments indicate that starlings that fly by day use the sun as a compass and actually adjust their course to the sun's changes in position. Other day fliers are capable of using landmarks such as rivers and mountains especially as they near their destination. Night fliers such as Old World warblers navigate by the stars; they seem to have an innate time clock or gyroscope which allows them to automatically know the right direction and to adjust their course during the night's flight. During adverse weather conditions when the stars are not visible, these animals become confused and their migration comes to a temporary halt. The center that controls these delicate responses and the orientation of these animals still eludes investigators.

The following statements are related to the information presented above. Based on the information given, select:
(A) if the statement is *supported by* the information given.
(B) if the statement is *contradicted by* the information given.
(C) if the statement is *neither supported nor contradicted by* information given.

24. The mystery of migration has been solved.

25. Long before man learned how, birds were already flying by the sun and stars.

26. All migrating birds use the same navigational guides.

27. The fall migration is triggered by exogenous factors.

28. Migration involves every member of a species.

29. The brightest star is probably utilized by night fliers to guide them.

30. Migration routes of all species have been mapped and studied by investigators.

31. Day fliers halt their migration during bad weather.

The temporomandibular joint is characterized as a bilateral diarthroidal articulation; that is, it is capable of both rotary (hinge) and translatory (gliding) motion. This range of motion permits movement both bodily (side) and in an anterior-posterior direction of the mandibular condyle within the glenoid fossa or cavity of this joint. The functional articulation atually occurs when each condyle contacts the articular eminence of the squamous part of the temporal bone. Both the right and left joints function as one unit, but each may move somewhat independently.

Interposed between the condyle and fossa and eminence is an articular disk or meniscus which is attached to the head of the condyle posteriorly and to the joint capsule laterally. This arrangement produces upper and lower joint compartments lined by synovium. The disk consists of dense collagenous connective tissue or may be fibrocartilaginous in nature. It fuses with the joint capsule that is composed of dense fibroelastic connective tissue. This capsule is attached to the concave surface of the fossa, the convex surface of the eminence, and inferiorly to the neck of the condyle. The thickened lateral part of the capsule forms the temporomandibular ligament.

The temporomandibular ligament functions to prevent excessive retraction of the mandible and thus limits border movements. Other ligaments attached to the joint include the sphenomandibular, the stylomandibular, and the tiny (pinto's). The sphenomandibular ligament functions to limit closure of the jaws. It becomes taut if the vertical dimension is decreased. The stylomandibular ligament functions to limit extreme mandibular protrusion and over closure of the jaws. The tiny ligament, attached to the capsule, disk, and sphenomandibular ligament, inserts on the malleus of the ear. Tension on it may cause some change in position of the malleus.

Each synovial compartment is lined with a vascular layer of connective tissue. In areas not exposed to pressure the synovial membrane is thrown into numerous folds. There are two kinds of cells comprising the membrane. Type A cells are phagocytic in nature and are found among Type B cells that are secretory in nature. The cavity is filled with synovial fluid, a transparent, yellowish, viscous material. The fluid is a dialysate of plasma and lymph consisting of a protein-mucopolysaccharide complex. Debris is removed from this lubricating and nutritional fluid by the type A cells of the membrane.

32. The main topic of this passage is
(A) the unlimited movement capabilities of the temporomandibular joint.
(B) the description of the functional anatomy of the joint.
(C) the role of the ligaments in movements of the joint.
(D) the histological characterization of various anatomic controls.
(E) the joint is vital for the normal activity of life.

33. According to the passage, the meniscus is best described as
(A) the layer internal to the synovial compartments.
(B) the connective tissue separating the lower compartment from the condyle.
(C) the fibrocartilage positioned above the upper synovial cavity.
(D) the attachment for the head of the condyle.
(E) none of the above.

34. Unlike the articular disk, the joint capsule
(A) contains some connective tissue.
(B) forms laterally into ligamentous tissue.
(C) makes attachment with the joint.
(D) consists of fibers and cells.
(E) attaches to the tiny ligament.

35. It can be concluded from the passage that
(A) border movements made by the mandible are restricted by ligamentous attachments.
(B) overclosure of the jaws occurs frequently.
(C) slack in one of the ligaments leads to tension in other ligaments.
(D) protrusion involves movement of the mandible posteriorly.
(E) retraction is common during wide opening of the mouth.

36. According to the passage, the following are correct EXCEPT which one?
(A) Phagocytes remove foreign material from the synovial fluid.
(B) Only Type B cells produce the synovial fluid.
(C) Pressure flattens areas of the synovial membrane.
(D) Blood vessels are found among the connective tissue of synovial compartments.
(E) The composition of synovial fluid is complex.

A considerable body of knowledge concerning headaches has accumulated over the years. Progress in treatment has been largely due to the increased information from differential diagnosis of the various syndromes and types of headaches. Pain, the universal denominator, may be due to a multitude of organic and psychological disturbances and usually is the symptom that drives the sufferer to seek help. Pain may be present at the site of the lesion or it may present itself as referred pain in a distant area of the body. This phenomenon can be partly explained on the basis that the afferent components of the central nervous system at a particular spinal cord level are overloaded and at times cannot distinguish visceral pain, which travels with the autonomics, from somatic pain; therefore, pain is felt over an area that is supplied by general somatic nerves. In a differential diagnosis, the location, the nature, the frequency, the time of day or night, the severity, the duration, response of pain to drugs, and type of pain are important factors. All this information must be gathered during a thorough physical examination which includes a detailed history of the patient and his family. Once the facts have been determined, the good physician is not satisfied with the control of pain but must pry on and determine the causative factors. Most headaches are transient but the ones that drive a patient to seek help might be caused by an underlying systemic infection, head injury, tumor, eye problems, sinus infection and vascular disturbances. Often the physician is ill-equipped to handle headache problems because of lack of adequate preparation in this area of medical training. After a thorough examination several tests might be in order; these may include a radiographic examination of the skull and cervical vertebral column, an electroencephalogram, an arteriogram, a lumbar puncture, and biopsies of organs. Headaches which occur rarely may, of course, be associated with fatigue or emotional stress; headaches associated with organic disease usually are intermittent but occur daily while headaches that persist for weeks on end might be associated with psychological disturbances. Treatment should be directed toward the cure of the underlying problem. Analgesics are among the safest of drugs; tranquilizers, etc., however, must be effectively monitored.

The following statements are related to the information presented above. Based on the information given, select:
(A) if the statement is *supported by* the information given.
(B) if the statement is *contradicted by* the information given.
(C) if the statement is *neither supported nor contradicted by* information given.

37. The majority of headaches are of vascular origin.
38. Before using any drug the patient should be checked for contraindications.
39. Aspirins will cure most headaches.
40. Analgesics are absolutely safe.
41. Pain usually stimulates the patient to seek help.
42. Acupuncture should be considered in the treatment of headaches.
43. A thorough history is essential to the treatment of the patient.
44. The concept of referred pain was fully explained.
45. Most common headaches are transient and probably never require a physician's treatment.
46. A radiographic examination of the skull might demonstrate a tumor.
47. All headaches that occur daily are associated with organic disease.
48. Psychological factors must be considered.

Blood transfusion has developed through the centuries from the primitive stage to the art as it is practiced today. While whole blood is still the major type of transfused product, component therapy is being increasingly practiced in order to minimize risk to the patient. Whole blood is indicated for transfusion when the patient is both anemic and hypovolemic, while packed cells are indicated only in anemic conditions. Because of supply and demand problems, most blood transfusions utilize stored blood rather than fresh blood. During storage, however, changes take place which are detrimental to the qualities of blood, such as potassium leakage into plasma, decreasing pH, increasing ammonia concentration, and increasing hemolysis of the red blood cells. The most important changes, however, are decreasing ATP and 2,3-DPG concentrations. ATP is concerned with membrane stability, and its loss is associated with increasing membrane fragility. 2,3-DPG, a glycolytic metabolite, is associated with oxygen affinity of the red cell, in that decreasing 2,3-DPG levels are associated with increasing oxygen affinity of the red blood cells. With this increased affinity, however, less tissue oxygenation occurs because the A-V (arterio-venous) O_2 concentration difference is less, and, therefore, less oxygen is liberated to the tissues. Advanced technology, however, now enables us to raise 2,3-DPG and ATP to their normal levels by biochemical alteration so that red blood cells with normal or decreased oxygen affinity can now be supplied to patients. Because of this accomplishment, tissue oxygenation immediately after transfusion is increased over that which would occur if the red cells had not been altered. This enables delivery of superior blood to the patient at a time of critical need.

49. According to the reading selection 2,3-DPG levels are
(A) normal in stored blood.
(B) not involved in tissue oxygenation.
(C) able to be manipulated experimentally.
(D) of no concern in transfusion therapy.
(E) concerned with membrane stability.

50. It can be inferred from the reading selection that tissue oxygenation
(A) is an object of transfusion therapy.
(B) is not altered by 2,3-DPG levels.
(C) does not depend on RBC oxygen affinity.
(D) has no relation to length of storage of blood.
(E) is of little concern.

51. It can be inferred from the reading selection that anemia is
(A) best treated by whole blood.
(B) influenced by quality of the RBC.
(C) unrelated to tissue oxygenation.
(D) best left untreated.
(E) found more often in older persons.

52. It can be inferred from the reading selection that ATP
(A) is directly related to 2,3-DPG levels.
(B) doesn't decrease with time in storage.
(C) has only a minimal effect on membrane stability.
(D) is necessary to prevent hemolysis of the RBC.
(E) is of no concern.

53. It can be inferred from the reading selection that patients should receive blood
(A) with high plasma potassium levels.
(B) consisting of only packed cells.
(C) with high 2,3-DPG levels.
(D) only if anemic.
(E) only if it has not been stored.

There are probably more myths associated with the drinking of alcohol than with any other form of human behavior. The use of alcoholic beverages can be traced to prehistoric times and today 85% of the adults drink without apparent ill effects. Ethyl alcohol which is commonly consumed is nonpoisonous; it is quickly oxidized and degraded. Methyl alcohol is oxidized into a poison that damages the nervous system and often leads to blindness and death of the consumer; ethyl alcohol is oxidized in the liver to acetaldehyde which is oxidized into acetic acid and on into carbon dioxide and water.

The most pronounced physiological effect of alcohol is exerted upon the nervous system; the extent depends on the concentration in the blood and tissues. Two to three ounces (0.05% in the blood) depresses the centers of inhibition, restraint and judgement; five to six ounces (blood level of 0.1%) depresses the somewhat lower motor areas concerned with locomotion. After a consumption of ten ounces (blood level of 0.2%) the entire motor area is affected and the consumer is unable to walk; also the midbrain where emotional behavior is largely controlled is influenced and rage and tears are easily elicited. After drinking a pint (blood level of 0.3%) man is still conscious but stupified, but when the level in the blood reaches 0.4 to 0.5% the complete perception areas of the brain are suppressed and coma results. When the concentration reaches 0.6 to 0.7%, the autonomic centers that control the heart and respiratory centers are affected and death ensues rapidly.

Ethyl alcohol may owe its toxic properties in part to its adsorption on the oxidative enzyme machinery of the brain cells which then results in the suppression of normal metabolic processes. Competition for these surfaces between ethyl alcohol and normal metabolites would be proportional to the concentration of ethyl alcohol in the system. Tissues show first an increased oxygen uptake, which normalizes relatively quickly and then starts to decrease. It is assumed that during the first phase ethyl alcohol is adsorbed on the oxidizing surfaces hitherto unoccupied, and therefore does not interfere with other metabolites, resulting in a net increase in the rate of oxygen uptake. When saturation is approached, competition with other metabolites begins and alcohol wins out because of its high concentration and easier permeability of the cell membranes, resulting in a fall in the rate of oxygen uptake.

The following statements are related to the passage above. Based on the information given, select:

(A) if the statement is *supported by* the information in the passage.
(B) if the statement is *contradicted by* the information in the passage.
(C) if the statement is *neither supported nor contradicted by* information in the passage.

54. Ethyl alcohol is a stimulant in small doses.

55. Ethyl alcohol usually exerts a depressant effect on man.

56. It is suggested that the drug acts on certain specific brain cells preferentially.

57. The rate of oxygen uptake is decreased because of the slow oxidation of ethyl alcohol.

58. The concentration of ethyl alcohol in the blood is a determining factor of the outcome of alcohol consumption.

59. The vascular system is directly responsible for the effects of ethyl alcohol.

60. Lower areas of the nervous system seem to be affected earlier.

61. Man can consume a pint of ethyl alcohol.

Questions 62-64:

62. You are assigned by your local newspaper to cover a symposium entitled "The Biology of Oncogenic Viruses." From this title you can assume that
(A) the symposium will cover problems concerning heart attacks.
(B) no speaker will be concerned with nucleic acids.
(C) the symposium will be concerned with the etiology of cancer.
(D) the symposium will be directed toward solving problems resulting from air pollution.

63. In order to gain some background information before attending, you decide to go to the university library and do some reading. Among the sources you will NOT consult is
(A) a monograph on the synthesis of nucleic acids.
(B) a recent immunology textbook.
(C) an article in a scientific journal on cholesterol metabolism.
(D) a review paper concerned with protein synthesis in cancer cells.

64. Despite the fact that you have prepared yourself well, as the symposium proceeds several terms are used which you do not understand. Which of the following groups of scientists would be most likely to be able to help you?
(A) immunologist, biochemist
(B) physicist, anesthesiologist
(C) civil engineer, sociologist
(D) electrical engineer, statistician

Following the work of Chalmers and others, 831 geriatric and orthopedic patients in west London were reviewed for osteomalacia. History, relevant blood tests (calcium, phosphate, alkaline phosphatase, 24-hour urinary calcium), and radiology were assessed. Thirty-eight bone biopsies were performed. Thrity-three were positive (32 female, 1 male). Average age was 73.4 years. None had a history of gastric surgery. Twenty-eight were widows living alone. Three were sisters (spinsters) living together. Twenty-two lived on their own property. Average weekly income was \$23.8. Average weekly food bill, \$3.1 (mostly bread, canned meat, and canned fruit). The minimum for a balanced diet was thought to be \$6.5. Average milk consumption ⅔ pint per week. None of the patients cooked regularly. Twenty-six never cooked at all. None had sought the assistance of any of the welfare organizations, either through pride, ignorance, or apathy. All showed subjective and objective improvement following Vitamin D supplementation and dietary improvement.

65. Osteomalacia
(A) has a predilection for males.
(B) occurs more frequently in females.
(C) can only be diagnosed by bone biopsy.
(D) has a predilection for apartment dwellers.

66. The average weekly income did not allow these people to buy more food.
(A) True.
(B) False.
(C) They needed to save for their old age.
(D) They spent their money on the little luxuries of life.

67. From these data we may conclude that
(A) homeowners are more likely to develop osteomalacia than are renters.
(B) spinsters will not develop osteomalacia if they live alone.
(C) consumption of bread is a causative factor in development of osteomalacia.
(D) there seems to be a correlation between an unbalanced diet, irregular meal consumption, and osteomalacia.

68. Given a greater income, these individuals would have
(A) eaten more nutritious meals.
(B) cooked at least two meals each day.
(C) spent a greater percentage of their income for food.
(D) none of the above.

STOP. If you finish before the time limit is up, go over your work for this section. DO NOT look at any other sections of the model examination. When your time limit is up, go on to the next section.

SKILLS ANALYSIS: QUANTITATIVE

85 MINUTES
68 QUESTIONS

The following questions are to be answered based on your knowledge of basic mathematical principles and relationships.

DIRECTIONS: Read each passage carefully, study each table or chart, then answer the questions following it. Consider only the material presented in answering the questions. Eliminate those choices that you think to be incorrect and mark the letter of your choice on the answer sheet.

Blood samples from two groups of rats were assayed for LH luteinizing hormone in two separate radioimmunoassays. Half the rats were intact and half were orchidectomized. Some samples in each group were collected in the morning and some were collected in the afternoon. The data are summarized in the following table:

Assay 1				Assay 2			
#	Intact or Orchid X.	Sampled AM or PM	LH ng/ml	#	Intact or Orchid X.	Sampled AM or PM	LH ng/ml
1	I	AM	5.0	11	I	PM	7.5
2	O	AM	50	12	O	PM	75
3	I	PM	4.8	13	I	AM	7.7
4	O	PM	480	14	O	AM	770
5	I	AM	5.2	15	I	PM	7.3
6	O	AM	52	16	O	PM	250
7	I	PM	5.1	17	I	AM	7.4
8	O	PM	350	18	O	AM	100
9	I	AM	4.9	19	I	PM	7.6
10	O	AM	100	20	O	PM	640

The following statements are related to the information presented above. Based on the information given, select:

(A) if the statement is *supported by* the information given.
(B) if the statement is *contradicted by* the information given.
(C) if the statement is *neither supported nor contradicted by* information given.

1. Orchidectomy is followed by increased levels of LH in the blood.

2. Blood LH levels are higher in the afternoon than in the morning.

3. Assays 1 and 2 are measuring different molecules.

4. The differences between LH values in these 2 assays are probably explained by interassay variations since the ratios between intact and orchidectomized levels are similar.

5. LH release in the orchidectomized rats may be occurring episodically.

6. The results of the 2 assays could be compared more precisely if some of the samples had been included in both assays.

7. Larger volumes of blood were assayed in Assay 1 than in Assay 2.

8. A significant change in LH release would be seen in intact rats had samples been taken at noon.

9. The testes are responsible for the production of LH.

10. The ovaries are responsible for the production of LH.

Ovulation in the rat can be blocked by systemic administration of drugs which depress neural function. However, ovulation depends on the response of the ovaries to LH released from the pituitary gland. In the following experiment drug X was injected subcutaneously at 13:45 hours into several groups of rats and the presence or absence of ova in the oviduct determined on the following morning. In order to pinpoint the site of action of the drug attempts were made to restore ovulation by stimulation of the brain, injection of LRF, the hormone which causes pituitary LH release, and injection of LH which induces ovulation. The results are summarized below.

Treatment	Number of Rats Treated	Number of Rats Ovulating
Drug X	10	1
Drug X + LRF	10	5
Drug X + LH	10	5
Drug X + Brain Stimulation	10	1

The following statements are related to the information presented. Based on the information given, select:

(A) if the statement is *supported by* the information given.
(B) if the statement is *contradicted by* the information given.
(C) if the statement is *neither supported nor contradicted by* information given.

11. Drug X may be blocking the release of LRF from the brain and thereby preventing the activation of pituitary LH release.

12. Drug X may be preventing pituitary LH release in response to LRF.

13. Drug X appears to interfere with the ovarian response to LH.

14. Drug X does not affect the brain since stimulation of the brain does not restore ovulation.

15. Injection of drug X at 21:00 hours would be equally effective since its effect is at the ovary.

16. The effect of drug X on the brain is greater than its effect on the ovary.

17. Drug X would be a useful oral contraceptive in the human.

18. Drug X functions as a competitive inhibitor of LH action on the ovary.

Use the following table as a reference to answer questions 19-21:

Country	Crude Birth Rate	Crude Death Rate
Lebanon	54	26
Egypt	50	26
India	50	25
Pakistan	49	26
USSR	43	18
East Germany	18	10
West Germany	16	16
France	35	11
Spain	19	7
Holland	45	8
Luxemburg	17	11.8
Japan	15	13

19. Which of the countries in the table shows the most rapid population growth?
(A) Spain
(B) Holland
(C) USSR
(D) Lebanon
(E) Japan

20. Which country can claim the lowest rate of population growth?
(A) East Germany
(B) Luxemburg
(C) Japan
(D) West Germany
(E) India

21. Which country has the longest doubling time?
(A) India
(B) East Germany
(C) Japan
(D) France
(E) Lebanon

Female albino rats weighing between 170 and 230 gm were housed in pairs in wire bottom cages and received a standard diet of rat pellets and chlorinated water *ad libitum*. Unanesthetized rats were restrained and shielded with lead so that only the head and neck regions were exposed. The animals received 6400 R of X-radiation in a single dose. Following irradiation careful check was maintained on the water and food consumption. Also, at varying intervals after exposure the animals were killed and the wet weights of their parotid salivary glands were determined. The results of these follow-ups are depicted below:

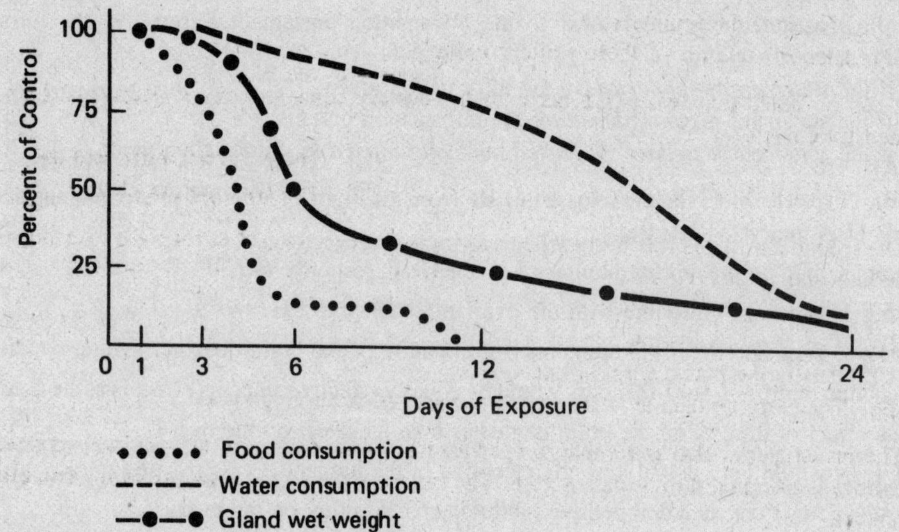

22. These experiments were designed to determine if
(A) variation in sex causes differences in rodent salivary glands.
(B) exposure to X-radiation causes premature death in female rats.
(C) chlorinated water *ad libitum* determines the wet weight of parotid glands.
(D) X-radiation causes alteration in water consumption and volume of salivary glands in rats.

23. The first parameter measured in this experiment which was affected by 6400 R X-radiation was
(A) percent of chlorinated water given to the animals.
(B) water consumption.
(C) wet weight of the glands.
(D) food intake.

24. Which of the following statements is true concerning the data obtained from this experiment?
(A) The animals continued to consume large quantities of water up to the time of death.
(B) An alteration in food consumption was already evident at 3 days after radiation.
(C) Even though drinking and eating declined, the weights of the salivary glands remained unaffected until time of death.
(D) Water consumption and wet weight of the glands first began to vary from control values at 8 days.

Levels of estrogens in the urine of the human female during the menstrual cycle, pregnancy, and the post-menopausal period were obtained from women during some routine work-ups during their visits to the ob-gyn clinic. The following data were obtained.

Time	Estriol µg/24 hr.	Estrone µg/24 hr.	Estradiol µg/24 hr.
Onset of menstruation	9	7	3
Ovulation peak	30	24	10
Luteal peak	20	18	9
Pregnancy, 150 days	10	1	.5
Pregnancy, term	35	4	2
Postmenopause	2	2	1

25. The object of the experiment was to
(A) develop a technique for estrogen assay.
(B) see if females possessed estrogens in urine.
(C) obtain meaningful data concerning estrogen excretion during various reproductive phases of the female.
(D) keep the records of these patients complete.

26. It can be noted that two peaks occur in the urinary concentration of estrogens during the menstrual cycle.
(A) True.
(B) False.
(C) There are not sufficient data.
(D) The data are not clear.

27. The second rise in all probability reflects an increased secretion of estrogens by the theca luteal cells of the corpus luteum.
(A) This is a good assumption.
(B) This is a bad assumption.
(C) This is the purest speculation.
(D) There are no data available at all to make such an assumption.

28. The investigators also were able to speculate as to the source of the minimal quantities of estrogens excreted during menopause. The organs most likely responsible for this estrogen are the
(A) testes.
(B) uterus.
(C) adrenals (cortex).
(D) vagina.

Twenty male New Zealand albino rabbits were divided into four groups of 5 animals each and treated as follows:

Group 1: Received a subcutaneous injection of 10×10^{-6} sheep red blood cells at two week intervals for a total of three injections.

Group 2: Received an intradermal injection of 10×10^{-6} sheep red blood cells at two week intervals for a total of three injections.

Group 3: Received a subscapular injection of 10×10^{-6} sheep red blood cells at two week intervals for a total of three injections.

Group 4: Received an intravenous injection of 10×10^{-6} sheep red blood cells at two week intervals for a total of three injections.

During the six week immunization period antibody titers against sheep red blood cells were measured and the following results obtained:

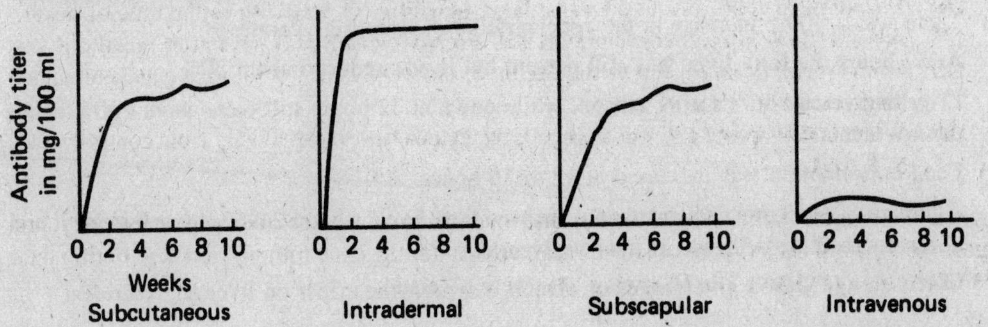

29. The purpose of this study was to
   (A) assay the rate of antigen clearance from immunized animals.
   (B) determine the effect of different routes of administration on antibody titer.
   (C) determine the effect of sheep red blood cells on total I_gG content of serum.
   (D) determine the effect of different antigen dosage on antibody titer.

30. These data show that
   (A) there is little difference in the results produced by the various routes of administration.
   (B) there is little difference between subscapular and subcutaneous injection routes.
   (C) the animals receiving intravenous red blood cells were immunologically incompetent.
   (D) antigen clearance was most rapid in the animals receiving intradermal injections.

31. It may also be seen that
   (A) intravenous administration of antigen leads to anaphylactic shock.
   (B) subscapular administration produces delayed hypersensitivity.
   (C) subcutaneous administration produces a generalized Arthus reaction.
   (D) intradermal administration produces the highest antibody titer.

An experimental drug, S24953, may maintain hepatic fatty acid oxidation at a normal rate in ethanol-treated rats. The following groups were studied at 8, 16, and 32 hours after administration of ethyl alcohol and glucose. Biochemically speaking a fatty liver is the end result of ethanol consumption.

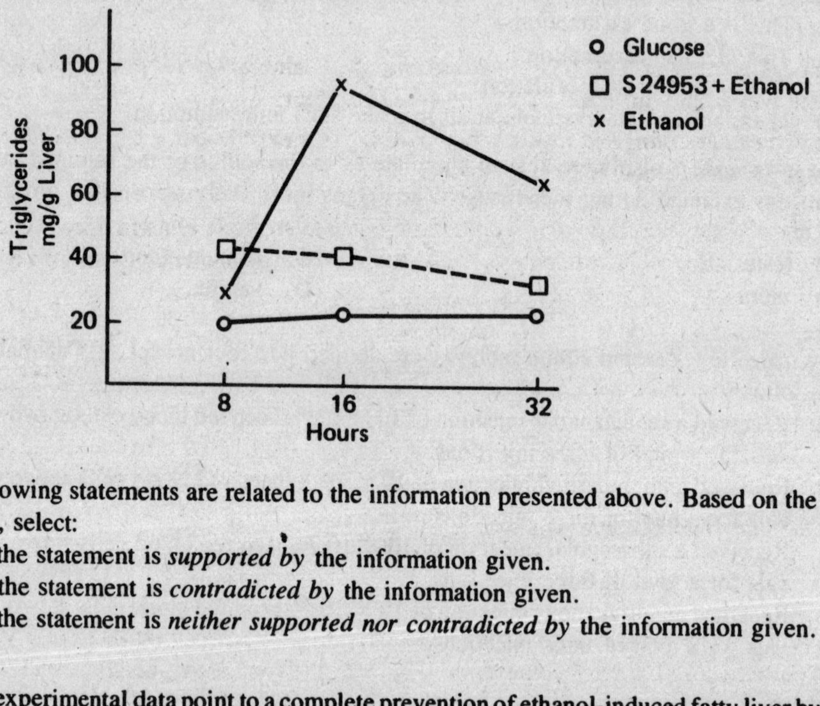

The following statements are related to the information presented above. Based on the information given, select:
   (A) if the statement is *supported by* the information given.
   (B) if the statement is *contradicted by* the information given.
   (C) if the statement is *neither supported nor contradicted by* the information given.

32. The experimental data point to a complete prevention of ethanol-induced fatty liver by S24953.
33. The peak of the ethanol-induced fatty liver was observed around 16 hours after consumption.
34. There was a 300% increase in the concentration of liver triglycerides.
35. At 32 hours the fatty liver was still present but it was reduced about 30%.
36. Liver triglyceride levels after ethanol while down at 32 hours still were about 100% above control levels.
37. Food consumption was increased at 12 to 16 hours.
38. Although S24953 prevents an ethanol-induced fatty liver, when S24953 is given alone it produces an absolute decrease in liver triglycerides.
39. Glucose and S24953 given together exhibit a synergistic effect on liver triglycerides.

A blood sample was taken from a test subject. Then a masked man came in with a gun and appeared to murder 2 persons. The test subject was visibly upset. After 30 seconds, the "victims" stood up. The subject was told of the hoax, and blood samples were taken over a period of time for counting red blood cells (RBC).

Time	RBC/mm³ of Blood
Control (before "murder")	5.5 million
30 seconds after "murder"	5.9 million
6.5 minutes after "murder"	7.0 million
14.5 minutes after "murder"	5.6 million
18.5 minutes after "murder"	5.5 million

The following statements are related to the information presented above. Based on the information given, select:

(A) if the statement is *supported by* the information given.
(B) if the statement is *contradicted by* the information given.
(C) if the statement is *neither supported nor contradicted by* information given.

40. There was an increase in the RBC/mm³ of blood of the test subject a few minutes after he thought he witnessed murder.

41. A larger change in the RBC/mm³ of blood would have been noted if the test subject had been placed in greater fear for his own life.

42. Having changed from the control value, there was no return to the control value for over 20 minutes.

43. Although a return of RBC/MM³ of blood to control value was noted, a rebound would be expected within an hour after the end of the experiment.

44. The *percentage change* in RBCs in blood during this experiment is less than the *percentage change* in white blood cells in the blood.

Production of organic compounds by photosynthesis was studied in Puerto Rico. The results are given in the table below with the theoretical yield based on percentage of light captured by the plant.

	Carbohydrate Production (tons/acre)		
Plants	**Present**	**Theoretical**	**Percentage of Sunlight Captured by Plant**
Kelp	2.0	14	15
Cane	0.7	0.9	1.0
Plant Z	4.1	18	20

45. The protein yield per acre would be greatest from
(A) kelp.
(B) cane.
(C) plant Z.
(D) no basis for comparison.

46. It would be expected that doubling the incident light on an acre of cultivated kelp would cause it to ______________ as compared with an acre of plant Z on which the incident light is unchanged.
(A) surpass the carbohydrate yield per acre
(B) approach the carbohydrate yield per acre
(C) surpass the protein yield per acre
(D) surpass the percentage of incident light captured

47. It is decided that sugar syrup for sweetening purposes will be made from each of the plants. When the carbohydrate content is equal, the sugar syrup from plant Z is not accepted by the tasters. This might be because of
(A) impurities with bad tastes.
(B) a large percentage of the carbohydrate of this plant is not sweet.
(C) A and/or B.
(D) none of the above.

48. Without changing the incident sunlight, the largest percentage increase that is theoretically possible is predicted for
(A) plant Z.
(B) kelp.
(C) cane.

Use the following table as a reference to answer questions 49-54:

MIDDLE INCOME PEOPLE

	Food Consumed Predominantly			Type of Tooth Decay (percent)			Type of Toothpaste Used (grams/brushing)	
Samples	Starchy Foods	Meaty Foods	Liquids	I	II	III	I	II
1	79	6.6	8	69	61	7	23	27
2	38	27	12	35	31	7	6	7
3	9	26	40	9	5	1	2	3

The following statements are related to the information presented above. Based on the information given, select:
(A) if the statement is *supported by* the information given.
(B) if the statement is *contradicted by* the information given.
(C) if the statement is *neither supported nor contradicted by* information given.

49. Considering the group classified as starch eaters, there does not seem a noticeable difference between the types of tooth decay and the sample of population.
50. The average diet consumed results in less tooth decay.
51. As shown in sample 3, the less tooth paste that was used the fewer the cavities.
52. Sample 3 exhibited less tooth decay.
53. The type of tooth decay can be correlated and based on a particular diet.
54. Amount of tooth paste used significantly influences dental problems.

Use the following graphs to answer questions 55-57:

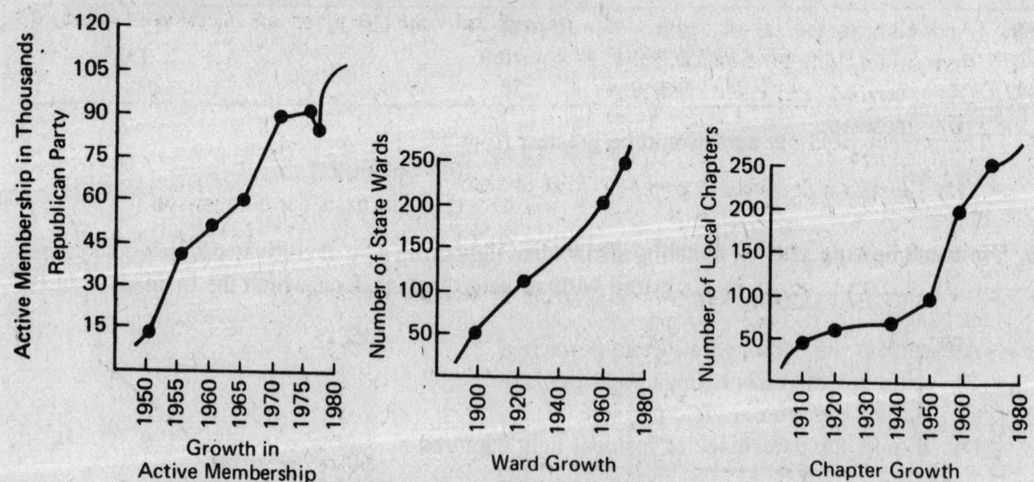

55. Based solely on the size of the membership trend and size of membership the Republican party seems to be strong.
(A) True
(B) False
(C) Not enough information

56. The total number of wards and chapters, like total membership, is at an all-time high.
(A) True
(B) False
(C) Not enough information

57. There is every reason to believe that given a change in leadership this growth can be maintained and steadily increased.
(A) True
(B) False
(C) Not enough information

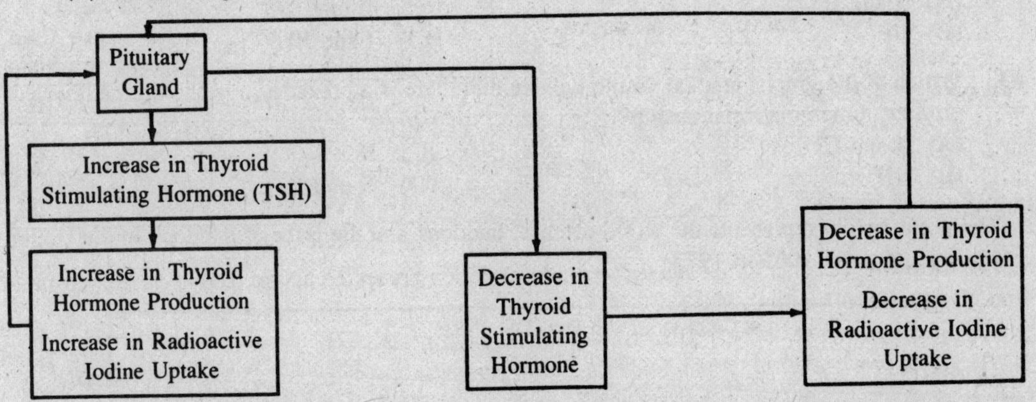

The pituitary gland is responsible for the secretion of thyroid stimulating hormone (TSH), which elicits an increased production of thyroid hormone from the gland; this thyroid hormone then may inhibit the pituitary via a negative feedback. Under hyperthyroid conditions, the following tests would give elevated values:

1. Basal metabolic rate (BMR)
2. Protein bound iodine (PBI)
3. Radioactive iodine uptake (RAI)

58. When TSH secretion falls, the secretion by the thyroid of thyroid hormone
(A) stays the same.
(B) increases.
(C) decreases.
(D) will feed back upon the pituitary.

59. According to the schema given, if a normal individual is given an injection of TSH, his thyroid hormone production will first
(A) show no noticeable change.
(B) increase.
(C) decrease.
(D) lead to a decrease in pituitary TSH output.

Use the following graphs to answer questions 60-63:

RAI Uptake After Administration of Thyroid Hormones

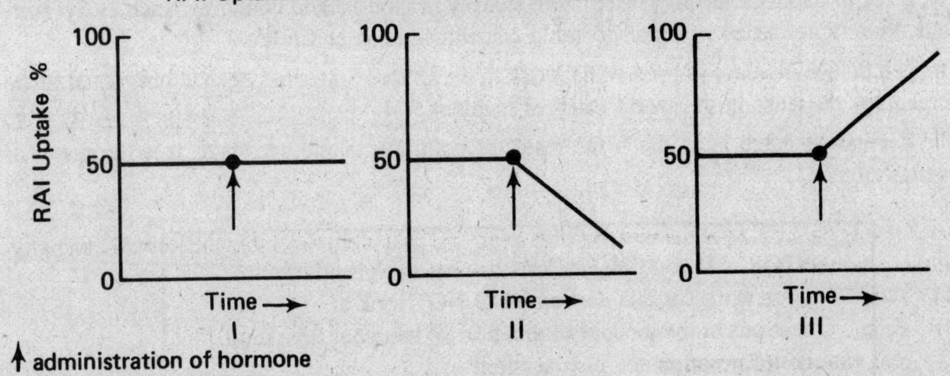

60. Utilizing the information of the flow chart, paragraph, and graphs, in which of the graphs is there evidence of thyroid malfunction?
(A) I
(B) I and II
(C) I and III
(D) III

61. Which graph (s) probably represent (s) the case of a typical hyperthyroid person?
(A) II
(B) I
(C) I and III
(D) II and III

62. Which graph (s) probably represent (s) the case of normal individuals?
(A) I and II
(B) II
(C) II and III
(D) I and III

63. Which of the graphs lead (s) you to believe that there is a breakdown in the normal thyroid-pituitary functional relationship?
(A) I and III
(B) III
(C) II
(D) II and III

The graph below represents the world catch of haddock and the price of haddock in the United States for the years 1965 to 1972.

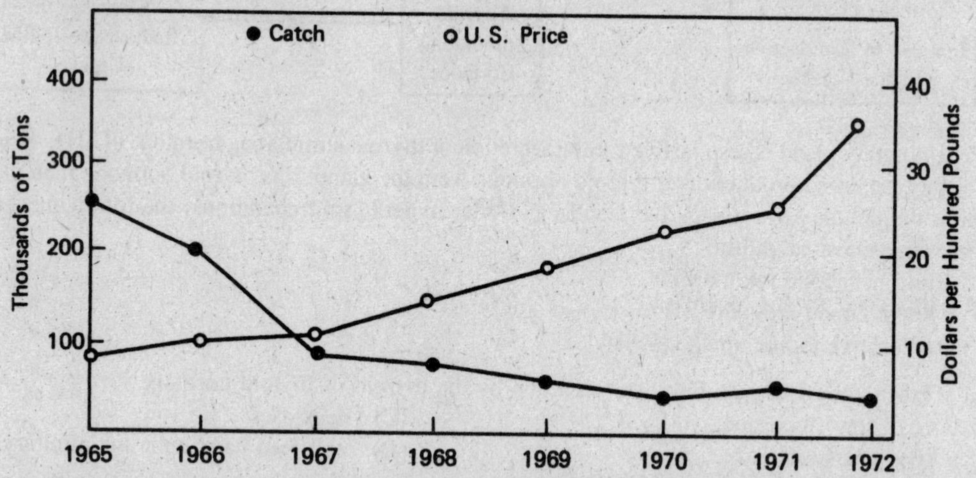

The following statements concern the information printed in the graph above. Based on information in the graph, select:
(A) if the statement is *supported by* the information given.
(B) if the statement is *contradicted by* the information given.
(C) if the statement is *neither supported nor contradicted by* information given.

64. From 1968 to 1972 the price of haddock in the United States has more than doubled.

65. The price of haddock has increased in the United States at a rate similar to the increase in Mexico between 1966 and 1971.

66. The price of haddock has increased more sharply in land-locked countries, such as Switzerland, than in countries with considerable coastlines, such as Chile.

67. The percentage increase in price of haddock in the United States has been almost equal to the percentage decrease in the world catch of haddock.

68. The decreasing catch is as much the result of pollution of the oceans as it is the result of overfishing.

STOP. If you finish before the time limit is up, go over your work for this section. DO NOT look at any other sections of the model examination. When your time limit is up, go on to the next section.

Model Test A Answers*

SCIENCE KNOWLEDGE

Biology

1. A	9. C	17. C	25. B	32. A
2. A	10. B	18. B	26. E	33. C
3. C	11. A	19. B	27. B	34. A
4. D	12. B	20. A	28. B	35. A
5. B	13. A	21. B	29. E	36. E
6. D	14. C	22. B	30. C	37. C
7. E	15. B	23. C	31. B	38. A
8. C	16. A	24. B		

Chemistry

1. D	11. B	21. A	31. D	41. B
2. D	12. B	22. A	32. A	42. D
3. A	13. C	23. C	33. B	43. E
4. C	14. A	24. B	34. C	44. C
5. B	15. B	25. B	35. E	45. B
6. B	16. A	26. D	36. E	46. B
7. A	17. B	27. C	37. D	47. B
8. C	18. A	28. D	38. D	48. C
9. A	19. E	29. A	39. D	49. E
10. D	20. A	30. D	40. C	

Physics

1. D	9. C	17. D	25. C	32. D
2. B	10. B	18. A	26. C	33. B
3. A	11. D	19. E	27. B	34. E
4. C	12. E	20. B	28. D	35. A
5. D	13. B	21. D	29. E	36. D
6. A	14. A	22. D	30. D	37. B
7. A	15. D	23. E	31. A	38. D
8. C	16. C	24. E		

*Explanations for science answers can be found on p. 135.

SCIENCE PROBLEMS

1. B	15. C	29. C	43. C	57. A
2. C	16. D	30. E	44. E	58. B
3. C	17. B	31. E	45. A	59. C
4. B	18. C	32. A	46. A	60. C
5. C	19. D	33. C	47. C	61. D
6. A	20. D	34. D	48. A	62. A
7. A	21. C	35. A	49. B	63. B
8. D	22. A	36. E	50. B	64. B
9. B	23. B	37. D	51. A	65. A
10. B	24. B	38. A	52. A	66. E
11. C	25. D	39. B	53. A	
12. A	26. C	40. B	54. B	
13. D	27. E	41. C	55. B	
14. E	28. A	42. E	56. E	

SKILLS ANALYSIS: READING

1. B	15. B	29. C	43. A	57. B
2. C	16. D	30. B	44. B	58. A
3. A	17. C	31. C	45. A	59. B
4. A	18. D	32. B	46. C	60. A
5. A	19. B	33. A	47. B	61. A
6. C	20. A	34. B	48. A	62. C
7. C	21. B	35. A	49. C	63. C
8. A	22. B	36. B	50. A	64. A
9. B	23. B	37. C	51. B	65. B
10. C	24. B	38. C	52. D	66. B
11. B	25. C	39. C	53. C	67. D
12. C	26. B	40. B	54. C	68. D
13. B	27. A	41. A	55. A	
14. B	28. C	42. C	56. B	

SKILLS ANALYSIS: QUANTITATIVE

1. A	15. C	29. B	43. C	57. C
2. B	16. C	30. B	44. C	58. C
3. C	17. C	31. D	45. D	59. B
4. A	18. C	32. A	46. B	60. C
5. A	19. B	33. A	47. C	61. B
6. A	20. D	34. A	48. B	62. B
7. C	21. C	35. A	49. C	63. A
8. C	22. D	36. A	50. B	64. A
9. B	23. D	37. C	51. C	65. C
10. C	24. B	38. C	52. A	66. C
11. A	25. C	39. C	53. C	67. B
12. B	26. A	40. A	54. C	68. C
13. A	27. A	41. C	55. A	
14. A	28. C	42. B	56. A	

Explanation of Answers for Science Questions-Model Test A

SCIENCE KNOWLEDGE

Biology

1. (A) Chorionic gonadotropin is produced by the placenta and acts with other reproductive hormones to maintain pregnancy.

2. (A) Relaxin is a product of the ovaries and placenta and functions in relaxing the pelvic ligaments during parturition.

3. (C) Cortisol is produced by the adrenal and is active in the conversion of proteins to carbohydrates.

4. (D) Ptyalin (salivary amylase) is found in saliva and initiates starch digestion.

5. (B) Vasopressin (ADH) elaborated by the hypothalamus has an antidiuretic action on the kidney tubules.

6. (D) Maltase, a component of saliva, participates in starch digestion.

7. (E) Chitin, mucus, and keratin are products elaborated by epithelial cells.

8. (C) The striated muscle fiber is multinucleated.

9. (C) The tsetse fly transmits African sleeping sickness to humans.

10. (B) Complete metamorphosis comprises the following sequence:
    egg → larva → pupa → adult

11. (A) One of the distinguishing features of chordates is a dorsal tubular nerve cord.

12. (B) The cell is the basic unit of structure and function and the basis of all life; all cells come from preexisting cells.

13. (A) Ribosomes can be free floating or they may be attached to the endoplasmic reticulum which is then called rough endoplasmic reticulum (RER).

14. (C) Lysosomes contain hydrolytic enzymes and are also known as digestive bags, etc.

15. (B) The pituitary gland is located within the sella tursica.

16. (A) Ectoderm is the germ layer of origin of the nervous system.

17. (C) Stress and strain will have a pronounced influence on the output of epinephrine and norepinephrine by the adrenal medulla. Activation of the sympathetic portion of the autonomic nervous system will result in increased activity by the adrenal medulla which can be considered the site of the postganglionic cell bodies of that segment of the sympathetics.

18. (B) Mesoderm is the germ layer of origin of the skeletal system.

19. (B) Connective tissue, cartilage, and bone are basically supporting tissues. An abundance of nonliving-formed substance is the feature that is common to the group as a whole. Cells are interspersed in the intercellular substance and fibers are a constituent of the formed substance. Fibers and ground substance are called matrix.

20. (A) Human sperm and ova are similar in the respect that they both carry a haploid chromosomal complement. After fertilization the diploid composition is again found.

21. (B) A group of nerve cell bodies is commonly considered to be the site of a nucleus.

22. (B) The neurolemma of an axon is a part of the Schwann cell (outer membrane).

23. (C) CO_2 and O_2 exchange takes place in the alveoli of the lung.

24. (B) Sweat glands, salivary glands, and sebaceous glands are all exocrine glands.

25. (B) The appendix is a blind sac originating from the cecum of the ascending colon (large intestines).

26. (E) Active transport requires energy and allows a cell to move material from a point of lower concentration to a point of higher concentration.

27. (B) The internal structure of a cilium or flagellum is composed of 9 outer and 2 inner pairs of tubules.

28. **(B)** It is the reproductive system that is highly specialized in the tapeworm.

29. **(E)** Sodium fluoride (or other fluoride salts) is added to drinking water in very small amounts in order to reduce the incidence of tooth decay.

30. **(C)** Treatment of municipal water supplies with chlorine (i.e., chlorination) is commonly practiced to kill harmful organisms.

31. **(B)** During metaphase of mitosis the centrioles with asters are at the opposite poles; the chromosomes move to the equator of the cell and duplicate.

32. **(A)** Cilia are utilized by planaria for movement.

33. **(C)** In an open circulatory system blood is not always enclosed within well defined blood vessels.

34. **(A)** The corpus callosum connects the two cerebral hemispheres in the mammal; association fibers cross in this bundle.

35. **(A)** A heterotroph is an organism that cannot make all the complex organic molecules necessary for the metabolic machinery of the system from simple molecules such as CO_2, H_2O, etc. Man gets these complex molecules from other living organisms. Photosynthetic organisms are autotrophs.

36. **(E)** It is generally agreed that in order for speciation to occur we need genetic isolation and time.

37. **(C)** The peculiar features of renal circulation, such as the renal arteries originating directly from the aorta, the glomerulo-capillary arrangement, and differences in the calibers of the afferent and efferent vessels, indicate that blood pressure is of great functional significance for the production of urine. The vascular component probably plays an important role in the filtration process.

38. **(A)** Salivary secretions come readily into contact with the host when the latter is bitten by an insect, and parasites can be transmitted via this mode.

Chemistry

1. **(D)** Double replacement reactions involve a double exchange; compounds react chemically to form two new compounds.

2. **(D)** See explanation for question 1.

3. **(A)** In a synthesis reaction two or more elements can unite to form a single compound.

4. **(C)** In a single replacement reaction a more active element reacts with a compound to replace a less active one. A new element and a new compound are the result.

5. **(B)** In a decomposition reaction a compound is broken into simpler compounds or into its elements.

6. **(B)** A saturated fatty acid has the structure $CH_3(CH_2)_nCOOH$ or the empirical formula $C_nH_{2n}O_2$.

7. **(A)** A carbohydrate approximates the empirical formula of $C_m(H_2O)_n$, and this accounts for the name.

8. **(C)** A saturated hydrocarbon has the formula of C_nH_{2n+2}.

9. **(A)** A reaction that requires energy is an endergonic reaction while one that liberates energy is an exergonic reaction.

10. **(D)** This configuration: $\underset{\underset{\displaystyle O}{\|}}{-C}-OH$

is characteristic of carboxyl groups. A hydroxyl group is identified by — OH.

11. **(B)** The anode is a positive electrode attracting negatively charged particles while the cathode is the negative electrode attracting positively charged particles.

12. **(B)** In the absence of peroxides Markovnikov's rule would predict 2-bromobutane as the major product. HBr adds with the opposite orientation in the presence of peroxides, apparently by a free-radical mechanism rather than ionic mechanism.

13. **(C)** The gain of electrons is known as reduction, while the loss of electrons is classified as oxidation.

14. **(A)** This is basically a definition of eutectic temperature.

15. **(B)** The other half-cell reaction must release the electrons required by the first half-cell reaction $Zn \rightarrow Zn^{++} + 2e^-$.

16. **(A)** $K_{sp} = 6.2 \times 10^{-12} = [Ag^+]^2[CO_3^=]$

$$[Ag^+]^2 = \frac{6.2 \times 10^{-12}}{[CO_3^=]} = \frac{6.2 \times 10^{-12}}{6.2 \times 10^{-6}} = 1 \times 10^{-6}$$

$$[Ag^+] = \sqrt{1 \times 10^{-6}} = 1 \times 10^{-3} \text{ moles/liter}$$

17. **(B)** The K_{sp} of NiS is 1×10^{-26}
$K_{sp} = [Ni^{++}]\,[S^=]$

$$[S^=] = \frac{1 \times 10^{-26}}{1 \times 10^{-20}} = 1 \times 10^{-6}$$

18. **(A)** Pyrolysis of dry acetic acid in the presence of ThO_2 produces acetone and CO_2. Longer chain acids produce higher ketones.

19. **(E)** There are 4 asymmetric centers, $2^4 = 16$. The best answer given is 17.

20. **(A)** Anabolism is the synthetic phase and catabolism is the breakdown phase of metabolism.

21. **(A)** Hydrofluoric acid reacts with glass, resulting in etching. Carbolic acid is a common name for phenol.

22. **(A)** Sulfur trioxide, SO_3, is often produced by the oxidation of any fuel that contains sulfur.
$SO_3 + H_2O \rightarrow H_2SO_4$ (sulfuric acid)
$SO_2 + H_2O \rightarrow H_2SO_3$ (sulfurous acid)

23. **(C)** The atomic number represents the number of protons in the nucleus and (in the uncharged atom) the number of electrons in the shells surrounding the nucleus. Neutrons are found in the nucleus but have no charge.

24. **(B)** An atom which has lost 2 electrons has a charge of +2; an atom which is electrically neutral has equal numbers of protons and electrons.

25. **(B)** Oparin believed that the early atmosphere lacked free oxygen. The atmosphere consisted mainly of water vapor, carbon dioxide, nitrogen and compounds such as ammonia and methane. Hydrogen, oxygen, carbon and nitrogen make up over 99% of the tissues of living things.

26. **(D)** This is an example of the Wurtz-Fittig (or Fittig-Wurtz) Reaction. The two rings will be joined, and halogen will be lost.

27. (C) $ØCH_2Cl + Ø \xrightarrow{AlCl_3} Ø—CH_2—Ø$
Friedel-Crafts Reaction
$ØCH_2Cl + Na \longrightarrow Ø—CH_2CH_2—Ø$
Wurtz Reaction

28. **(D)** The question has listed the general properties of organic compounds.

29. **(A)** Remember that nitro groups are deactivating, meta-directing substituents and that halogens are deactivating, ortho, para-directing substituents. If bromination precedes nitration, then very little meta-bromonitrobenzene will result.

30. **(D)** Halogen on adjacent carbon atoms may be removed by heating with zinc duct in alcohol, yielding an alkene. Treatment of the 1,2-dihalide with alcoholic KOH would have produced the alkyne.

31. **(D)** Charles Goodyear discovered the process of vulcanization (the chemical reaction of rubber with sulfur) in 1839. Vulcanization produces a material with greater toughness and elasticity than natural rubber. This is so because sulfur adds to the double bonds in such a manner that the chains of rubber molecules are bound together, resulting in large, cross-linked molecules.

32. **(A)** This is the classic Diels-Alder condensation between a diene and a dienophile:

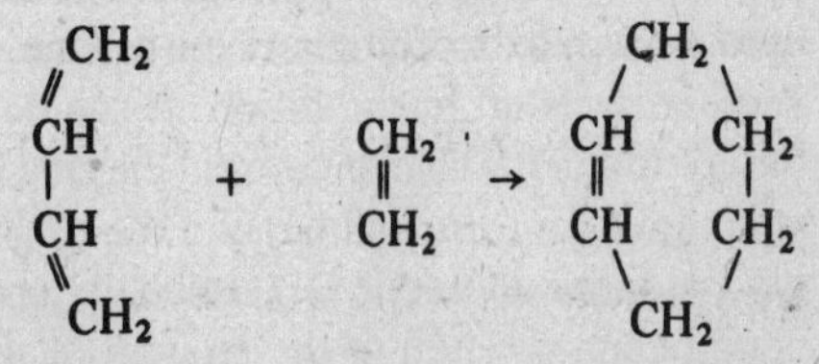

1,3-butadiene (diene) ethylene (dienophile) cyclohexene

33. **(B)** The *K* shell (1*s*) is filled with 2 electrons. The *L* shell (subshells 2*s* and 2*p*) is filled with 8 electrons. This element, fluorine, is a nonmetal that is most likely to gain one electron and fill the *L* shell.
This will give the atom a charge (and valence) of −1.

34. **(C)** See explanation for question 33.

35. **(E)** A nonmetal oxide reacts with water to form an acid.
$P_2O_3 + 3H_2O \rightarrow 2H_3PO_3$ (Phosphorus Acid)

36. **(E)** The two sugars found in the nucleotides of nucleic acids are D-deoxyribose and D-ribose.

37. **(D)** $CH_3-\overset{\overset{O}{\|}}{C}-Cl$ is a mixed anhydride.
$Cl-CH_2-\overset{\overset{O}{\|}}{C}-OH$ is simply chloroacetic acid. The other two formulas are for acetic anhydride and the anhydride of phosphoric acid.

38. **(D)** HCl ionizes to form H^+ and Cl^-. The other compounds contain only covalent bonds.

39. **(D)** C.A. de Coulomb was a French physicist after whom the coulomb was named; a coulomb is a unit of quantity of electricity. A coulomb is the quantity transferred by one ampere in one second. The other scientists in the question are properly matched to their contributions. The magnetic lines of force around a current-carrying wire were described by Oersted.

40. **(C)** Addition of a crystal is commonly employed to induce crystal formation and precipitation in a supersaturated solution.

41. **(B)** Polytetrafluoroethylene is highly prized for its chemical inertness. It is also used as a dry lubricant. One of its tradenames is Teflon.

42. **(D)** Enzymes decrease the activation energy and thereby decrease the time to reach equilibrium. The equilibrium constant is not affected.

43. **(E)** Change of specific rotation of plane polarized light as a result of conversion of one anomer to another is called mutarotation. It can occur only if the compound is able to go from the ring form to the straight chain form and back to the ring form. In a glycoside the anomeric OH is tied up, and the compound cannot return to the straight chain form.

44. **(C)** The Lobry de Bruyn-van Ekenstein Transformation in very dilute alkali will primarily convert an aldose to its 2-epimer or to a 2-ketose. This is thought to involve a 1,2-enediol intermediate. Thus D-glucose could be converted to its 2-epimer (i.e., D-mannose) or to the 2-ketose (i.e., D-fructose).

45. **(B)** The iron in hemoglobin and the magnesium in chlorophyll are held in place by chelation in a so-called clawlike structure.

46. **(B)** Although nitrates are usually colored, and many are important fertilizers, the major use of trinitrotoluene (TNT) is as an explosive.

47. **(B)** Phenolphthalein is colorless in solution at low pH and changes to red at a pH of about 8 to 10. It is quite useful in determining the equivalence point in a titration such as that of a strong acid by a strong base.

48. **(C)** Sodium bisulfite reacts with aldehydes and unhindered methyl ketones to produce a sparingly soluble bisulfite addition compound.

49. **(E)** Schiff bases are formed by the reaction between aromatic aldehydes and primary amines.

Physics

1. **(D)** Mathematical expression of Ohm's law.

2. **(B)** Mathematical expression of Charles' law.

3. **(A)** Mathematical expression of Graham's law of diffusion.

4. **(C)** Mathematical expression of centripetal force.

5. **(D)** If two forces act upon each other at right angles, the following formula should be used:

$$R = \sqrt{(\text{Force } 1)^2 + (\text{Force } 2)^2}$$
$$R = \sqrt{(12)^2 + (16)^2}$$
$$R = \sqrt{144 + 256}$$
$$R = \sqrt{400}$$
$$R = 20 \text{ lb.}$$

6. **(A)** Any combination of forces acting upon the same object in the same direction will result in an addition of the forces and the result will be equal to the sum of the forces.

7. **(A)** The formula for determining pressure is $\text{Pressure} = \frac{\text{Force}}{\text{Area}}$. In the example the man's weight of 185 pounds is the force and the area of the shoe sole is 13 inch². Applying the formula

$$P = \frac{185 \text{ lbs.}}{13 \text{ in.}^2} = 14.23 \text{ lb./in.}^2$$

8. **(C)** Specific gravity is usually expressed as the weight of an object in air divided by the loss of weight when weighed in water. In our example:

$$\text{Sp. G} = \frac{\text{Weight in Air}}{\text{Loss of Weight}} = \frac{720 \text{ g}}{360 \text{ g}} = 2$$

9. **(C)** If 0.5 remains after 1 cm, then $(0.5)^3$ will remain after 3 cm.
$(0.5)^3 = 0.125$ or 12.5%
100% − 12.5% = 87.5% stopped

10. **(B)** $v = rw$ where v = linear velocity, r = radius, and w = angular velocity in radians/time (there are 2π radians/rev).
$v = 10\ (2\pi \times 1000)$
$v = 20{,}000\ \pi$ cm/min.
$v = 62{,}800$ cm/min.

11. **(D)** In the northern hemisphere winds circulate about a high pressure area in a clockwise direction. In the southern hemisphere winds circulate about a high pressure area in a counterclockwise direction.

12. **(E)** The image in a plane mirror appears to be the same size as the object and as far behind the mirror as the object is in front.

13. **(B)** Work is equal to force times distance. A mass of 120 lb. exerts a force of 120 lb. with our gravitational acceleration.
120 lb. × 40 ft. = 4800 ft.-lb.

14. **(A)** $\frac{P_1V_1}{T_1} = \frac{P_2V_2}{T_2}$ where P is pressure, V is volume, T is temperature in °K. STP (standard temperature and pressure) is 273°K and 1 atm pressure.

$$\frac{1 \times 16}{273} = \frac{4V_2}{819°\text{K}}$$
$$V_2 = 12$$

15. **(D)** Boyle's law states that the product of volume and pressure of a gas is a constant at constant temperature.
$P_1V_1 = P_2V_2$

$V_2 = \frac{P_1}{P_2} V_1$

If the pressure is doubled $\frac{P_1}{P_2} = ½$. Thus $V_2 = ½ V_1$

16. **(C)** S, the distance, equals zero when the object has returned. V_0, the initial velocity, equals 128 ft./sec., and g, the acceleration of gravity, equals 32 ft./sec.^{2}

$0 = 128t - \frac{32t^2}{0} = 128t - 16t^2$

$16t^2 - 128t = 0$

Factoring, $t(16t - 128) = 0$

When the product equals zero, one of the factors must equal zero.

Either $t = 0$ (not valid)

or $165 - 128 = 0$

and $t = \frac{128}{16} = 8$ sec.

17. **(D)** The boiling point of a liquid is the temperature at which the vapor pressure of a liquid equals the external pressure to which the system is subjected.

18. **(A)** The volume of the particles is equal to the increase in liquid level (i.e., 125 − 100 = 25)

$\frac{50g}{25 \text{ ml}} = 2$ g/ml

19. **(E)** Neither the wave nor the particle theory alone explains the properties of light, which are best explained by a combination of the two theories.

20. **(B)** $S = V_0t + ½ g t^2$
$S = (0)t + ½ (32) (8)^2$
$S = 0 + 16 (64) = 1024$ ft.

21. **(D)** $V = at$; $t = 60$ sec. $= \frac{60}{3600}$ hr.

$800 = a \frac{60}{3600} = \frac{a}{60}$

$a = 48{,}000$ mi./hr.^{2}

22. **(D)** The resultant force is the difference between the two forces and, therefore, the two forces must be directly opposing each other (i.e., at 180°).

23. **(E)** Heat is the energy of molecular activity. Conduction is the molecular disturbance through a substance due to the collisions of neighboring molecules. Convection is the transfer of heat from one substance to another by the actual migration of the hot material. Radiant energy may be absorbed and then converted into heat. Evaporation is the formation of vapor by a liquid at its surface only.

24. **(E)** Celsius and Fahrenheit conversions utilize the following formulas:
F = 9/5C + 32°
C = 5/9 (F − 32°)

25. **(C)** If the half-life is 21 days, then 42 days would represent two half-lives. In the first half-life 50% will be lost, and in the second half-life 50% of the remainder will be lost.

Remainder = 0.5^n and n = number of half-lives.
Remainder = $(0.5)^2 = 0.25$ or 25%

26. **(C)** Surface tension explains this phenomenon. Because of surface tension the pin may be floated on water even though the metal is denser.

27. **(B)** 1 kilogram = 2.205 pounds, avoirdupois

Therefore, $\frac{165 \text{ lb.}}{2.205 \text{ lb./kg}} = 74.8$ kg

28. **(D)** The acceleration is the change in speed divided by the time factor necessary to achieve the change.

$a = \frac{50 \text{ mi./hr.} - 10 \text{ mi./hr.}}{20 \text{ sec.}} = \frac{40 \text{ mi./hr.}}{20 \text{ sec.}}$

$a = 2$ mi./hr. per sec.

29. **(E)** If the elevator did not move, the man would be at equilibrium and the floor would exert a force of 200 lb. upon him. To move upward *additional force* is required.

$F = \frac{W}{g}a = \frac{(200 \text{ lb.}) (10 \text{ ft./sec.}^2)}{32 \text{ ft./sec.}^2} = 62.5$ lb.

The total force exerted upon the man is $F = 200 + 62.5$ lb. $= 262.5$ lb.

30. **(D)** Air resistance decreases the speed, the maximum height attained and the range of a projectile.

31. **(A)** $F = \mu N$ or $\mu = \frac{F}{N}$

$\mu = \frac{F}{N} = \frac{300 \text{ lb.}}{20{,}000 \text{ lb.}} = 0.013$

32. **(D)** Friction has to be neglected in this case. Potential Energy (PE) = Weight (W) times the Height (h) to which the sack was transported, (i.e., the amount of work done in the transporting). Hence,

$PE = Wh$
$PE = (50 \text{ lb.}) (160 \text{ ft.})$
$PE = 8000$ ft.-lb.

33. **(B)** $P = \frac{F}{A} = \frac{400 \text{ lb.}}{144 \text{ in.}^2} = 2.8$ lb./in.^{2}

34. **(E)** $V = IR$
15 amp × 36 ohms = 540 volts

35. **(A)** $W = VIt$
$W =$ (110 volts) (5.0 amp) (1800 sec.)
$W = 5.0 \times 10^6$ joules

36. **(D)** All of the substances listed are light sensitive and used in the production of photoelectric tubes.

37. **(B)** The question gives a definition of the depth of field.

38. **(D)** The basic constituent of all electricity is the electron.

SCIENCE PROBLEMS

1-3. **(1-B) (2-C) (3-C)** The answers to questions *1-3* are self-explanatory.

4-6. **(4-B) (5-C) (6-A)** The answers to questions *4-6* are self-explanatory.

7. **(A)** The atmospheric pressure that will support a column of mercury 760 mm high will support the same weight of water.
760 × 14 = 10640 or 1.0×10^4

8. **(D)** Since $P_1V_1 = P_2V_2$, a decreased pressure leads to an increased volume. The balloon will become larger; only if the volume change is large enough will the balloon explode.

9. **(B)** This is essentially the converse of the above question. Since the pressure has increased, the volume must decrease. This can occur in this case only by the crumpling of the can.

10. **(B)**

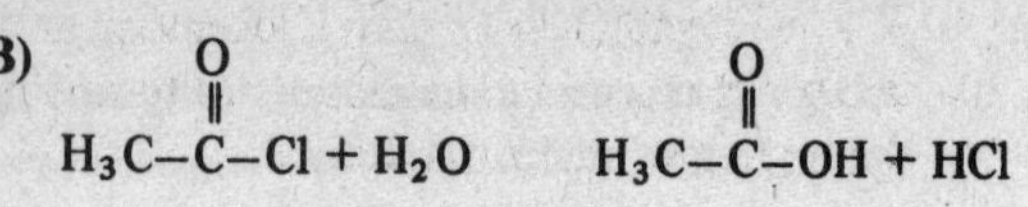

Both of the products are acids.

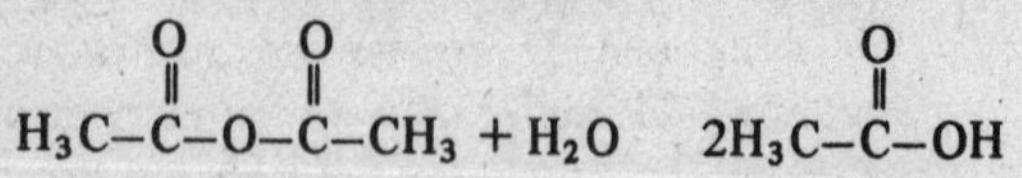

Two moles of product are formed from one mole of starting material, but there is only one product

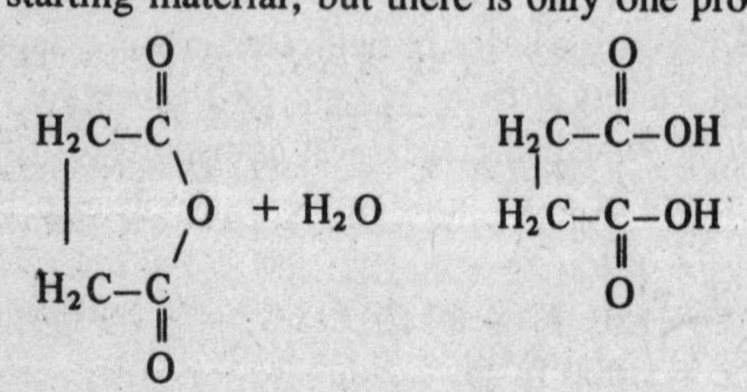

11. **(C)** See the previous explanation.

12. **(A)** See the explanation above.

13. **(D)** Since the solutions are of equal molarity, there will be equal numbers of molecules. But, NaCl produces one particle (ion) per molecule; glucose does not ionize and thus gives only one particle per molecule; $Ba(NO_3)_2$ produces three particles per molecule; and HCl produces two ions per molecule. With a greater number of particles the $Ba(NO_3)_2$ solution will have the greater osmotic pressure.

14. **(E)** Since $P = cRT$, a one degree rise in T will produce the same percentage increase in all these solutions.

15. **(C)** See the answer to question 13. The value of R does not change unless we wish to change the units in which R and the remaining parts of the equation are expressed.

16. **(D)** Purebred white (bb) Rough coat (RR) mated to purebred black (BB) smooth coat (rr).

male bbRR × BBrr female
↓
Sperms bR × Br eggs
↓
F_1 BbRr all black with rough coats

BbRr × BbRr

sperm Br, Br, bR, br × eggs BR, Br, bR, br

17. **(B)** Four types of offspring.

18. **(C)** Black-rough 9; black-smooth 3; white rough 3; white-smooth 1.

19. **(D)** From 27 to 30°C the Δt is 3°C.
$\Delta L = \alpha L_i$, $\Delta t = \alpha L_i$ (3) or 3 αL_i.

20. **(D)** $\Delta L = \alpha L_i \, \Delta t$
cm = α (cm) (°C)

$$\alpha = \frac{\text{cm}}{(\text{cm})(^\circ\text{C})} = \frac{1}{^\circ\text{C}} + {}^\circ\text{C}^{-1}$$

21. **(C)** The greatest increase in length will occur with the greatest coefficient of linear expansion. This will cause the joined strip to curve away from the metal with greatest α.

22. **(A)** In beaker (1)

$$[Ba^{++}] = \frac{2 \times 10^{-6}}{[F^-]^2} = \frac{2 \times 10^{-6}}{(1 \times 10^{-2})^2} = \frac{2 \times 10^{-6}}{1 \times 10^{-4}}$$
$$= 2 \times 10^{-2}$$

In beaker (2)

$$[Ba^{++}] = \frac{7 \times 10^{-9}}{[CO_3^{=}]} = \frac{7 \times 10^{-9}}{7 \times 10^{-5}} = 1 \times 10^{-4}$$

23. **(B)** With F^-

$$[Ba^{++}] = \frac{2 \times 10^{-6}}{(0.1)^2} = \frac{2 \times 10^{-6}}{1 \times 10^{-2}} = 2 \times 10^{-4}$$

With $CO_3^=$

$[Ba^{++}] = \frac{7 \times 10^{-9}}{0.01} = \frac{7 \times 10^{-9}}{1 \times 10^{-2}} = 7 \times 10^{-7}$

24. **(B)** In beaker (5)

$[F^-]^2 = \frac{2 \times 10^{-6}}{[Ba^{++}]} = \frac{2 \times 10^{-6}}{1 \times 10^{-1}} = 2 \times 10^{-3}$

and $[F^-] = 4.5 \times 10^{-3}$.

In beaker (7)

$[CO_3^=] = \frac{7 \times 10^{-9}}{[Ba^{++}]} = \frac{7 \times 10^{-9}}{1 \times 10^{-1}} = 7 \times 10^{-8}$

Thus, beaker (7) would have the lower concentration of the α anion in question. (In beaker (5) the calculations indicate there will be no precipitation of F^- under these conditions.)

25. **(D)** One mole of iodine (254 gm) will react with one mole of fatty acid having one double bond; two moles of iodine (508 gm) will react with one mole of fatty acid having two double bonds.

For compounds (1) and (2):

$\frac{254}{254} = \frac{x}{100}$ $x = 100$ for iodine number

Compound (3) does not react with iodine and thus has an iodine number of zero. For compound (4) with two double bonds

$\frac{504}{280} = \frac{x}{100}$ $x = 180$ for iodine number

26. **(C)** See answer above.

27. **(E)** See answer above. Compounds (1) and (2) have equal iodine numbers, but this combination is not one of the answers given.

28-30. **(28-A) (29-C) (30-D)** Four primary blood groups are found in man. They are 0 (47%), A (41%), B (9%), and AB (3%). These blood groups are based on the presence or absence of antigens (agglutinogens) on red blood cells and antibodies (agglutinins) in the serum.

31. **(E)** The force exerted upon the bottom is calculated in the following fashion:

$(20 + 50)$ cm $\times$ 2.8 gm/cm^3 $\times$ (50 cm)^2 = 490,000 gm = 490 kg

32. **(A)** The area of the top exposed to hexabromoethane is derived as follows:

(50 cm)^2 − 15 cm^2 = 2485 cm^2

33. **(C)** The force exerted upon the top is derived as follows:

20 cm $\times$ 2.8 gm/cm^3 $\times$ 2485 cm^2 = 139,160 gm = 139.2 kg

34. **(D)** Since hydrogen gas is a diatomic molecule, one gram atomic weight will occupy a volume of $\frac{22.4}{2} = 11.2$ liters. 0.1 mole of lithium will produce $11.2 \times 0.1 = 1.12$ l of hydrogen.

35. **(A)** See above. 0.001 mole potassium produces 0.001 gram atomic weights of hydrogen or 0.0005 moles.

$2H_2 + O_2 \rightarrow 2H_2O$

0.0005/2 = 0.00025 moles oxygen

22.4 l $\times$ 2.5×10^{-4} = 5.6×10^{-3} l = 5.6 ml

36. **(E)** One mole of any of these will produce 0.5 mole of hydrogen, and 0.001 mole of either of the three will produce 0.0005 mole of hydrogen.

37. **(D)** The density of this piece of steel is arrived at in the following manner:

8.0 $\times$ density of water = 8.0 $\times$ 1 g/cm^3 = 8.0 g/cm^3

38. **(A)** Now we use the same reasoning and substitute for 1 g/cm^3 the value 62.4 lb./ft.^{3}:

8.0 $\times$ 62.4 lb./ft.^{3} = 499 lb./ft.^{3}

39. **(B)** The weight of 35 ft.^{3} of this steel is arrived at as follows:

35 ft.^{3} $\times$ 499 lb./ft.^{3} = 17465 lb.

40. **(B)** On oxidation of one mole the compound represented by structure (1) will produce 2 moles of acetaldehyde; *that represented by structure (2) will produce one mole each of acetaldehyde and propionaldehyde;* and that represented by structure (3) will produce one mole of hexanedial. In the latter case the ring prevents the formation of two moles after oxidation, but there is an aldehyde functional group on each end of the chain.

41. **(C)** See explanation above. Remember that although compound (1) produces only one product, there are two moles produced.

42. **(E)** See explanations above. Both compound (1) and compound (3) produce only one product. Disregarding the earlier data on the number of moles of product from one mole of reactant, this could be either compound (1) or (3).

43. **(C)** $F = mg$. 10 kg $\times$ 9.8 m/sec.^{2} = 98 kg − m/sec.^{2} = 98 N. The acceleration of gravity is 32 ft./sec.^{2}. This may be converted to acceleration in the Mks system by working out a conversion factor

$\frac{2.54 \text{ cm}}{\text{in.}} \times 12 = 30.48$ cm/ft. = 0.30 m/ft.

32 $\times$ 0.30 = 9.6 m/sec.^{2}

The smaller number results from rounding, but this is close enough.

44. **(E)** The volume of the glass may be calculated as follows:

$$10{,}000 \text{ gm} \times \frac{1 \text{ cm}^3}{6 \text{ gm}} = 1666 \text{ cm}^3$$

45. **(A)** $1666 \text{ cm}^3 \times \frac{1 \text{ gm}}{\text{cm}^3} = 1666 \text{ gm of } H_2O$

$1.7 \text{ kg } H_2O \times 9.8 \text{ m/sec.}^2 = 16.66 \text{ N}$

Therefore 100 N
minus 17 N
83 N

46. **(A)** $v = \frac{336}{6} = 56$ mi./hr.

47. **(C)** $a = \frac{v_2 - v_1}{t}$

$$a = \frac{58 \text{ mi./hr.} - 23 \text{ mi./hr.}}{3.5 \text{ sec.}} = \frac{35 \text{ mi./hr.}}{3.5 \text{ sec.}} =$$

10 mi./hr. per sec.
Or, since 35 mi./hr. = 51 ft./sec.

$$a = \frac{51 \text{ ft./sec.}}{3.5 \text{ sec.}}$$

$a = 12.7 \text{ ft./sec.}^2$

48. **(A)** $v = \frac{v_1 + v_2}{2}$

$v = \frac{1}{2}(23 + 58)$ mi./hr.
$v = 40.5$ mi./hr.

$$v = 40.5 \times \frac{5280 \text{ ft./mi.}}{3600 \text{ sec./hr.}}$$

$v = 59.4$ ft./sec.
$X = 59.4 \text{ ft./sec.} \times 3.5 \text{ sec.}$
$X = 208$ ft.

49. **(B)** Only the #2 carbon of this compound is asymmetric. $2^1 = 2$

50. **(B)** Only the #3 carbon of this compound is asymmetric. $2^1 = 2$

51. **(A)** There are no asymmetric carbon atoms in this compound. $2^0 = 1$

52-54. **(52-A) (53-A) (54-B)** If a cell is placed in a hypertonic solution, water from within it will cross the semipermeable membrane, leave the cell and it will shrink. If a cell is placed in a hypotonic solution, water from without will enter the cell and it will swell. In an isotonic solution, as many molecules of water will enter as will leave the cell and the cell remain the same.

55. **(B)** 0.01 molar = 1×10^{-2}
$\log(1 \times 10^{-2}) = -2$
$pH = -\log(1 \times 10^{-2}) = 2$

56. **(E)** 0.001 molar = 1×10^{-3}
$[H^+](1 \times 10^{-3}) = 10^{-14}$
$[H^+] = 10^{-14}/10^{-3} = 10^{-11}$
$\log 10^{-11} = -11$
$pH = -\log 10^{-11} = 11$

57. **(A)** $pOH = -\log[OH^-]$
As calculated above, $[OH^-] = 10^{-3}$
$\log 10^{-3} = -3$
$pOH = -\log 10^{-3} = 3$

58-60. **(58-B) (59-C) (60-C)** the answers to 58-60 can be found in the flow diagram of the question.

61. **(D)** The alkyne, 2-butyne, is converted to *trans*-2-butene.

62. **(A)** Reaction of Cl_2 produces addition across the double bond to produce 2,3-dichlorobutane.

63. **(B)** Alcoholic KOH reacts to produce 2-butyne. If we had desired 2-butene, we could have reacted the dichloro compound with zinc.

64. **(B)** Presumably H_3Y ionizes to produce 3H + Y. Therefore, 270/3 = 90

65. **(A)** Three OH^- are produced from $Z_3(OH)_3$. 180/3 = 60.

66. **(E)** One mole of each is 3 equivalents. Equal numbers of equivalents of strong acid and strong base mixed together will produce a neutral solution.

Answer Sheet–Model Test B

SCIENCE KNOWLEDGE

Biology

1. Ⓐ Ⓑ Ⓒ Ⓓ Ⓔ
2. Ⓐ Ⓑ Ⓒ Ⓓ Ⓔ
3. Ⓐ Ⓑ Ⓒ Ⓓ Ⓔ
4. Ⓐ Ⓑ Ⓒ Ⓓ Ⓔ
5. Ⓐ Ⓑ Ⓒ Ⓓ Ⓔ
6. Ⓐ Ⓑ Ⓒ Ⓓ Ⓔ
7. Ⓐ Ⓑ Ⓒ Ⓓ Ⓔ
8. Ⓐ Ⓑ Ⓒ Ⓓ Ⓔ
9. Ⓐ Ⓑ Ⓒ Ⓓ Ⓔ
10. Ⓐ Ⓑ Ⓒ Ⓓ Ⓔ
11. Ⓐ Ⓑ Ⓒ Ⓓ Ⓔ
12. Ⓐ Ⓑ Ⓒ Ⓓ Ⓔ
13. Ⓐ Ⓑ Ⓒ Ⓓ Ⓔ
14. Ⓐ Ⓑ Ⓒ Ⓓ Ⓔ
15. Ⓐ Ⓑ Ⓒ Ⓓ Ⓔ
16. Ⓐ Ⓑ Ⓒ Ⓓ Ⓔ
17. Ⓐ Ⓑ Ⓒ Ⓓ Ⓔ
18. Ⓐ Ⓑ Ⓒ Ⓓ Ⓔ
19. Ⓐ Ⓑ Ⓒ Ⓓ Ⓔ
20. Ⓐ Ⓑ Ⓒ Ⓓ Ⓔ
21. Ⓐ Ⓑ Ⓒ Ⓓ Ⓔ
22. Ⓐ Ⓑ Ⓒ Ⓓ Ⓔ
23. Ⓐ Ⓑ Ⓒ Ⓓ Ⓔ
24. Ⓐ Ⓑ Ⓒ Ⓓ Ⓔ
25. Ⓐ Ⓑ Ⓒ Ⓓ Ⓔ
26. Ⓐ Ⓑ Ⓒ Ⓓ Ⓔ
27. Ⓐ Ⓑ Ⓒ Ⓓ Ⓔ
28. Ⓐ Ⓑ Ⓒ Ⓓ Ⓔ
29. Ⓐ Ⓑ Ⓒ Ⓓ Ⓔ
30. Ⓐ Ⓑ Ⓒ Ⓓ Ⓔ
31. Ⓐ Ⓑ Ⓒ Ⓓ Ⓔ
32. Ⓐ Ⓑ Ⓒ Ⓓ Ⓔ
33. Ⓐ Ⓑ Ⓒ Ⓓ Ⓔ
34. Ⓐ Ⓑ Ⓒ Ⓓ Ⓔ
35. Ⓐ Ⓑ Ⓒ Ⓓ Ⓔ
36. Ⓐ Ⓑ Ⓒ Ⓓ Ⓔ
37. Ⓐ Ⓑ Ⓒ Ⓓ Ⓔ
38. Ⓐ Ⓑ Ⓒ Ⓓ Ⓔ

Chemistry

1. Ⓐ Ⓑ Ⓒ Ⓓ Ⓔ
2. Ⓐ Ⓑ Ⓒ Ⓓ Ⓔ
3. Ⓐ Ⓑ Ⓒ Ⓓ
4. Ⓐ Ⓑ Ⓒ Ⓓ Ⓔ
5. Ⓐ Ⓑ Ⓒ Ⓓ
6. Ⓐ Ⓑ Ⓒ Ⓓ Ⓔ
7. Ⓐ Ⓑ Ⓒ Ⓓ Ⓔ
8. Ⓐ Ⓑ Ⓒ Ⓓ
9. Ⓐ Ⓑ Ⓒ Ⓓ Ⓔ
10. Ⓐ Ⓑ Ⓒ Ⓓ Ⓔ
11. Ⓐ Ⓑ Ⓒ Ⓓ Ⓔ
12. Ⓐ Ⓑ Ⓒ Ⓓ Ⓔ
13. Ⓐ Ⓑ Ⓒ Ⓓ Ⓔ
14. Ⓐ Ⓑ Ⓒ Ⓓ Ⓔ
15. Ⓐ Ⓑ Ⓒ Ⓓ
16. Ⓐ Ⓑ Ⓒ Ⓓ Ⓔ
17. Ⓐ Ⓑ Ⓒ Ⓓ Ⓔ
18. Ⓐ Ⓑ Ⓒ Ⓓ Ⓔ
19. Ⓐ Ⓑ Ⓒ Ⓓ Ⓔ
20. Ⓐ Ⓑ Ⓒ Ⓓ Ⓔ
21. Ⓐ Ⓑ Ⓒ Ⓓ Ⓔ
22. Ⓐ Ⓑ Ⓒ Ⓓ Ⓔ
23. Ⓐ Ⓑ Ⓒ Ⓓ Ⓔ
24. Ⓐ Ⓑ Ⓒ Ⓓ Ⓔ
25. Ⓐ Ⓑ Ⓒ Ⓓ Ⓔ
26. Ⓐ Ⓑ Ⓒ Ⓓ Ⓔ
27. Ⓐ Ⓑ Ⓒ Ⓓ Ⓔ
28. Ⓐ Ⓑ Ⓒ Ⓓ Ⓔ
29. Ⓐ Ⓑ Ⓒ Ⓓ Ⓔ
30. Ⓐ Ⓑ Ⓒ Ⓓ Ⓔ
31. Ⓐ Ⓑ Ⓒ Ⓓ Ⓔ
32. Ⓐ Ⓑ Ⓒ Ⓓ Ⓔ
33. Ⓐ Ⓑ Ⓒ Ⓓ Ⓔ
34. Ⓐ Ⓑ Ⓒ Ⓓ Ⓔ
35. Ⓐ Ⓑ Ⓒ Ⓓ Ⓔ
36. Ⓐ Ⓑ Ⓒ Ⓓ Ⓔ
37. Ⓐ Ⓑ Ⓒ Ⓓ Ⓔ
38. Ⓐ Ⓑ Ⓒ Ⓓ Ⓔ
39. Ⓐ Ⓑ Ⓒ Ⓓ Ⓔ
40. Ⓐ Ⓑ Ⓒ Ⓓ Ⓔ
41. Ⓐ Ⓑ Ⓒ Ⓓ Ⓔ
42. Ⓐ Ⓑ Ⓒ Ⓓ Ⓔ
43. Ⓐ Ⓑ Ⓒ Ⓓ Ⓔ
44. Ⓐ Ⓑ Ⓒ Ⓓ Ⓔ
45. Ⓐ Ⓑ Ⓒ Ⓓ Ⓔ
46. Ⓐ Ⓑ Ⓒ Ⓓ Ⓔ
47. Ⓐ Ⓑ Ⓒ Ⓓ Ⓔ
48. Ⓐ Ⓑ Ⓒ Ⓓ Ⓔ
49. Ⓐ Ⓑ Ⓒ Ⓓ Ⓔ

Physics

1. Ⓐ Ⓑ Ⓒ Ⓓ Ⓔ
2. Ⓐ Ⓑ Ⓒ Ⓓ Ⓔ
3. Ⓐ Ⓑ Ⓒ Ⓓ Ⓔ
4. Ⓐ Ⓑ Ⓒ Ⓓ Ⓔ
5. Ⓐ Ⓑ Ⓒ Ⓓ Ⓔ
6. Ⓐ Ⓑ Ⓒ Ⓓ Ⓔ
7. Ⓐ Ⓑ Ⓒ Ⓓ Ⓔ
8. Ⓐ Ⓑ Ⓒ Ⓓ Ⓔ
9. Ⓐ Ⓑ Ⓒ Ⓓ Ⓔ
10. Ⓐ Ⓑ Ⓒ Ⓓ Ⓔ
11. Ⓐ Ⓑ Ⓒ Ⓓ Ⓔ
12. Ⓐ Ⓑ Ⓒ Ⓓ Ⓔ
13. Ⓐ Ⓑ Ⓒ Ⓓ Ⓔ
14. Ⓐ Ⓑ Ⓒ Ⓓ Ⓔ
15. Ⓐ Ⓑ Ⓒ Ⓓ Ⓔ
16. Ⓐ Ⓑ Ⓒ Ⓓ Ⓔ
17. Ⓐ Ⓑ Ⓒ Ⓓ Ⓔ
18. Ⓐ Ⓑ Ⓒ Ⓓ Ⓔ
19. Ⓐ Ⓑ Ⓒ Ⓓ Ⓔ
20. Ⓐ Ⓑ Ⓒ Ⓓ Ⓔ
21. Ⓐ Ⓑ Ⓒ Ⓓ Ⓔ
22. Ⓐ Ⓑ Ⓒ Ⓓ Ⓔ
23. Ⓐ Ⓑ Ⓒ Ⓓ Ⓔ
24. Ⓐ Ⓑ Ⓒ Ⓓ Ⓔ
25. Ⓐ Ⓑ Ⓒ Ⓓ Ⓔ
26. Ⓐ Ⓑ Ⓒ Ⓓ Ⓔ
27. Ⓐ Ⓑ Ⓒ Ⓓ Ⓔ
28. Ⓐ Ⓑ Ⓒ Ⓓ Ⓔ
29. Ⓐ Ⓑ Ⓒ Ⓓ Ⓔ
30. Ⓐ Ⓑ Ⓒ Ⓓ Ⓔ
31. Ⓐ Ⓑ Ⓒ Ⓓ Ⓔ
32. Ⓐ Ⓑ Ⓒ Ⓓ Ⓔ
33. Ⓐ Ⓑ Ⓒ Ⓓ Ⓔ
34. Ⓐ Ⓑ Ⓒ Ⓓ Ⓔ
35. Ⓐ Ⓑ Ⓒ Ⓓ Ⓔ
36. Ⓐ Ⓑ Ⓒ Ⓓ Ⓔ
37. Ⓐ Ⓑ Ⓒ Ⓓ Ⓔ
38. Ⓐ Ⓑ Ⓒ Ⓓ Ⓔ

SCIENCE PROBLEMS

1. Ⓐ Ⓑ Ⓒ Ⓓ Ⓔ
2. Ⓐ Ⓑ Ⓒ Ⓓ Ⓔ
3. Ⓐ Ⓑ Ⓒ Ⓓ Ⓔ
4. Ⓐ Ⓑ Ⓒ Ⓓ Ⓔ
5. Ⓐ Ⓑ Ⓒ Ⓓ Ⓔ
6. Ⓐ Ⓑ Ⓒ Ⓓ Ⓔ
7. Ⓐ Ⓑ Ⓒ Ⓓ Ⓔ
8. Ⓐ Ⓑ Ⓒ Ⓓ Ⓔ
9. Ⓐ Ⓑ Ⓒ Ⓓ Ⓔ
10. Ⓐ Ⓑ Ⓒ Ⓓ Ⓔ
11. Ⓐ Ⓑ Ⓒ Ⓓ Ⓔ
12. Ⓐ Ⓑ Ⓒ Ⓓ Ⓔ
13. Ⓐ Ⓑ Ⓒ Ⓓ Ⓔ
14. Ⓐ Ⓑ Ⓒ Ⓓ Ⓔ
15. Ⓐ Ⓑ Ⓒ Ⓓ Ⓔ
16. Ⓐ Ⓑ Ⓒ Ⓓ Ⓔ
17. Ⓐ Ⓑ Ⓒ Ⓓ Ⓔ
18. Ⓐ Ⓑ Ⓒ Ⓓ Ⓔ
19. Ⓐ Ⓑ Ⓒ Ⓓ Ⓔ
20. Ⓐ Ⓑ Ⓒ Ⓓ Ⓔ
21. Ⓐ Ⓑ Ⓒ Ⓓ Ⓔ
22. Ⓐ Ⓑ Ⓒ Ⓓ Ⓔ
23. Ⓐ Ⓑ Ⓒ Ⓓ Ⓔ
24. Ⓐ Ⓑ Ⓒ Ⓓ Ⓔ
25. Ⓐ Ⓑ Ⓒ Ⓓ Ⓔ
26. Ⓐ Ⓑ Ⓒ Ⓓ Ⓔ
27. Ⓐ Ⓑ Ⓒ Ⓓ Ⓔ
28. Ⓐ Ⓑ Ⓒ Ⓓ Ⓔ
29. Ⓐ Ⓑ Ⓒ Ⓓ Ⓔ
30. Ⓐ Ⓑ Ⓒ Ⓓ Ⓔ
31. Ⓐ Ⓑ Ⓒ Ⓓ Ⓔ
32. Ⓐ Ⓑ Ⓒ Ⓓ Ⓔ
33. Ⓐ Ⓑ Ⓒ Ⓓ Ⓔ
34. Ⓐ Ⓑ Ⓒ Ⓓ Ⓔ
35. Ⓐ Ⓑ Ⓒ Ⓓ Ⓔ
36. Ⓐ Ⓑ Ⓒ Ⓓ Ⓔ
37. Ⓐ Ⓑ Ⓒ Ⓓ Ⓔ
38. Ⓐ Ⓑ Ⓒ Ⓓ Ⓔ
39. Ⓐ Ⓑ Ⓒ Ⓓ Ⓔ
40. Ⓐ Ⓑ Ⓒ Ⓓ Ⓔ
41. Ⓐ Ⓑ Ⓒ Ⓓ Ⓔ
42. Ⓐ Ⓑ Ⓒ Ⓓ Ⓔ
43. Ⓐ Ⓑ Ⓒ Ⓓ Ⓔ
44. Ⓐ Ⓑ Ⓒ Ⓓ Ⓔ
45. Ⓐ Ⓑ Ⓒ Ⓓ Ⓔ
46. Ⓐ Ⓑ Ⓒ Ⓓ Ⓔ
47. Ⓐ Ⓑ Ⓒ Ⓓ Ⓔ
48. Ⓐ Ⓑ Ⓒ Ⓓ Ⓔ
49. Ⓐ Ⓑ Ⓒ Ⓓ Ⓔ
50. Ⓐ Ⓑ Ⓒ Ⓓ Ⓔ
51. Ⓐ Ⓑ Ⓒ Ⓓ Ⓔ
52. Ⓐ Ⓑ Ⓒ Ⓓ Ⓔ
53. Ⓐ Ⓑ Ⓒ Ⓓ Ⓔ
54. Ⓐ Ⓑ Ⓒ Ⓓ Ⓔ
55. Ⓐ Ⓑ Ⓒ Ⓓ Ⓔ
56. Ⓐ Ⓑ Ⓒ Ⓓ Ⓔ
57. Ⓐ Ⓑ Ⓒ Ⓓ Ⓔ
58. Ⓐ Ⓑ Ⓒ Ⓓ Ⓔ
59. Ⓐ Ⓑ Ⓒ Ⓓ Ⓔ
60. Ⓐ Ⓑ Ⓒ Ⓓ Ⓔ
61. Ⓐ Ⓑ Ⓒ Ⓓ Ⓔ
62. Ⓐ Ⓑ Ⓒ Ⓓ Ⓔ
63. Ⓐ Ⓑ Ⓒ Ⓓ Ⓔ
64. Ⓐ Ⓑ Ⓒ Ⓓ Ⓔ
65. Ⓐ Ⓑ Ⓒ Ⓓ Ⓔ
66. Ⓐ Ⓑ Ⓒ Ⓓ Ⓔ

SKILLS ANALYSIS: READING

1. Ⓐ Ⓑ Ⓒ
2. Ⓐ Ⓑ Ⓒ
3. Ⓐ Ⓑ Ⓒ
4. Ⓐ Ⓑ Ⓒ
5. Ⓐ Ⓑ Ⓒ
6. Ⓐ Ⓑ Ⓒ
7. Ⓐ Ⓑ Ⓒ
8. Ⓐ Ⓑ Ⓒ
9. Ⓐ Ⓑ Ⓒ
10. Ⓐ Ⓑ Ⓒ
11, Ⓐ Ⓑ Ⓒ
12. Ⓐ Ⓑ Ⓒ
13. Ⓐ Ⓑ Ⓒ Ⓓ
14. Ⓐ Ⓑ Ⓒ Ⓓ
15. Ⓐ Ⓑ Ⓒ Ⓓ
16. Ⓐ Ⓑ Ⓒ Ⓓ
17. Ⓐ Ⓑ Ⓒ
18. Ⓐ Ⓑ Ⓒ
19. Ⓐ Ⓑ Ⓒ
20. Ⓐ Ⓑ Ⓒ
21. Ⓐ Ⓑ Ⓒ
22. Ⓐ Ⓑ Ⓒ
23. Ⓐ Ⓑ Ⓒ
24. Ⓐ Ⓑ Ⓒ
25. Ⓐ Ⓑ Ⓒ
26. Ⓐ Ⓑ Ⓒ
27. Ⓐ Ⓑ Ⓒ
28. Ⓐ Ⓑ Ⓒ
29. Ⓐ Ⓑ Ⓒ
30. Ⓐ Ⓑ Ⓒ Ⓓ Ⓔ
31. Ⓐ Ⓑ Ⓒ
32. Ⓐ Ⓑ Ⓒ
33. Ⓐ Ⓑ Ⓒ
34. Ⓐ Ⓑ Ⓒ
35. Ⓐ Ⓑ Ⓒ
36. Ⓐ Ⓑ Ⓒ
37. Ⓐ Ⓑ Ⓒ
38. Ⓐ Ⓑ Ⓒ
39. Ⓐ Ⓑ Ⓒ
40. Ⓐ Ⓑ Ⓒ
41. Ⓐ Ⓑ Ⓒ
42. Ⓐ Ⓑ Ⓒ
43. Ⓐ Ⓑ Ⓒ
44. Ⓐ Ⓑ Ⓒ
45. Ⓐ Ⓑ Ⓒ
46. Ⓐ Ⓑ Ⓒ
47. Ⓐ Ⓑ Ⓒ
48. Ⓐ Ⓑ Ⓒ
49. Ⓐ Ⓑ Ⓒ
50. Ⓐ Ⓑ Ⓒ
51. Ⓐ Ⓑ Ⓒ
52. Ⓐ Ⓑ Ⓒ
53. Ⓐ Ⓑ Ⓒ
54. Ⓐ Ⓑ Ⓒ
55. Ⓐ Ⓑ Ⓒ
56. Ⓐ Ⓑ Ⓒ
57. Ⓐ Ⓑ Ⓒ
58. Ⓐ Ⓑ Ⓒ
59. Ⓐ Ⓑ Ⓒ
60. Ⓐ Ⓑ Ⓒ
61. Ⓐ Ⓑ Ⓒ
62. Ⓐ Ⓑ Ⓒ
63. Ⓐ Ⓑ Ⓒ
64. Ⓐ Ⓑ Ⓒ
65. Ⓐ Ⓑ Ⓒ
66. Ⓐ Ⓑ Ⓒ
67. Ⓐ Ⓑ Ⓒ
68. Ⓐ Ⓑ Ⓒ

SKILLS ANALYSIS: QUANTITATIVE

1. Ⓐ Ⓑ Ⓒ Ⓓ
2. Ⓐ Ⓑ Ⓒ Ⓓ
3. Ⓐ Ⓑ Ⓒ Ⓓ
4. Ⓐ Ⓑ Ⓒ Ⓓ
5. Ⓐ Ⓑ Ⓒ Ⓓ
6. Ⓐ Ⓑ Ⓒ Ⓓ
7. Ⓐ Ⓑ Ⓒ Ⓓ
8. Ⓐ Ⓑ Ⓒ Ⓓ
9. Ⓐ Ⓑ Ⓒ
10. Ⓐ Ⓑ Ⓒ
11, Ⓐ Ⓑ Ⓒ
12. Ⓐ Ⓑ Ⓒ
13. Ⓐ Ⓑ Ⓒ
14. Ⓐ Ⓑ Ⓒ Ⓓ
15. Ⓐ Ⓑ Ⓒ Ⓓ
16. Ⓐ Ⓑ Ⓒ Ⓓ
17. Ⓐ Ⓑ Ⓒ Ⓓ
18. Ⓐ Ⓑ Ⓒ
19. Ⓐ Ⓑ Ⓒ
20. Ⓐ Ⓑ Ⓒ
21. Ⓐ Ⓑ Ⓒ
22. Ⓐ Ⓑ Ⓒ
23. Ⓐ Ⓑ Ⓒ
24. Ⓐ Ⓑ Ⓒ
25. Ⓐ Ⓑ Ⓒ
26. Ⓐ Ⓑ Ⓒ
27. Ⓐ Ⓑ Ⓒ
28. Ⓐ Ⓑ Ⓒ
29. Ⓐ Ⓑ Ⓒ
30. Ⓐ Ⓑ Ⓒ Ⓓ Ⓔ
31. Ⓐ Ⓑ Ⓒ Ⓓ Ⓔ
32. Ⓐ Ⓑ Ⓒ Ⓓ Ⓔ
33. Ⓐ Ⓑ Ⓒ Ⓓ Ⓔ
34. Ⓐ Ⓑ Ⓒ Ⓓ Ⓔ
35. Ⓐ Ⓑ Ⓒ
36. Ⓐ Ⓑ Ⓒ
37. Ⓐ Ⓑ Ⓒ
38. Ⓐ Ⓑ Ⓒ
39. Ⓐ Ⓑ Ⓒ
40. Ⓐ Ⓑ Ⓒ
41. Ⓐ Ⓑ Ⓒ
42. Ⓐ Ⓑ Ⓒ
43. Ⓐ Ⓑ Ⓒ
44. Ⓐ Ⓑ Ⓒ
45. Ⓐ Ⓑ Ⓒ
46. Ⓐ Ⓑ Ⓒ
47. Ⓐ Ⓑ Ⓒ
48. Ⓐ Ⓑ Ⓒ
49. Ⓐ Ⓑ Ⓒ
50. Ⓐ Ⓑ Ⓒ
51. Ⓐ Ⓑ Ⓒ
52. Ⓐ Ⓑ Ⓒ
53. Ⓐ Ⓑ Ⓒ
54. Ⓐ Ⓑ Ⓒ
55. Ⓐ Ⓑ Ⓒ
56. Ⓐ Ⓑ Ⓒ
57. Ⓐ Ⓑ Ⓒ
58. Ⓐ Ⓑ Ⓒ
59. Ⓐ Ⓑ Ⓒ
60. Ⓐ Ⓑ Ⓒ
61. Ⓐ Ⓑ Ⓒ
62. Ⓐ Ⓑ Ⓒ
63. Ⓐ Ⓑ Ⓒ
64. Ⓐ Ⓓ Ⓞ
65. Ⓐ Ⓑ Ⓒ
66. Ⓐ Ⓑ Ⓒ
67. Ⓐ Ⓑ Ⓒ
68. Ⓐ Ⓑ Ⓒ

The New MCAT Model Examination B*

SCIENCE KNOWLEDGE

135 MINUTES
125 QUESTIONS

The following questions are based on your knowledge of science. The questions are varied; therefore, you are advised to pay careful attention to the instructions for each portion.

Biology

DIRECTIONS: Each of the statements or questions is followed by five suggested completions or answers. Choose the one that best completes the statement or answers the question, and mark the letter of your choice on the answer sheet.

1. The gastric juice in the stomach
   (A) has a neutral pH.
   (B) is alkaline.
   (C) is acidic.
   (D) contains trypsin.
   (E) contains insulin.

2. Rh-related hemolytic anemia of the newborn (erythroblastosis foetalis) may result when the
   (A) father, mother, and fetus are all Rh negative.
   (B) father and mother are Rh positive, but the fetus is Rh negative.
   (C) mother is Rh negative and the fetus is Rh positive.
   (D) mother is Rh positive and the fetus is Rh negative.
   (E) father, mother, and fetus are all Rh positive.

3. The region of the retina where vision is most acute is known as the
   (A) ciliary body.
   (B) vitreous humor.
   (C) conjunctiva.
   (D) fovea centralis.
   (E) aqueous humor.

4. If a cell is viewed under low power and then under high power, and no fine adjustment is necessary to see it clearly, the microscope is considered
   (A) achromatic.
   (B) bifocal.
   (C) parfocal.
   (D) unifocal.
   (E) apochromatic.

5. During the follicular phase of a normal menstrual cycle ovarian changes occur which are due to pituitary secretions of
   (A) FSH only.
   (B) LH only.
   (C) oxytocin.
   (D) vasopressin.
   (E) FSH and LH.

*Explanations for science answers can be found on p. 191.

6. Which of the following patterns would you expect to find in the blood one hour after a rich meal?

	Blood Sugar	Insulin
(A)	high	low
(B)	low	low
(C)	high	high
(D)	low	high
(E)	no change	no change

7. Which of the following type(s) of lens(es) is used to correct the vision of a near-sighted individual?
(A) convex
(B) biconvex
(C) biconcave
(D) none of the above
(E) all of the above

8. The developing embryo is a hollow sphere of cells, one cell thick during the ____________ stage.
(A) blastula
(B) gastrula
(C) polar body
(D) morula
(E) cleavage

9. The experiments of Miller and Urey enhanced the validity of Oparin's theory on the origin of life. They essentially
(A) found fossil remnants in meteorites.
(B) were able to produce a simple form of living organism after placing DNA in a mixture of hydrogen and oxygen and irradiating it.
(C) were able to produce simple viruses.
(D) discharged electricity into a medium consisting of water vapor, methane, ammonia, and hydrogen.
(E) were able to produce bacteria.

10. Characteristics which are common to the Arthropod, Mollusk, Echinoderm, and Chordate lines are a(an)
(A) coelom and a parietal eye.
(B) endoskeleton and a coelom.
(C) segmentation and a coelom.
(D) compound eye and segmentation.
(E) endoskeleton and a parietal eye.

11. Man can become infected with trichinosis by
(A) drinking unpasteurized milk.
(B) cutting himself while dressing wild game.
(C) wading in polluted water or eating raw fish.
(D) eating poorly cooked pork.
(E) eating poorly cooked beef.

12. Characteristics of epithelial tissues may include
(A) protection.
(B) secretion.
(C) absorption.
(D) all of the above.
(E) none of the above.

13. The relationship of two organisms living together for their mutual benefit is classified as
(A) symbiosis.
(B) commensalism.
(C) saprophytism.
(D) parasitism.
(E) civilization.

14. The contractile vacuole of protozoa functions to
(A) remove undigested food materials.
(B) digest food materials.
(C) regulate the pH of the internal milieu.
(D) secrete proteins.
(E) remove surplus water.

15. A hog breeder would use a backcross to
(A) produce a bigger and healthier strain.
(B) produce a larger number of offspring.
(C) maintain a pure line of desirable traits.
(D) determine if a particular hog is genotypically pure.
(E) eliminate chances of congenital malformations.

16. The state of a continuously mild or partial contraction of a muscle is denoted as
(A) tetanus.
(B) tonus.
(C) an "all or none" contraction.
(D) a twitch.
(E) a reflex contraction.

17. The cell bodies of the motor neurons are located in the spinal cord in
(A) intermediolateral cell column.
(B) dorsal root ganglia.
(C) dorsal horn (gray matter).
(D) ventral horn (gray matter).
(E) ventral root ganglia.

18. Body temperature is regulated by the
(A) thalamus.
(B) medulla.
(C) pons.
(D) cerebellum.
(E) hypothalamus.

19. When a physician informs a patient that his blood pressure reading is 160/90, she refers respectively to
(A) systolic blood pressure of the left ventricle.
(B) blood pressure in the veins of the arm.
(C) systolic and diastolic pressures of the brachial artery.
(D) systolic pressure of the aorta and diastolic pressure in the superior vena cava.
(E) systolic pressure of the right ventricle.

20. Mesoderm, one of the germ layers, gives rise to a group of structures in animals. Which group includes structures of exclusively mesodermal origin?
(A) bone, lens of the eye, pars distalis, gall bladder
(B) muscle, outer layer of digestive tract, cartilage, bone
(C) skin, brain, bladder, vagina
(D) trachea, lungs, stomach, skin
(E) none of the above

21. Vigorous exercise will cause muscle fatigue which is primarily due to
(A) the utilization and exhaustion of ATP.
(B) the accumulation of ADP.
(C) the accumulation of lactic acid.
(D) the accumulation of carbon dioxide.
(E) a sodium and potassium imbalance.

22. A patient awaiting selective surgery presents the following symptoms. Which of them indicate(s) a heightened activity of the sympathetic portion of his autonomic nervous system?
(A) a yearning for water due to a dry mouth
(B) sweaty palms
(C) pale skin
(D) all of the above
(E) none of the above

23. The stimulus that induces migration in animals is
(A) hydrotrophic.
(B) photoperiodic.
(C) geotrophic.
(D) hydroperiodic.
(E) chemotrophic.

24. Follicle-stimulating hormone is to estrogen as luteinizing hormone is to
(A) progesterone.
(B) testosterone.
(C) vasopressin.
(D) luteotrophic hormone.
(E) androgen.

25. Which of the following structures are NOT considered modifications of the cell membrane?
(A) basement membrane
(B) terminal bars
(C) desmosomes
(D) intercalated discs
(E) microvilli

26. Administration of which of the following compound(s) increases clotting time?
(A) heparin
(B) aspirin
(C) dicumarol
(D) all of the above
(E) none of the above

27. The functional role an organism plays in a community is referred to as its
(A) habitat.
(B) home range.
(C) niche.
(D) environment.
(E) ecosystem.

28. All of the following may be considered as secondary sex characteristics of the male EXCEPT
(A) increase in sex drive.
(B) external genitalia.
(C) pattern of hair and beard growth.
(D) development of a deeper voice.
(E) skin pigmentation patterns.

29. In an auto accident the driver suffers complete sectioning of several anterior (ventral) roots of spinal nerves. What would be the result of such a lesion to the regions supplied by those spinal nerves?
(A) no neural deficit
(B) loss of motor activity
(C) loss of sensation
(D) loss of sensation and motor activity
(E) loss of temperature and pain sensation

30. The reflex arc is of utmost importance to human beings. Which of the following is NOT a component of the reflex arc?
(A) medulla
(B) dendrite (receptor)
(C) synapse
(D) ventral horn cell (effector)
(E) axon

31. An aggregation of nerve cell bodies inside the CNS (central nervous system) is typically called a
(A) clone.
(B) colony.
(C) Nissl zone.
(D) tract.
(E) nucleus.

32. The vital centers for control of heart rate, respiratory rate, and blood pressure are located in the
(A) pons.
(B) medulla.
(C) cerebellum.
(D) hypothalamus.
(E) midbrain.

33. The most numerous leukocytes are the
(A) lymphocytes.
(B) monocytes.
(C) eosinophils.
(D) neutrophils.
(E) basophils.

34. Bile, which is important in the digestion of fats, is produced by the
(A) stomach.
(B) liver.
(C) duodenum.
(D) gall bladder.
(E) lacteals.

35. The primitive condition of the cyclostomata is indicated by their
(A) possession of scales.
(B) jawless mouth.
(C) asexual reproduction.
(D) surface slime.
(E) toothless jaws.

36. The plasma membrane of animal cells
(A) may not be seen by any microscope.
(B) contains two layers of lipid between layers of protein.
(C) is *not* selectively permeable.
(D) lies just interior to the cell wall.
(E) can only be visualized with the aid of the electron microscope.

37. A sustained contraction is called
(A) tonus.
(B) recovery period.
(C) tetany.
(D) contraction period.
(E) all or none contraction.

38. A mink breeder finds that 50% of the offspring are aa. What genotype were their parents?
(A) aa x aa
(B) Aa x Aa
(C) AA x aa
(D) Aa x aa
(E) Aa x AA

STOP. If you finish before the time limit is up, go over your work for this section. DO NOT look at any other sections of the model examination. When your time limit is up, go on to the next section.

Chemistry

DIRECTIONS: Each of the statements or questions is followed by four or five suggested completions or answers. Choose the one that best completes the statement or answers the question, and mark the letter of your choice on the answer sheet.

1. Fatty acid is to fat as glucose is to
(A) starch.
(B) glycogen.
(C) cellulose.
(D) all of the above.
(E) none of the above.

2. The reaction of sodium alkoxide with an alkyl halide is often used to produce
(A) an ether.
(B) an acetal.
(C) an ester.
(D) a sodium halide.
(E) none of the above.

3. The most acidic compound listed below is

(A) CH_3OH

(B) 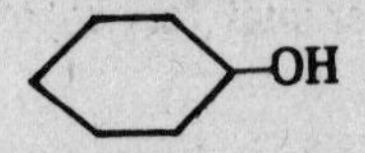

(C) 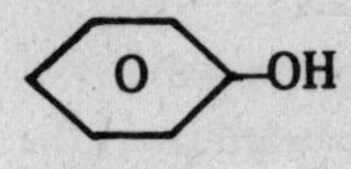

(D) 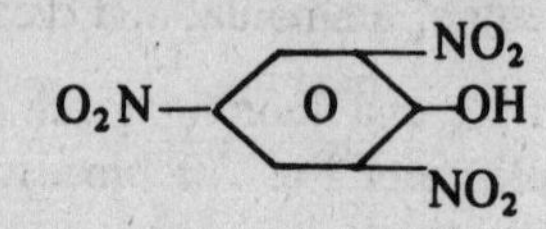

(E) $HOCH_2—CH_2OH$

4. Of the compounds listed below, the one that reacts best with ethers is

(A) HCl.
(B) HBr.
(C) HI.
(D) HF.
(E) $NaNO_3$.

5. The Hell-Volhard-Zelinsky reaction utilizes Br_2 and PBr_3 to convert a carboxylic acid to

(A) $R{-}CH_2{-}C(=O){-}Br$

(B) $R{-}CH(Br){-}COBr$

(C) $R{-}CH(PBr_2){-}COBr$

(D) $R{-}CH_2{-}C(=O){-}PBr_2$

(E) a glycol

6. Glucose is NOT a (an)

(A) aldose.
(B) reducing sugar.
(C) disaccharide.
(D) sugar possessing optical activity.
(E) monosaccharide.

7. The Tollens silver mirror test (ammoniacal silver nitrate) does not give a positive test with

(A) $H_3C-C(=O)-H$

(B) $H_3C-CH_2-C(=O)-H$

(C) $H_3C-CH_2-C(=O)-CH_3$

(D) 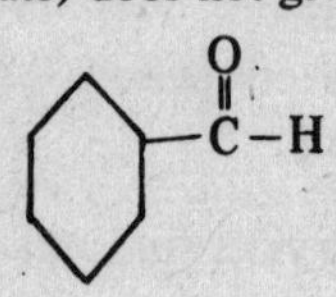

(E) any of the above

8. HIO_4 will oxidize all of the following except

(A) 1,3-propanediol.
(B) ethylene glycol.
(C) glycerol.
(D) 1,2-cyclopentanediol.
(E) B and C

9. Alcohols have higher boiling points than do alkyl halides of the same chain lengths because

(A) alcohols are more polar.
(B) alcohols have higher molecular weights.
(C) alcohols form ethers.
(D) alcohols form intermolecular hydrogen bonds.
(E) of all of the above.

10. Catalysts

(A) are changed and consumed during a reaction.
(B) have virtually no effect on the overall rate of the reaction.
(C) must be present in high concentrations.
(D) are changed but not consumed during a reaction.
(E) speed up the rate of the reaction.

11. Which of the following are nitrogenous metabolic waste products?

(A) sodium chloride, potassium phosphate, and water
(B) urea, ammonia, and creatinine

(C) amino acids, ammonia, and DNA
(D) glucosamine, creatine, and RNA
(E) sugar, ammonia, and creatine

12. Margarine and shortening are made from vegetable oils and animal fats by treatment to decrease rancidity. The process is known as
(A) oxidation.
(B) hydrogenation.
(C) esterification.
(D) hydrolysis.
(E) reduction.

13. The process referred to in the previous question
(A) removes high molecular weight glycerides.
(B) increases the number of free carboxylic acids.
(C) removes high molecular weight alcohols.
(D) raises the melting point of the mixture.
(E) decreases the melting point of the mixture.

14. One mole of methyl magnesium bromide will react with one mole of substrate to give the indicated product upon hydrolysis.
(A) acetaldehyde → primary alcohol
(B) carboxylic acid → tertiary alcohol
(C) ester → ketone
(D) ketone → secondary alcohol
(E) acetaldehyde → secondary alcohol

15. If solution A is less concentrated in dissolved particle content than solution B, then solution A is said to be
(A) hypertonic.
(B) hypotonic.
(C) isoosmotic.
(D) isotonic.
(E) supersaturated.

16. Two moles of carbon dioxide contain ______________ more molecules than one mole of oxygen.
(A) 25×10^6
(B) 12.04×10^{46}
(C) 6.02×10^{23}
(D) 12.04×10^{23}
(E) 6.02×10^6

17. An example of a fatty acid is
(A) $CH_3(CH_2)_{16}CH_2OH$
(B) $CH_2—COOH$
$\quad|$
$CH—COOH$
$\quad|$
$CH_2—COOH$
(C) $CH_3(CH_2)_{12}COOH$
(D) $CH_3(CH_2)_{14}COOH_3$
(E) $\phi—OH$

18. Which one of the following acids does not commonly form acid salts?
(A) $HC_2H_3O_2$
(B) H_2SO_4
(C) H_2CO_3
(D) H_3PO_4
(E) HOOC—COOH

19. One mole of acetal may be synthesized from the quantitative reaction of
(A) one mole of alcohol and two moles of aldehyde.
(B) two moles of alcohol and one mole of aldehyde.
(C) one mole each of alcohol and aldehyde.
(D) one mole each of aldehyde and ketone.
(E) one mole each of aldehyde, ketone, and alcohol.

20. An atom undergoing neutron capture and negatron decay will produce an atom of
(A) smaller atomic number.
(B) greater atomic number.
(C) greater atomic weight.
(D) greater atomic weight and smaller atomic number.
(E) greater atomic weight and greater atomic number.

21. Which of the statements listed below is false?
(A) An aqueous solution in which $(H^+) > 1 \times 10^{+7}$ is said to be acidic.
(B) Ions are atoms or groups of atoms that have lost or gained one or more electrons.
(C) HCl is a Bronsted acid because it furnishes H^+ ion in solution.
(D) NaOH is called a base because it furnishes Na^+ ions in solution.

22. Cholesterol is an intermediate in the biosynthesis of
(A) essential fatty acids.
(B) steroid hormones.
(C) essential amino acids.
(D) prostaglandins.
(E) thyroglobulin.

23. The essential fatty acids are required in the human body in the biosynthesis of
(A) ascorbic acid
(B) bile acids.
(C) estrogens.
(D) prostaglandins.
(E) androgens.

24. 2-Butyne + $H_2 \xrightarrow{Pd}$
(A) *trans*-2-butene
(B) *cis*-2-butene
(C) 1,3-butadiene
(D) 1-butyne
(E) no reaction

25. A compound which is insoluble in concentrated sulfuric acid is
(A) 1-pentyne.
(B) 1,3-pentadiene.
(C) 2-pentyne.
(D) *n*-pentane.
(E) none of the above.

26. Which reaction would yield 1-butene as the major product?
(A) $CH_3—CH_2—CH_2—CH_2—Br$ + alcoholic KOH $\xrightarrow{heat}$
(B) $CH_3—CH_2—\underset{}{\overset{\displaystyle Br}{\overset{|}{C}}}H—CH_3$ + alcoholic KOH $\xrightarrow{heat}$
(C) $CH_3CH_2CH_2CH_2—OH + H_2SO_4 \xrightarrow{heat}$
(D) $CH_3C \equiv C—CH_3 + H_2 \xrightarrow{Pt}$
(E) $CH_3—CH_2—CH_3—CH_3$ + Na

27. In the chlorination of nitrobenzene the product recovered in greatest yield is
(A) *o*-chloronitrobenzene.
(B) *m*-chloronitrobenzene.
(C) *p*-chloronitrobenzene.
(D) *p*-dichlorobenzene.
(E) *o*-dichloronitrobenzene.

28. The nitro group present on the benzene ring in the above question is
(A) activating, meta-directing.
(B) activating, para-directing.
(C) deactivating, meta-directing.
(D) none of the above.

29. An atom undergoing beta decay will initially produce an atom of
(A) greater atomic number.
(B) smaller atomic number.
(C) greater atomic weight.
(D) greater atomic weight and greater atomic number.
(E) equal atomic number.

30. In the decomposition of $KClO_3$ to generate oxygen gas, MnO_2 is added in order to
(A) increase the volume of oxygen obtained from the $KClO_3$.
(B) produce oxygen of higher purity.
(C) reduce the temperature at which decomposition of $KClO_3$ takes place.
(D) decrease the volume of Cl_2 produced.
(E) increase the temperature at which decomposition of $KClO_3$ takes place.

31. The name applied to a substance such as MnO_2 used in the reaction above is a (an)
(A) enzyme.
(B) catalyst.
(C) isotope.
(D) free radical scavenger.
(E) cofactor.

32. Large ring compounds are difficult to prepare because
(A) these rings are stable but the two ends of the chain must be brought close together to effect ring closure.
(B) these rings are flat and their bond angles exceed 109.5°.
(C) both large and small rings are highly strained.
(D) these rings are puckered and their bond angles are compressed to less than 109.5°.
(E) these rings are extremely unstable.

33. The species which acts as the electrophile in the bromination of benzene is
(A) benzene.
(B) Br^-.
(C) $Br\cdot$.
(D) Br^+.
(E) $-Br^+$

34. The ionization constant for an acid, HA, may be designated as K_a. It is equal to
(A) $\dfrac{(H^+)\quad(A^-)}{(HA)}$
(B) $\dfrac{(H^+)}{(HA)\quad(A^-)}$
(C) $\dfrac{(HA)}{(H^+)\quad(A^-)}$
(D) $\dfrac{(H^+)^2}{(HA)}$

35. Gasoline having the same combustion characteristics as a mixture of 95% iso-octane and 5% n-heptane (by volume) will have an octane number of
(A) 5.
(B) 50.
(C) 89.
(D) 100.
(E) 95.

36. Which of the following compounds would NOT exhibit optical activity?
(A) 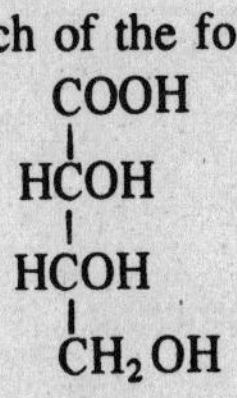
(B) 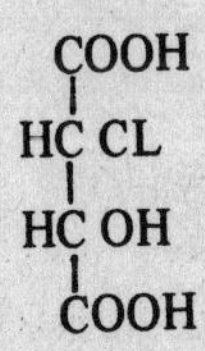
(C) 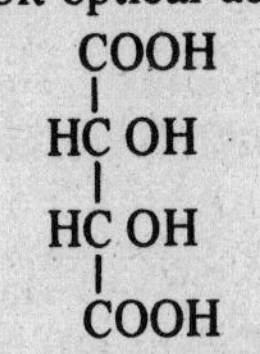
(D) 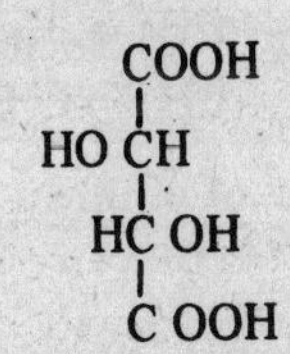

37. A racemic mixture contains dextrorotatory and levorotatory isomers in the proportion of
(A) 2:1.
(B) 10:1.
(C) 3:1.
(D) all of the above.
(E) none of the above.

38. All of the following are true EXCEPT
(A) pH + pOH = 14
(B) $(H^+)(OH^-) = 10^{-14}$
(C) $pH = \log \dfrac{1}{(H^+)}$
(D) the stronger acid has the larger pK_a
(E) the weaker acid has the larger pK_a

39. Ammoniacal silver nitrate was added to a solution of an unknown compound. If a silver mirror was formed, the unknown compound was NOT
(A) benzaldehyde.
(B) 2-butanone.
(C) formaldehyde.
(D) 2-methylpropanal.

40. Which of the following reactions CANNOT be used to form salts?
(A) the reaction of an acid anhydride and a metal oxide
(B) the reaction of a nonmetal and oxygen

(C) the reaction of an acid and a metal
(D) the reaction of a metal oxide and an acid

41. The most polar of the following bonds is
(A) N—F.
(B) F—F.
(C) C—F.
(D) O—F.
(E) F—Cl.

42. A gas cylinder contains an equimolar mixture of C_2H_4 and CO_2. If the gas is allowed to exit for a short time through a pinhole, the gas remaining in the cylinder will contain
(A) an equimolar mixture of the two gases.
(B) more CO_2 than C_2H_4 molecules.
(C) more C_2H_4 than CO_2 molecules.
(D) pure C_2H_4.
(E) pure CO_2.

43. If phosphoric acid, H_3PO_4, reacts with excess sodum hydroxide, the product is
(A) Na_3HPO_4
(B) Na_3PO_3
(C) NaH_2PO_4
(D) Na_3PO_4
(E) H_2

44. The oxidation of foods in the body provides part of the water supply. The largest amount of water per gram is formed by the oxidation of
(A) glucose.
(B) fat.
(C) protein.
(D) lactic acid.
(E) polysaccharides.

45. Loss or gain of an orbital electron by an atom produces a (an)
(A) molecule.
(B) polymer.
(C) ion.
(D) isotope.
(E) radioactive compound.

46. The atomic number of an element refers to the number of
(A) isotopes.
(B) neutrons.
(C) protons in the nucleus.
(D) beta particles.
(E) electrons in the nucleus.

47. Fats
(A) contain the three elements: carbon, hydrogen, and oxygen.
(B) are greasy or oily, making them relatively insoluble in water.
(C) contain more calories per gram than do carbohydrates.
(D) All of the above are correct statements.
(E) None of the above are correct statements.

48. Brownian movement is a result of
(A) diffusion.
(B) molecular bombardment of suspended particles.
(C) meniscus formation.
(D) acid-base balance.
(E) adhesion.

49. Which of the following compounds will NOT react with CH_3MgBr to give CH_4 as a gas?
(A) $HC\equiv CH$
(B) HCOOH
(C) H_3C–CH_2OH
(D) H_3C–C(H)=O
(E) ϕ—OH

STOP. If you finish before the time limit is up, go over your work for this section. DO NOT look at any other sections of the model examination. When your time limit is up, go on to the next section.

Physics

DIRECTIONS: Each of the statements or questions is followed by four or five suggested completions or answers. Choose the one that best completes the statement or answers the question, and mark the letter of your choice on the answer sheet.

1. A 200-lb. highdiver climbed a tower 60 ft. tall. How much work did he do against gravitational forces?
(A) 1200 ft.-lb.
(B) 260 ft.-lb.
(C) 12,000 ft.-lb.
(D) 1.2×10^6 ft.-lb.
(E) 3.3 ft.-lb.

2. A gas occupies a volume of 4 liters at STP. It is heated to 546°C and compressed to 2 atm. It now occupies a volume of
(A) 4 liters.
(B) 2 liters.
(C) 6 liters.
(D) 12 liters.
(E) 8 liters.

3. If the absolute pressure on a gas is doubled at constant temperature, the volume
(A) is doubled.
(B) is halved.
(C) is unchanged.
(D) decreases to one-fourth its previous volume.
(E) is quadrupled.

4. An object is thrown upward with a vertical velocity of 65 ft./sec. It will return in
(A) 2 sec.
(B) 4 sec.
(C) 16 sec.
(D) 120 sec.
(E) 1 sec.

5. The boiling point of any liquid at atmospheric pressure is
(A) 2(760) 2/3 Celsius molecular weight + 273.
(B) the temperature at which as many molecules leave the liquid as return to it.
(C) a function of the shape of the vessel holding the liquid.
(D) dependent on the energy used to heat it.
(E) the temperature at which the vapor pressure is equal to atmospheric pressure.

6. According to the kinetic molecular theory, the average kinetic energy of gaseous molecules depends on the
(A) temperature and the identity of the gas molecules.
(B) identity of the gas molecules and is independent of temperature.
(C) third root of the absolute pressure under which the gas molecules are contained.
(D) pressure and the identity of the gas molecules.
(E) temperature without regard to the identity of the gas molecules.

7. Small particles (90 g) of a new alloy are added to a graduated cylinder containing 30 ml of water. After the addition the volume reads 45 ml. The density of the alloy is
(A) 6 g/ml.
(B) 7.5 g/ml.
(C) 9 g/ml.
(D) 3 g/ml.
(E) 15 g/ml.

8. In the absence of friction, raising a 60 kg mass to a height of 6 m directly requires
(A) less work than in moving the same mass to the same vertical height on a 45° plane.
(B) more work than in moving the same mass to the same vertical height on a 45° plane.
(C) the same quantity of work as in moving the same mass to the same vertical height on a 30° plane.
(D) more work than in moving a 70 kg mass to the same vertical height on a plane 15° to the vertical.
(E) more work than the potential energy derived from the system.

9. The properties of light are explained by
(A) wave theory.
(B) particle theory.
(C) propagation theory.
(D) conduction theory.
(E) both wave and particle theories.

10. An object dropped from the top of a tower hits the ground 4 sec. later. How high is the tower?
(A) 4 ft.
(B) 16 ft.
(C) 64 ft.
(D) 256 ft.
(E) 128 ft.

11. During a game of chance a gambler tossing a coin has a string of nine "heads" appearing in succession. His chances of getting another "head" on his next toss are
(A) 1/1
(B) 9/10
(C) 1/2
(D) 3/4
(E) 9/1

12. A test pilot who is accelerated from rest to 600 mi./hr. in 30 sec. would be subjected to an acceleration of
(A) 1200 mi./hr.^{2}.
(B) 20 mi./hr.^{2}.
(C) 72,000 mi./hr.^{2}.
(D) 1200 ft./sec.^{2}.
(E) 18,000 mi./hr.^{2}.

13. In a plane two forces of 4 newtons and 6 newtons are acting on an object to produce a resultant force of 2 newtons. They must be oriented at ________ with respect to each other.
(A) 45°
(B) 90°
(C) 180°
(D) 360°
(E) 270°

14. A twenty-pound cannonball is shot from a cannon horizontally at a height of three feet from the ground at the same time that an identical cannonball is dropped from a height of three feet. The cannonball which is dropped will
(A) strike the ground with a greater vertical velocity than the other cannonball.
(B) reach the ground at the same time as the other cannonball.
(C) reach the ground after the other cannonball.
(D) reach the ground before the other cannonball.
(E) strike the ground with a lesser vertical velocity than the other cannonball.

Questions 15, 16, 17, 18:

Object X (mass 50 gm) is moving at a speed of 0.2 m/sec. along a frictionless horizontal surface. When it strikes object Z (mass 10 gm), the two objects stick together. Object Z was at rest prior to the collision.

15. The momentum of the system prior to the collision is
(A) 10 gm-m/sec.
(B) 12 gm-m/sec.
(C) 6 gm-m/sec.
(D) 250 gm-m/sec.
(E) 100 gm-m/sec.

16. The momentum of the system after the collision is
(A) 10 gm-m/sec.
(B) 12 gm-m/sec.
(C) 6 gm-m/sec.
(D) 25 gm-m/sec.
(E) 60 gm-m/sec.

17. The velocity of the objects after they are stuck together is
(A) 0.2 m/sec.
(B) 0.32 m/sec.
(C) 0.17 m/sec.
(D) 0.38 m/sec.
(E) 0.01 m/sec.

18. The kinetic energy of the new XZ object after they are stuck together is
(A) 1.2 gm-m²/sec./sec.²
(B) 0.87 gm-m²/sec.²
(C) 0.38 gm-m²/sec.²
(D) in excess of 4 gm-m²/sec.²
(E) none of the above.

19. If a radioactive isotope of silver has a half-life of about 7.5 days, at the end of 15 days ____________ of the original radioactive isotope will remain.
(A) 25%
(B) 15%
(C) 7.5%
(D) none
(E) 50%

20. The velocity of sound in a vacuum is ____________ in air.
(A) greater than
(B) less than
(C) the same as
(D) none of the above

21. A steel needle may be carefully floated on the surface of water
(A) because steel is less dense than water.
(B) because of surface tension.
(C) only if the water is at a temperature of about 4°C.
(D) only if the water contains detergent.
(E) because steel is more dense than water.

22. An approaching locomotive sounds its horn. The frequency of the tone (as compared with the tone of the horn when it is stationary) will appear
(A) to be higher.
(B) to be lower.
(C) to be unchanged.
(D) to be outside the frequency range of the human ear.

23. A 0.5 kg object attached to a nylon cord outside a space vehicle is travelling in a circular orbit of 20 m diameter at a speed of 2m/sec. The cord is subjected to a force of
(A) 0.2 newtons.
(B) 4.0 newtons.
(C) 5.0 newtons.
(D) 0.1 newtons.
(E) 20.0 newtons.

24. A nuclear reactor that is used for the production of electricity by a power company serves to
(A) generate electricity directly by the photoelectric effect.
(B) produce wind currents that turn generators.
(C) produce heat for the generation of steam.
(D) vaporize carbon to turn air turbines.
(E) transform uranium into electrons.

25. A microscope with an eyepiece magnification of 10X and an objective of 97X would magnify an object on the stage
(A) 19.7X.
(B) 107X.
(C) 197X.
(D) 97X.
(E) 970X.

26. The critical temperature of a compound is
(A) the temperature at which a sustained chain reaction begins.
(B) the highest temperature at which the gas may be liquefied.
(C) the temperature at which the shell of a nuclear reactor is strongest.
(D) none of the above.
(E) all of the above.

27. A direct current circuit is wired with resistances of 3 ohms, 6 ohms, and 2 ohms in series. They could be replaced by one resistor of ______________ to produce the same equivalent resistance.
(A) 11 ohms
(B) 6 ohms
(C) 1 ohm
(D) none of the above
(E) 36 ohms

28. If the above question had used the individual resistances (i.e., 3 ohms, 6 ohms, and 2 ohms) in parallel instead of in series, the equivalent resistance would be
(A) 11 ohms.
(B) 6 ohms.
(C) 1 ohm.
(D) 17 ohms.
(E) 36 ohms.

29. If white light is dispersed by a prism, one sees a series of colors. Which listing of colors below is out of order?
(A) red, yellow, green, blue
(B) red, orange, green, blue
(C) red, yellow, violet, blue
(D) orange, yellow, green, violet
(E) none of the above

30. A battery of 20 volts is attached to a circuit containing resistances of 2 ohms, 3 ohms, and 5 ohms. The current in the circuit is
(A) 2 amps.
(B) 3 amps.
(C) 5 amps.
(D) 10 amps.
(E) 30 amps.

31. Utilizing radioactive decay, people have been able to date the oldest rocks, etc. These methods employ radioactive decay of
(A) rubidium-87.
(B) potassium-40.
(C) carbon-14.
(D) none of the above.
(E) all of the above.

32. You have determined that a certain laboratory bench measures 78 cm in length. The carpenter, however, wants to know how many inches in length the new formica top should be. You tell him ______________ inches.
(A) 39.0
(B) 30.7
(C) 26.0
(D) 36.1
(E) 78.0

33. The strength of an electromagnet may be increased by
(A) increasing current supply.
(B) adding more coiled wire.
(C) increasing the size of the iron core.
(D) all of the above.
(E) none of the above.

34. The heat energy of food ingested by people is measured in units called
(A) B.T.U.'s.
(B) degrees C.
(C) degrees F.
(D) calories.
(E) coulombs.

35. The weather forecaster has just announced that Europe experienced one of its hottest days ever recorded. The temperature in Frankfurt, Germany, hit 45°C. This would equal ______________ F.
(A) 135°
(B) 100°
(C) 113°
(D) 105°
(E) 180°

36. At the end of one second a falling object will attain a velocity of ______________ feet/sec.
(A) 16
(B) 36
(C) 32
(D) 8
(E) 4

37. During this one second of falling, an object previously at rest will have covered a distance of
(A) 16 ft.
(B) 36 ft.
(C) 32 ft.
(D) 8 ft.
(E) 4 ft.

38. All objects, whether a lead weight or a Ping-Pong ball, will drop at the same rate if they
(A) are dropped from an airplane at 30,000 ft. or above.
(B) are in a vacuum.
(C) possess identical weights.
(D) are of equal volume.
(E) are of the same shape and elicit equal friction.

STOP. If you finish before the time limit is up, go over your work for this section. DO NOT look at any other sections of the model examination. When your time limit is up, go on to the next section.

SCIENCE PROBLEMS

85 MINUTES
66 QUESTIONS

The following questions require you to use your knowledge of science to solve problems.

DIRECTIONS: The following questions are in groups. Preceding each series of questions is a paragraph or a short explanatory statement, a formula or set of formulas, or a definition. Read the written material and then answer the questions. Eliminate those choices that you think to be incorrect and mark the letter of your choice on the answer sheet.

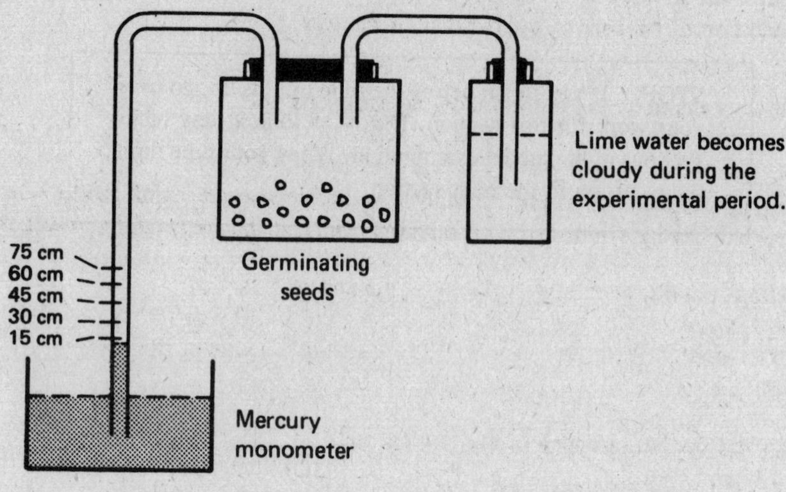

1. The process demonstrated by this experiment is
(A) osmosis.
(B) respiration.
(C) metabolism.
(D) photosynthesis.
(E) titration.

2. The gas produced as indicated by the clouding of the lime water is
(A) CO_2.
(B) O_2.
(C) N_2.
(D) CO.
(E) H_2.

3. If the germinating seeds used up all the air (gases) available, the mercury manometer would rise to a level of
(A) 15 cm.
(B) 30 cm.
(C) 45 cm.
(D) 4 cm.
(E) 76 cm.

Ethanol has a boiling point of 78.3°C. When a mixture of ethanol and water is distilled, a product with a boiling point of 78.15°C is collected. This product is 95.6% ethanol by weight. If benzene is added to the initial mixture, distillation produces a ternary mixture (7.4% water, 18.5% ethanol, and 74.1% benzene) with a boiling point of 64.85°C.

4. Distillation of one kilogram of a 50% mixture (by weight) of ethanol and water would produce __________ pure ethanol.
(A) 500 g of
(B) 478 g of
(C) 22 g of
(D) 92.5 g of
(E) no

5. Distillation of one kilogram of a 50% (by weight) mixture of ethanol and water would produce ________________ pure water.
   (A) 23 g of
   (B) 477 g of
   (C) 500 g of
   (D) 92.5 g of
   (E) no

6. Increasing the amount of pure ethanol produced in the distillation of ethanol and water may be accomplished by
   (A) more efficient fractionating column.
   (B) redistillation of the product.
   (C) addition of benzene to the product.
   (D) removal of water by phase separation.
   (E) addition of benzene to the distillation mixture.

In uniformly accelerated motion the following equations hold:

$$v = v_0 + at$$

$$x = v_0 t + \tfrac{1}{2}at^2$$

where v = velocity at time t, v_0 = initial velocity, x = displacement, t = time, and a = acceleration. A smooth steel ball having a mass of 1 kg is released from rest and starts falling toward the ground.

7. Neglecting friction, what is its velocity at the end of 1 second?
   (A) 4.9 m/sec.
   (B) 9.8 m/sec.
   (C) 14.7 m/sec.
   (D) 19.6 m/sec.
   (E) none of the above.

8. How far has the ball dropped in the first second?
   (A) 4.9 m
   (B) 9.8 m
   (C) 14.7 m
   (D) 19.6 m
   (E) none of the above

9. If the ball is originally 19.6 m above the ground, how long will it take to hit the ground?
   (A) 10 sec.
   (B) 8 sec.
   (C) 6 sec.
   (D) 4 sec.
   (E) 2 sec.

Buffer solutions are prepared from a salt of a weak acid and a weak acid. These solutions are resistant to changes in pH when acid or base is added. Buffers are generally effective within ±1 pH unit of the pK_a ($-\log K_a$) of the weak acid. According to the Henderson-Hasselbach equation

$$\text{pH} = \text{p}K_a + \log \frac{\text{salt}}{\text{weak acid}}$$

the pH of a buffer solution is defined by the pK_a and the ratio of the concentration of salt of a weak acid to the concentration of a weak acid.

10. When the salt is ten times that of the weak acid then the pH is
    (A) equal to the pK_a.
    (B) ten times the pK_a.
    (C) 1/10 the pK_a.
    (D) the pK_a plus 1.
    (E) the pK_a minus 1.

11. From the Henderson-Hasselbach equation, when pH = pK, then the salt is
    (A) zero.
    (B) equal to the weak acid.
    (C) greater than the acid concentration.
    (D) less than the acid concentration.
    (E) equal to one.

12. The pH of a 0.1 M solution of a strong acid is 1. What is the pH of a 0.1 M solution of a weak acid (pK_a 5) and 0.1 M salt?
(A) 1
(B) 5
(C) 7
(D) 9
(E) none of the above

Amino acids may be represented by the formula $R—\overset{\displaystyle H}{\underset{\displaystyle NH_2}{C}}—COOH$. A polypeptide is a polymer of amino acids in which the amino group of one amino acid is attached to the carboxyl of the neighboring amino acid in an amide (peptide) linkage. Ninhydrin will react with "free" amino groups (i.e., those not in amide or other linkage) to produce a purple product. In solution the intensity is proportional to the concentration of "free" amino groups.

13. Boiling a polypeptide solution in 1 N HCl prior to reacting with ninhydrin will
(A) increase the intensity of purple color compared to an equal amount of polypeptide not boiled in the presence of HCl.
(B) decrease the intensity of purple color compared to an equal amount of polypeptide not boiled in the presence of HCl.
(C) have no effect on the intensity of purple color compared to an equal amount of polypeptide not boiled in the presence of HCl.
(D) result in production of no purple color.
(E) cause reaction of ninhydrin with carboxyl groups to produce a green color.

14. Reacting a polypeptide solution with peptidase enzyme prior to reacting with ninhydrin will
(A) increase the intensity of purple color compared to an equal amount of polypeptide not reacted with peptidase.
(B) decrease the intensity of purple color compared to an equal amount of polypeptide not reacted with peptidase.
(C) have no effect on the intensity of purple color compared to an equal amount of polypeptide not reacted with peptidase.
(D) result in production of no purple color.
(E) cause reaction of ninhydrin with carboxyl groups to produce a green color.

15. The addition of an inhibitor of the peptidase enzyme to the peptide solution prior to adding the peptidase enzyme will ______________ as compared to a sample containing no inhibitor.
(A) increase the amount of purple color that will be produced on reacting with ninhydrin
(B) decrease the amount of purple color that will be produced on reacting with ninhydrin
(C) have no effect on the amount of purple color that will be produced on reacting with ninhydrin
(D) result in production of no purple color
(E) cause reaction of ninhydrin with carboxyl groups to produce a green color

Fatty acids may be defined as straight hydrocarbon chains terminating in a carboxyl group. The chains may be saturated or unsaturated. The unsaturation may consist of *cis* or *trans* double bonds, but the double bonds in the fatty acids of the fats of animals and higher plants are almost exclusively *cis*. *Trans* double bonds absorb light at 10.3 microns; saturated fatty acids and fatty acids containing *cis* double bonds do not absorb at this wavelength.

16. In a solution of fatty acid in solvent, absorption of light at 10.3 microns may be used to determine the concentrations of
(A) fatty acids.
(B) *cis* fatty acids.
(C) *trans* fatty acids.
(D) unsaturated fatty acids.
(E) saturated fatty acids.

17. Catalytic hydrogenation of a sample containing saturated fatty acids, *cis*-unsaturated fatty acids, and *trans*-unsaturated fatty acids will
    (A) decrease the absorption of light at 10.3 microns.
    (B) increase the absorption of light at 10.3 microns.
    (C) increase the amount of *cis*-unsaturated fatty acids.
    (D) have no effect on the absorption of light at 10.3 microns.
    (E) decrease the amount of saturated fatty acids.

18. Of the organisms listed below, the highest concentrations of *trans* fatty acids would be expected in the fats of
    (A) coconuts.
    (B) olives.
    (C) kangaroos.
    (D) bacteria.
    (E) crows.

The density of water is 1 gm/cm³ and that of mercury is 13.6 gm/cm³.

19. What is the mass in kg of a 30 cm³ volume of mercury?
    (A) 0.001 kg
    (B) 0.030 kg
    (C) 0.408 kg
    (D) 13.600 kg
    (E) 30.000 kg

20. What is the mass of the same volume of water?
    (A) 0.030 kg
    (B) 1.000 kg
    (C) 13.600 kg
    (D) 30.000 kg
    (E) none of the above

21. What is the specific gravity of the mercury?
    (A) 1
    (B) 13.6
    (C) 30.0
    (D) 48.0
    (E) none of the above

Ten milliliters of blood were removed from a patient, and centrifugation was utilized to separate 5 ml of plasma from the blood cells. A 3-ml sample of the plasma was extracted with 100 ml of an appropriate lipid solvent. The lipid solvent was then evaporated to 10 ml, and a 0.1 ml sample was analyzed for cholesterol. The color produced in the colorimetric analysis at 560 millimicrons was exactly equal to a standard in which 0.5 mg of cholesterol was known to be present.

22. The cholesterol concentration of the patient's plasma was
    (A) 200 mg cholesterol/100 ml plasma.
    (B) 295 mg cholesterol/100 ml plasma.
    (C) 867 mg cholesterol/100 ml plasma.
    (D) 1238 mg cholesterol/100 ml plasma.
    (E) 1665 mg cholesterol/100 ml plasma.

23. In order to make the above calculations it was NOT necessary to know
    (A) the volume of plasma separated from the blood.
    (B) the volume of plasma subjected to extraction.
    (C) the solvent volume after evaporation.
    (D) the volume of sample that was subjected to colorimetric analysis.
    (E) any of the above.

24. If the addition of twice the volume of standard produces more than twice the absorbance at 560 millimicrons, this is probably best explained by
    (A) exceeding the linear range of the method.
    (B) error in pipetting.
    (C) error in weighing to prepare the standard solution.
    (D) any or all of the above.
    (E) none of the above.

A generated water wave travels from its source with a period of 10 seconds and a wavelength of 50 meters.

25. What is the frequency of the wave?
(A) 1/10
(B) 1/50
(C) 1
(D) 5
(E) 1/5

26. Calculate the velocity of the wave.
(A) 5 m/sec.
(B) 10 m/sec.
(C) 1 m/sec.
(D) 1/2 m/sec.
(E) none of the above

27. The wave is generated at an angle to the shore such that portions of the wave nearest the shore have a decrease in velocity while the remaining portions maintain their velocity. This phenomenon is known as wave refraction and it tends to
(A) make wave trains normal to the shore.
(B) make wave trains parallel to the shore.
(C) not change the wave approach.
(D) decrease the wave height.
(E) none of the above.

The following graph illustrates several phenomena that develop while a muscle is being repetitively stimulated:

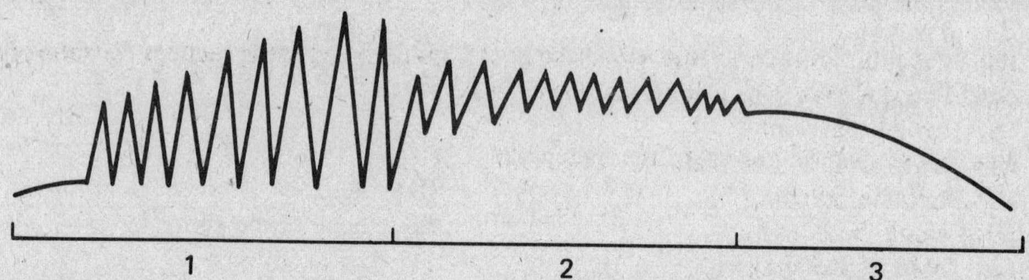

Match the numbered area of the graph with the appropriate lettered phenomenon.

28. (1) ______
29. (2) ______
30. (3) ______

(A) Treppe or staircase phenomenon
(B) Fatigue
(C) Physiological contracture

An enzyme, lactic dehydrogenase, catalyzes the oxidation of lactic acid to produce pyruvic acid. As lactic acid is oxidized, a coenzyme, NAD^+, is reduced to $NADH + H^+$. The normal serum enzyme activity is about 40-100 enzyme units/ml, but the enzyme activity is often increased after occlusion of a blood vessel which nourishes the heart.

31. If the rate of reduction of NAD^+ (in the presence of lactic acid) in the serum of a patient suspected of having a heart attack is decreased compared to pooled normal serum, this is
(A) evidence of a heart attack.
(B) definite proof of a heart attack.
(C) not evidence of a heart attack.
(D) proof that no heart attack occurred.
(E) proof of laboratory error.

32. The rate of production of $NADH + H^+$ by the lactic dehydrogenase in 0.1 ml of serum from patient B is 4 times the rate that is noted in 0.2 ml of serum from patient E. If the lactic dehydrogenase activity in patient E is 40 units/ml, then the activity in patient B's serum is
(A) 40 units/ml.
(B) 160 units/ml.
(C) 10 units/ml.
(D) 320 units/ml.
(E) 5 units/ml.

33. The rate of appearance of $NADH + H^+$ is ____________ the rate of disappearance of NAD^+ in the enzymatic reaction catalyzed by lactic dehydrogenase.
(A) unrelated to
(B) twice
(C) one-half
(D) one-fourth
(E) equal to

Given that the index of refraction is defined as the ratio of the speed of light in a vacuum to that of the speed of light in the medium ($n = C/S_m$), $C = 3.0 \times 10^8$ m/sec., and that the speed of light in water is about 2.25×10^8 m/sec.

34. Calculate the index of refraction of water.
(A) 0.75
(B) 1.00
(C) 1.33
(D) 6.25
(E) 6.75

35. If a beam of light strikes a water surface at an angle of 45° after leaving a vacuum, then
(A) $n_r/n_i = 1$.
(B) $n_r/n_i > 1$.
(C) $n_r/n_i < 1$.
(D) $n_r/n_i = 0$.
(E) none of the above.

36. If the direction of the beam is reversed and goes from the water to the vacuum, the ratio of n_r/n_i would be less than 1 indicating that the n_i beam would bend
(A) toward the normal.
(B) away from the normal.
(C) into the normal.
(D) along the boundary.
(E) none of the above.

The following diagram represents a graduated centrifuge tube containing 10 ml of blood following 15 to 20 min. of centrifugation at a speed of 2,500 rpm. The tube had been heparinized to prevent coagulation.

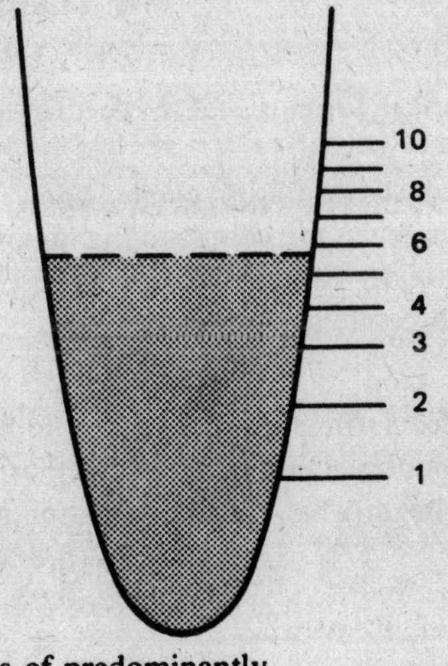

37. The lower 5.5 ml consists of predominantly
(A) fibrin clot material.
(B) platelets.
(C) white blood cells.
(D) red blood cells.

38. The hematocrit of the donor is
(A) 45%
(B) 55%
(C) 4.5 ml.
(D) 5.5 ml.
(E) 10 ml.

39. This situation deviates from the normal in such a way that it could be due to
(A) living at high altitude.
(B) sickle-cell anemia.
(C) pernicious anemia.
(D) excessive X-ray treatment.
(E) all of the above.

Hydrofluoric acid, HF, ionizes in water to produce H^+ and F^-. The ionization constant is 2×10^{-4}.

40. The pH of a 0.5 *M* aqueous solution of HF may be calculated to be
(A) 2.
(B) 4.
(C) 5.
(D) 8.
(E) 10.

41. Failure to consider the ionization of water in the above calculation of pH leads to an error of ____________ pH units.
(A) >0.5
(B) 0.4
(C) 0.2
(D) 0.09
(E) <0.01

42. The pH of a 0.5 *N* aqueous solution of HF may be calculated to be
(A) 2.
(B) 4.
(C) 5.
(D) 8.
(E) 10.

An unidentified compound is composed solely of carbon and hydrogen. Complete combustion of 0.100 g of the compound produced 0.677 g of CO_2 and 0.138 g of water.

43. The empirical formula of this compound is
(A) CH.
(B) CH_2.
(C) CH_3.
(D) C_2H_4.
(E) CH_4.

44. The molecular formula could be
(A) CH_4.
(B) C_2H_4.
(C) C_2H_2.
(D) C_2H_6.
(E) C_3H_6.

45. Having determined the empirical formula, the molecular formula can be determined by information derived from
(A) the amount of oxygen consumed during combustion.
(B) freezing point depression when the compound is dissolved in water.
(C) the amount of nitrogen oxides formed during combustion.
(D) the temperature at which combustion begins.
(E) all of the above.

To 100 ml of 0.1 *M* $AgNO_3$ is added sufficient solid Na_2SO_4 to begin precipitation.

46. Knowing that the solubility product constant for Ag_2SO_4 is 6.4×10^{-5}, it is possible to predict that precipitation will begin when the concentration of Na_2SO_4 reaches
(A) 6.4×10^{-7} *M*.
(B) 6.4×10^{-6} *M*.
(C) 6.4×10^{-3} *M*.
(D) 0.8 *M*.
(E) 0.08 *M*.

47. If Na_2SO_4 were a weakly ionized salt, the addition of $NaNO_3$ in the above problem would be expected to
(A) cause the precipitation of $AgNO_3$.
(B) decrease the concentration of Na_2SO_4 required for precipitation to begin.
(C) increase the concentration of Na_2SO_4 required for precipitation to begin.
(D) have no effect on precipitation.
(E) change the solubility product constant for Ag_2SO_4.

48. If NaCl were substituted for $NaNO_3$ in the above question, we would expect to
(A) prevent any precipitation.
(B) increase the precipitation of $NaNO_3$.
(C) decrease but not abolish the precipitation of $NaNO_3$.
(D) precipitate $AgNO_3$.
(E) precipitate AgCl.

Given the circuit diagram below where R_1 = 20 ohms; R_2 = 5 ohms; R_3 = 10 ohms; and R_4 = 15 ohms

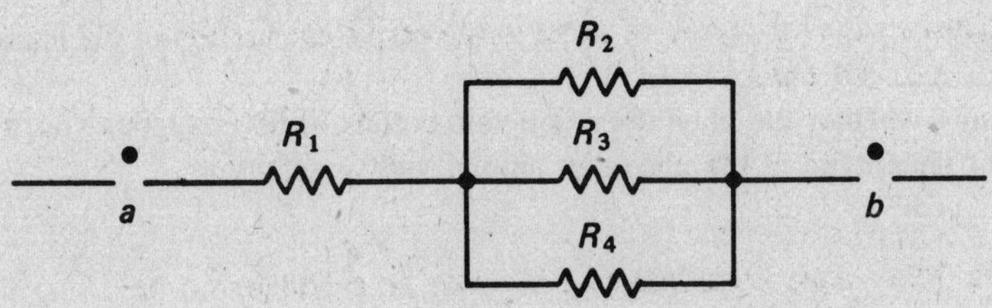

49. Calculate the resistance in the parallel resistors.
(A) 2.75 ohms
(B) 5.00 ohms
(C) 10.00 ohms
(D) 15.00 ohms
(E) 30.00 ohms

50. What is the total resistance in this circuit?
(A) 20.0 ohms
(B) 22.7 ohms
(C) 33.1 ohms
(D) 45.0 ohms
(E) 50.7 ohms

51. If the current through the circuit is 5 amperes, what is the potential difference from *a* to *b*?
(A) 100 volts
(B) 114 volts
(C) 220 volts
(D) 230 volts
(E) none of the above

In thermal expansion of solids, we can express a temperature coefficient of linear expansion (α) as $\alpha = \Delta L/L_0 \, \Delta T$ where ΔL = change of length, ΔT = change of temperature resulting in L change, and L_0 = original length.

52. If a platinum bar ($\alpha = 9 \times 10^{-6}$ per °C) is heated from an original temperature of 10°C to 20°C and its change in length was 1×10^{-2} cm, calculate the original length.
(A) 10 cm
(B) 80 cm
(C) 90 cm
(D) 100 cm
(E) 110 cm

53. If this bar is now cooled from 20°C to 0°C, what will its new length be?
(A) 9.99 cm
(B) 79.99 cm
(C) 89.99 cm
(D) 99.99 cm
(E) 109.99 cm

54. If one compares *volume* changes of solids and liquids, which of the statements below is best?
(A) The coefficient of volume expansion is constant over fairly wide temperature ranges for most solids and liquids.
(B) Nonisotropic substances expand equally in all directions.
(C) The coefficient of volume expansion is the same as the coefficient of linear expansion.
(D) The coefficient of volume expansion is almost always negative.
(E) None of the above.

Genetic ratios are probability ratios. If, for example, we mate (B = black dominant; b = gray recessive) two heterozygous black cows (Bb) and 4 offspring are produced, the ratio of 3 black and 1 gray should be possible. However, what are the chances of all black and all gray litters?

55. To produce all black cows our chances are
(A) 3/4.
(B) 1/4.
(C) 9/16.
(D) 81/256.
(E) 1/256.

56. To produce all gray cows our chances are
(A) 3/4.
(B) 1/4.
(C) 9/16.
(D) 81/256.
(E) 1/256.

57. To determine whether the phenotype is heterozygous or homozygous you would cross with a dominant phenotype of the above an animal with a genotype
(A) BB.
(B) Bb.
(C) bb.

One hundred ml of a 0.5 *N* aqueous solution of the acid HX is mixed with 100 ml of a 0.5 *N* aqueous solution of the base BOH.

58. The pH should approximate
(A) 2.
(B) 4.
(C) 7.
(D) 9.
(E) It is not possible to predict.

59. It was previously reported that the formula of the base was BOH, but it is now known that the formula is $B(OH)_2$. With this new information the pH in the previous question would be expected to be
(A) <2.
(B) between 2.5 and 5.
(C) between 8.5 and 10.
(D) 7.
(E) It is not possible to predict.

60. If we now know that the acid is HCl and the base is $Ca(OH)_2$, we will be able to predict that mixing 100 ml of 0.5 *N* solutions of each will produce a solution whose pH is
(A) <1.
(B) between 1.2 and 6.8.
(C) between 6.8 and 7.3.
(D) between 7.3 and 12.5.
(E) >12.7.

Use the following diagram to answer questions 61-63:

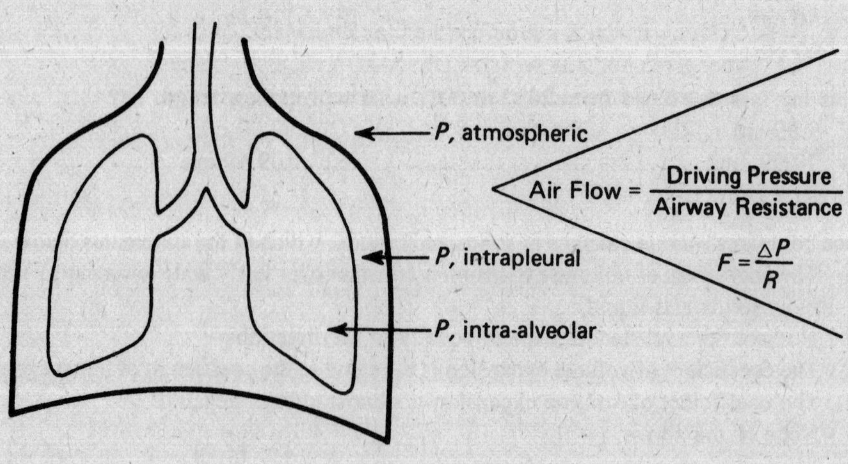

61. The driving pressure (ΔP) in breathing which causes air to flow into the lungs is
(A) atmospheric pressure (*Patm*).
(B) the intra-alveolar (intrapulmonary) pressure (*Palv*).
(C) atmospheric pressure minus the intra-alveolar pressure.
(D) the intrapleural pressure (*Ppl*).
(E) the intrapleural pressure minus the intra-alveolar pressure.

62. During inspiration, intra-alveolar pressure (*Palv*)
(A) transiently goes below atmospheric pressure (*Patm*).
(B) transiently goes above atmospheric pressure.
(C) equals atmospheric pressure.
(D) equals intrapleural pressure.
(E) transiently goes below intrapleural pressure.

63. The alveolar ventilation per minute refers to the amount of fresh air which reaches the alveoli of the lungs per minute. Alveolar ventilation per minute equals the
(A) functional residual capacity × frequency of breathing.
(B) physiologic dead space × frequency of breathing.
(C) anatomic dead space × frequency of breathing.
(D) tidal volume × frequency of breathing.
(E) (tidal volume − anatomic dead space) × frequency of breathing.

Complete catalytic hydrogenation of fatty acids containing double bonds produces saturated fatty acids. Complete catalytic hydrogenation of 1 mole (282.45 g) of a fatty acid produces a saturated fatty acid of molecular weight 284.47.

64. The number of double bonds in each molecule is
(A) 1.
(B) 2.
(C) 3.
(D) 4.
(E) 5 or more.

65. The double bond(s) prior to hydrogenation is (are)
(A) *cis*.
(B) *trans*.
(D) *cis*, *trans*, or a mixture of the two.
(E) conjugated.

66. A fatty acid of the same chain length but having two double bonds would have a molecular weight of
(A) 280.43.
(B) 286.49.
(C) 282.45.
(D) less than 279.
(E) more than 288.

STOP. If you finish before the time limit is up, go over your work for this section. DO NOT look at any other sections of the model examination. When your time limit is up, go on to the next section.

SKILLS ANALYSIS: READING

85 MINUTES
68 QUESTIONS

The following questions are to be answered based on your careful reading of selections from scientific writings.

DIRECTIONS: Read each passage carefully, then answer the questions following it. Consider only the material within the passage in answering the questions. Eliminate those choices that you think to be incorrect and mark the letter of your choice on the answer sheet.

As soon as any business becomes large enough for an owner to employ an assistant, a manager-subordinate relationship has been created. As the business grows even larger, we may find this subordinate having employees working for him or her so that the necessary duties are able to be performed.

The reason for having a subordinate is that the person supervising does not have the time, or in some cases, the ability to accomplish the tasks. The supervisor or manager must delegate part of his or her duties to another.

Delegation is made up of two parts—authority and responsibility. The manager or supervisor gives the subordinate the authority to do part of his or her duties so that he or she may be free to pursue other duties. The subordinate with this authority may then act independently without consulting the supervisor in the accomplishment of these tasks. Responsibility on the other hand, cannot be fully delegated. If the subordinate fails to carry out the tasks in a proper manner, it is the manager or supervisor who is held ultimately responsible for the failure.

Each level of supervision may create its own responsibility for getting the job accomplished. It can never fully be delegated, however, as there is still the upward reporting relationship back to the owner.

The important thing is to give a manager or supervisor the full authority within which to work if duties are to be delegated. Too many managers overlook this simple point and then wonder why the task is not accomplished. They also wonder why their supervisor is dissatisfied with the results over which they feel they have no control.

The following statements are related to the passage above. Based on the information given, select:
(A) if the statement is *supported by* the information in the passage.
(B) if the statement is *contradicted by* the information in the passage.
(C) if the statement is *neither supported nor contradicted by* information in the passage.

1. Managers often incompletely delegate to their subordinates freedom to carry out a total commitment.
2. Both authority and responsibility can and should be delegated to subordinates by their manager or supervisor.
3. Managers are held responsible for the acts of their employees.
4. Supervisors or managers may create their own responsibility as they delegate to their subordinates.
5. The only way to get a job accomplished is to do it yourself.
6. Responsibility and authority are the two components of delegation.

Wars have been won and lost. Men sent to the moon and back. Marriages made and divorces granted. All because of one little but very important, and often overlooked item—communication!

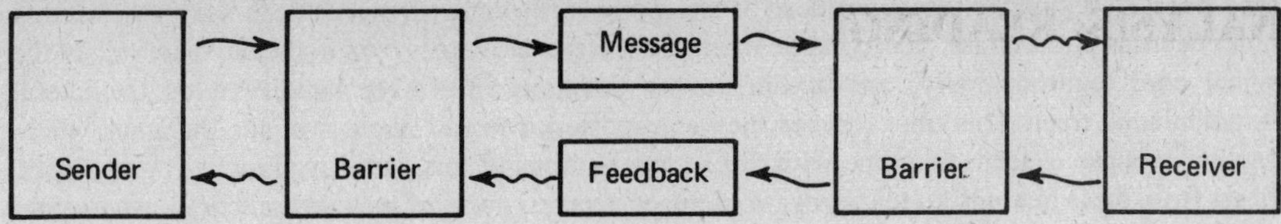

Senders will express a thought which will be influenced by their experiences, backgrounds, and personal needs. These barriers will change the way the message is expressed. The receiver is also influenced by experience, background, and personal interests; this will distort what is heard. Many times the thought expressed is completely different from what the receiver hears. By the same token, the reply that the receiver gives is influenced by these same barriers so that what is heard may be completely different from what was said. The end result could be conflict or at the very least, a misunderstanding.

When the receiver replies to the sender's statements, it becomes easier for the sender to determine if his or her message was understood. Many times this reply does not come forth. How can the sender make sure that he or she is understood? One can ask a clarifying question, but one must be careful not to phrase it "do you understand" as it is mostly likely the receiver will merely answer "yes." The sender will be more confident if he or she can phrase a question in a manner to elicit a response of "what do you understand?" that is understood. This clarification to the sender by the receiver is called "feedback." Unless the sender receives this positive feedback in one form or another, he or she can never be fully confident that the message was received as it was intended.

A simple example of how communications can break down without feedback is the parlor game where one person tells the person next to him a story. The second person repeats what was heard to the third and so on around the group until it gets back to the originator. Chances are, the story the originator receives back will be completely different from the one which was initiated.

In addition to verbal communications, there are several other types. One is physical communication. The pat on the back and handshake are examples of touch. A second type of physical communication is a visible movement of some part of the body. A nod of the head, the pointing of a finger, or a frown expresses this type of communication. Yet a third type would be symbols which we recognize. A flashing red light, newspapers or books, and traffic lights are common examples.

To summarize, we can say that communication is the transfer of some type of meaning from one person to another. Since we all wish to express ourselves, and be understood, communication becomes very important and our techniques must be continually practiced and improved.

The following statements are related to the passage above. Based on the information given, select:

(A) if the statement is *supported by* the information in the passage.

(B) if the statement is *contradicted by* the information in the passage.

(C) if the statement is *neither supported nor contradicted by* information in the passage.

7. Clear expression of a thought assures that it will be properly understood.

8. The best way to assure understanding by the receiver is to elicit feedback.

9. Communication is the interaction between individuals.

10. Our prejudices influence what we say and what we hear.

11. If the receiver returns the same message to the sender, one can always be sure that one has been understood.

12. "Feedback" is the clarification to the sender by the receiver of what the latter understood.

The sensation of pain and temperature is made possible in human beings by a neural pathway called the spinothalamic system. This system is composed of three neuron chains that extend from the spinal cord to the thalamus of the brain.

Various kinds of external receptors for pain and temperature relay impulses via myelinated and unmyelinated fibers to the first neuron in the chain that is located in the dorsal root ganglion of the dorsal (sensory) root of the spinal cord. No synapse occurs here, but these unipolar ganglion cells do send fibers to regions of the dorsal horn of the spinal cord where a synapse occurs with the second order neurons of the chain. Postsynaptic fibers from these cells cross over to the opposite side of the spinal cord (contralaterally) and ascend to the thalamus in a fiber bundle called the lateral spinothalamic tract. This tract reaches the ventroposterior lateral nucleus of the thalamus where another synapse is seen, this time with third-order neurons of this pathway. Finally, postsynaptic fibers from these neurons go to the region of the postcentral gyrus of the cerebral cortex where pain and temperature information is processed by the brain.

As one might expect, injury to the lateral spinothalamic tract results in contralateral loss of pain and temperature sensation below the level of the lesion. This fact is applied clinically since surgical sectioning of this tract is sometimes done to relieve persistent, intractable pain.

The following questions are based on the passage. Select the letter which corresponds to the best available answer.

13. Pain and temperature information reaches the postcentral gyrus of the cerebral cortex by which of the following route sequences?
(A) external receptors—dorsal root ganglion—lateral spinothalamic tract—ventroposterior nucleus of the thalamus—postcentral gyrus of cortex
(B) dorsal root ganglion—dorsal horn of spinal cord—lateral spinothalamic tract—medial ventroposterior nucleus of the thalamus—postcentral gyrus of cortex
(C) external receptors—dorsal root ganglion—contralateral lateral spinothalamic tract—ventroposterior lateral nucleus of the thalamus—postcentral gyrus of cortex
(D) external receptors—dorsal root ganglion—dorsal horn of spinal cord—contralateral lateral spinothalamic tract—ventroposterior lateral nucleus of the thalamus—postcentral gyrus of the cerebral cortex

14. The cell body of origin for fibers comprising the lateral spinothalamic tract is located in the
(A) dorsal root ganglion.
(B) dorsal horn of the spinal cord.
(C) external pain and temperature receptor organ.
(D) ventroposterior lateral nucleus of the thalamus.

15. The nucleus of termination for the lateral spinothalamic tract is found in
(A) the dorsal horn of the spinal cord.
(B) the postcentral gyrus of the cerebral cortex.
(C) the ventroposterior lateral thalamus.
(D) none of the above.

16. A lesion or injury to the left lateral spinothalamic tract would probably result in
(A) contralateral loss of pain and temperature sensation at the level of the lesion.
(B) loss of pain and temperature sensation from regions of the left side of the body supplied by spinal cord areas below the level of the lesion.
(C) contralateral loss of pain and temperature sensation from regions of the right side of the body supplied by spinal cord areas below the level of the lesion.
(D) none of the above.

In order for a thoracic surgeon to visualize the heart he or she must open up the pericardium which is a sac that covers the heart. A human heart is four-chambered and is composed of right and left atria which are separated by an interatrial septum that is frequently marred by defects. In the fetus the foramen ovale is an opening in this septum and blood passes from the right atrium to the left atrium so that the pulmonary circulation may be bypassed. A patent foramen ovale may contribute to the condition known as "blue baby." Two ventricles are also present; specifically we can speak of a right ventricle which pumps deoxygenated blood to the lungs and a left ventricle which pumps oxygenated blood to the tissues of the body. Between the ventricles is located the interventricular septum. As the surgeon approaches the heart from the anterior aspect he or she finds the atrioventricular sulcus which separates the atria from the ventricles and on the anterior side lodges the right coronary artery; while on the posterior side the coronary sinus, which is the confluence of most of the venous drainage of the heart, occupies this sulcus. The parts of the heart seen in an anterior view are mainly the right atrium and ventricle; only a portion of the left ventricle is seen in an anterior view. Between the right and left ventricle the surgeon finds the anterior interventricular sulcus which is continuous posteriorly as the posterior interventricular sulcus. In the anterior interventricular sulcus is lodged the anterior interventricular branch of the left coronary artery; while in the posterior the corresponding posterior interventricular branch of the right coronary artery can be found.

The superior and inferior vena cava and the coronary sinus empty into the right atrium. From here blood passes into the right ventricle to be pumped into the lungs via the pulmonary arteries. Blood from the lungs is returned to the left atrium by the pulmonary veins; it then passes into the left ventricle to leave upon its contraction via the aorta to supply the arterial system of the body. The heart alternately contracts and relaxes, and this cardiac cycle is repeated about 75 times per minute; the duration of one cycle is about 0.8 seconds. Atrial systole (contraction) which takes about 0.1 seconds is followed by ventricular systole lasting about 0.3 seconds and absolute diastole (relaxation) follows lasting about 0.4 seconds.

The heart has an automatic rhythmic beat, but it is also under the influence of nerves which, however, serve only to change the force or frequency of the contractions of the muscle in accordance with the physiologic needs of the organism. The modification of the intrinsic rhythmicity is by way of the two parts of the autonomic nervous system; stimulation occurs through the sympathetic portion while homeostatic maintenance is mainly a function of the parasympathetic portion. Stimulation through the sympathetic nerves increases the rate and force of the heart beat; while slowing and reduction in force are the result of parasympathetic stimulation. Vasodilation of the coronary arteries is brought about by sympathetic stimulation while vasoconstriction is elicited by parasympathetic stimulation.

The following statements are related to the passage. Based on the information given, select:

(A) if the statement is *supported by* the information in the passage.
(B) if the statement is *contradicted by* the information in the passage.
(C) if the statement is *neither supported nor contradicted by* information in the passage.

17. The paragraph deals mainly with the surgical anatomy of the heart.

18. At rest, the coronary circulation is dilated.

19. Most of the left side of the heart probably projects posteriorly.

20. The left ventricle is the main pumping chamber.

21. Most of the venous drainage of the heart enters the right atrium.

22. Venous blood brings deoxygenated blood back to the heart.

23. All chambers of the heart contract.

24. The actual period of rest for each chamber is 0.7 seconds for the atria and 0.5 seconds for the ventricles.

25. The heart is at rest longer than at work.

26. The parasympathetic portion of the autonomic nervous system slows down the activity of most organs of the body.

27. The automatic rhythmicity of the heart cannot be altered.

28. Heart rate may be controlled by neuronal stimulation.

29. A defect in the valvular system may be noticed as a murmur.

Graded or nongraded elementary schools? Educational authorities today are often in obvious disagreement as to which type of system produces the better student.

Many advocates of the nongraded approach are quick to argue that the time-honored practice of pupil classification by numerical grade levels is surely a pitfall for the school-age child. Under the graded system, a specified amount of progress is standard for the year's work. The content of the work to be covered and mastered, is laid out within the grade and the students are then manipulated to fit the mold. For example, children who are above average in ability are given the same materials as the average group, for whom the system was developed, in hopes that they will adapt themselves to the slower pace without turning the boredom they experience into a problem situation. The below-average child on the other hand, is pushed along and expected to master a slightly watered down version of the material. Failure to do so usually results in the child being forced to repeat the entire year using the same materials with the philosophy that a second-go-round will solve the problem.

Not so! cry educators who strongly defend the graded system and who predict that the pendulum is, in fact, swinging back to a more traditional approach for education.

Handled properly, the graded format provides for an organized, predictable program, in which teachers can be held accountable for imparting a specific amount of material within a given time frame. They are, however, by no means limited to the prescribed amount of material and are, therefore, able to accommodate all types of students through the use of supplementary as well as remedial programs.

What of the nongraded system? Traditionalists claim that while it is unique in theory, it more often than not causes serious problems when put into practice.

Organizationally, the nongraded approach is designed to provide continuous learning experiences for each pupil, which will allow the student to achieve success at every level of instruction. Movement from level to level occurs as fast as the individual student masters the content and skills at each level of achievement. The student will not experience failure; and boredom is eliminated even for the most gifted, as students are stimulated and challenged to move to new levels whenever they are ready to do so. Therein lies the main fallacy of the system, according to opponents, for who, they ask, will decide when the child is ready?

The argument of graded versus nongraded schools is likely to continue for some time to come. Who will be the judge of the better system? Most probably it will be the institutions of higher learning which receive the final products.

The following statements are related to the passage. Based on the information given, select:

(A) if the statement is *supported by* the information in the passage.
(B) if the statement is *contradicted by* the information in the passage.
(C) if the statement is *neither supported nor contradicted by* information in the passage.

30. Authorities always agree that the nongraded approach to education is superior, because it provides for every child's specific needs.

31. Once graduated from college or other institutions of higher learning, products of the nongraded system are able to acquire better jobs and hold them longer.

32. Advocates of the traditional method of education claim an organized, predictable frame work as one of the main strengths of a graded system.

33. The nongraded school system allows students to study whatever they want, whenever they choose.

34. Most school systems are swinging back to a more traditional educational philosophy, because they now realize that it suits the needs of the majority.

The pituitary (hypophysis) is a small gland at the base of the brain to which it is connected by the pituitary stalk. The pituitary, often referred to as the master gland, is composed of two lobes—the anterior lobe or adenohypophysis and the posterior lobe or neurohypophysis. The anterior pituitary secretes six major hormones while the neurohypophysis secretes two. Hormonal secretion by the pituitary is almost completely controlled by the hypothalamus which receives information from most of the nervous system. This incoming information then influences the regulatory control of the hypothalamus upon the pituitary. The hypothalamus synthesizes and secretes releasing factors which cause release of anterior pituitary hormones and, for three of these hormones, inhibiting factors as well. The hormones secreted by the anterior pituitary regulate metabolic functions of the body through their effect upon target glands. The target glands stimulated by the pituitary hormones subsequently release their products into the bloodstream, and the level of the products then, via a negative feedback loop, controls the output and activity of the pituitary. The anterior pituitary hormones are:

Growth hormone which stimulates body growth.

Thyrotropin which controls secretion of thyroxine by the thyroid gland. Thyroxine regulates the rates of most chemical reactions in the body.

Corticotropin regulates adrenal cortical hormone secretions which influence metabolism of proteins, carbohydrates and fats.

Follicle stimulating hormone, luteinizing hormone and *luteotrophic hormone*—all of which promote the growth and/or function of the gonads.

Two important hormones secreted by the posterior pituitary gland are synthesized directly in the hypothalamus. They are antidiuretic hormone, which regulates water excretion by the kidneys, and oxytocin, which promotes milk release during suckling. A few abnormalities of the pituitary may be agenesis (failure to develop), hyperplasia (growth to an abnormally large size), and tumors.

These anatomical deviations may result in hyperfunction or hypofunction of the pituitary gland and one or more of the target glands controlled by the specific hormone released in unusual quantities.

35. The main topic of this passage is the
(A) location and importance of the pituitary gland.
(B) role of the pituitary gland in endocrine function.
(C) major pituitary hormones and their target organs.

36. According to the passage,
(A) the glands in the body can function properly only if the pituitary secretion is normal.
(B) the anterior lobe of the pituitary is more important than the posterior pituitary because it secretes more hormones.
(C) any disease state affecting the pituitary could lead to dysfunction of endocrine glands controlled by the pituitary.

37. It cannot be inferred from the passage that
(A) the pituitary as the master gland is responsible for all glandular secretions.
(B) derangements in pituitary function may lead to extreme variations in size, e.g., giantism or dwarfism.
(C) hypersecretion of thyroxine by the thyroid may be caused by increased pituitary secretion of thyrotropin.

38. Corticotrophin influences electrolyte balance within the system.
(A) The statement is supported by the passage.
(B) The statement is contradicted by the passage.
(C) The statement is neither supported nor contradicted by the passage.

There is a great deal of independence exhibited in the manner in which many systems of the body perform their functions; in contrast the cellular organization and units of the nervous system are mutually dependent upon each other to carry out their complicated integrative activities. The functioning of the nervous system depends on its receptors, pathways, neurotransmitters, synaptic terminals, polarities, and effectors. An impulse perceived must be conducted and transmitted along a series of nerve cells; it must be interpreted and processed; and finally an effector organ response must be elicited. It is this complex arrangement among receiving, transmitting, integrating, and effector stimulation and response that results in the meaningful activities visualized and characterized as behavior. To clarify the highly complex operations of the system, research by neuroanatomists, neurophysiologists, and neuroendocrinologists is necessary. The neuroanatomist might be likened to the electrical engineer who traces the telephone wires of a city while the other two groups are perhaps more interested in the switching and relay stations. The course of the peripheral and central pathways and the functional significance of the many centers of the spinal cord and brain have been determined mainly by the study of animals and humans. Certain parts of their systems had been destroyed by disease, injury, the use of chemical or physical agents, or, in animals, by experimental lesions. In recent years scientific interest has turned to the hypothalamus since many of the body's physiological and endocrine functions seem to be influenced by its activities. It is an integrative center that controls behavior patterns and many of the organisms' basic life functions. The center is controlled and modulated by higher centers of the nervous system and via a direct and indirect feedback loop of the endocrine system which it influences. No direct neuronal connections exist between the hypothalamus and the pituitary gland and, therefore, hypothalamic humoral factors reach the anterior lobe of the pituitary via its blood supply. Most experts regard the hypophysial portal system as the critical link between the brain and the pituitary as far as the transport of neurosecretions are concerned. The hypothalamus secretes releasing factors or hormones which in turn elicit in the pituitary the production of pituitary trophic hormones which then influence target organs in the organism. We may illustrate this point by carrying out a subtotal thyroidectomy in an animal. We may reason that thyroid secretions should fall, thyroid hormone levels in the blood should drop, hypothalamic areas would be alerted, and the releasing factor output initiated. This then results in an increase of pituitary thyroid trophic hormone output which will lead to increased thyroid productivity and compensatory action. If, however, a subtotal thyroidectomy and electrolytic lesion in the proper hypothalamic area are carried out at the same time, the compensatory activity does not occur.

The following statements are related to the passage. Based on the information given, select:
(A) if the statement is *supported by* the information in the passage.
(B) if the statement is *contradicted by* the information in the passage.
(C) if the statement is *neither supported nor contradicted by* information in the passage.

39. Successful operation of the nervous system results from the combined activity of its cells.

40. All systems of the body can function independently of one another.

41. The pituitary gland is influenced by indirect neuronal connections of the hypothalamus.

42. The hypothalamus is under the influence of a feedback mechanism.

43. Neurosecretions reach the pituitary by means of the portal system.

44. The parts of the nervous system are mutually dependent upon each other.

45. Neurotransmitters are key elements in the transmission and integration of impulses.

46. Behavior might be considered the sum total of all nervous system activity.

47. The neuroanatomist is not interested in the transmission process of an impulse.

48. Disease processes lead only to destruction.

49. The hypophysial portal system begins as capillaries which form veins; these then break up into capillaries again.

50. Thyroidectomy leads to compensatory activity of the thyroid gland.

51. Electrolytic lesions may be used to study the functions of the nervous system.

The trigeminal nerve via its mandibular and maxillary divisions supplies innervation for general sensation to the anterior 2/3 of the tongue and the mandibular and maxillary teeth. Sensation from all the mandibular teeth is mediated by the inferior alveolar nerve, which is a branch of the mandibular division. The maxillary division gives rise to the posterior superior alveolar nerve which innervates the three maxillary molar teeth except the mesio-buccal root of the first molar. The infraorbital nerve, also a branch of the maxillary division, divides into middle and anterior superior alveolar nerves. The former innervates the first and second bicuspid teeth and the mesio-buccal root of the first molar. The remainder of the anterior teeth, the canines and incisors, are supplied by the anterior superior alveolar nerve. To provide local anesthesia to specific teeth, the nerve or nerves innervating them must be anesthetized by injecting an anesthetic drug.

The following statements are related to the passage above. Based on the information given, select:
(A) if the statement is *supported by* the information in the passage.
(B) if the statement is *contradicted by* the information in the passage.
(C) if the statement is *neither supported nor contradicted by* information in the passage.

52. The maxillary nerve must be anesthetized to block the sensory innervation of the hard palate.

53. The maxillary teeth can be blocked by anesthetizing the maxillary division of the trigeminal nerve.

54. Sensation from the mandibular incisor teeth is mediated via the inferior alveolar nerve.

55. The special sense of taste from the anterior 2/3 of the tongue is perceived by the facial nerve.
56. The trigeminal nerve divides into three divisions.
57. Sensation from the second maxillary molar tooth may be blocked by anesthetizing the posterior superior alveolar nerve.
58. Inadequate anesthesia of the maxillary incisors of one side may be due to overlapping innervation from the anterior superior alveolar nerve of the opposite side.
59. Innervation of the maxillary bicuspids can be blocked by anesthetizing the anterior superior alveolar nerve.
60. A mandibular block can be accomplished by using the lingula of the mandible as a landmark.
61. The mental nerve is a branch of the inferior alveolar nerve.

The orbit is a cone-shaped bony structure with an apex directed posteriorly and a large anterior opening. It may be described as having a floor, a roof, and medial and lateral walls. The roof is formed mainly by the frontal bone anterior to a small portion of the sphenoid bone. The floor of the orbit from anterior to posterior is composed of the zygomatic, maxillary, and palatine bones. The lateral wall consists of portions of the zygomatic bone anteriorly and the sphenoid bone posteriorly. The medial wall from anterior to posterior is formed by the frontal process of the maxilla, the lacrimal bone, the ethmoid bone, and the sphenoid bone. Besides the anterior opening, the orbit communicates with other regions via nine openings. The infraorbital nerve enters the orbit through the inferior orbital fissure, then lies in the infraorbital groove in the floor and exits anteriorly through the infraorbital foramen. On its medial wall the anterior and posterior ethmoidal foramina transmit the anterior and posterior ethmoidal nerves, respectively. Posteriorly, near the apex of the orbit, the optic nerve and the ophthalmic artery enter via the optic canal. Also located near the apex, the superior orbital fissure transmits the cranial nerves III, IV, and VI and the ophthalmic division of cranial nerve V.

The following statements are related to the passage above. Based on the information given, select:
(A) if the statement is *supported by* the information in the passage.
(B) if the statement is *contradicted by* the information in the passage.
(C) if the statement is *neither supported nor contradicted by* information in the passage.

62. The superior ophthalmic vein exits the orbit via the superior orbital fissure.
63. The orbit is formed by portions of seven bones.
64. The anterior margin, or entrance of the orbit, is bounded by parts of the frontal, zygomatic, and maxillary bones.
65. The lacrimal bone forms part of the lateral wall of the orbit.
66. The superior orbital fissure transmits the optic nerve.
67. The anterior ethmoidal foramen is located between the ethmoid and frontal bones.
68. The ophthalmic artery is a branch of the internal carotid artery.

> STOP. If you finish before the time limit is up, go over your work for this section. DO NOT look at any other sections of the model examination. When your time limit is up, go on to the next section.

SKILLS ANALYSIS: QUANTITATIVE

85 MINUTES
68 QUESTIONS

The following questions are to be answered based on your knowledge of basic mathematical principles and relationships.

DIRECTIONS: Read each passage carefully, study each table or chart, then answer the questions following it. Consider only the material presented in answering the questions. Eliminate those choices that you think to be incorrect and mark the letter of your choice on the answer sheet.

Ten adult male guinea pigs were housed in individual cages in a room at 37°C. Five of the guinea pigs were fed an ascorbic acid deficient diet while the other five were fed standard guinea pig diet. Both groups were allowed access to water *ad libitum*. At weekly intervals the serum concentration of gamma globulin and lymphocyte reactivity were measured in both the experimental and control groups. The following graphs illustrate data collected from this experiment.

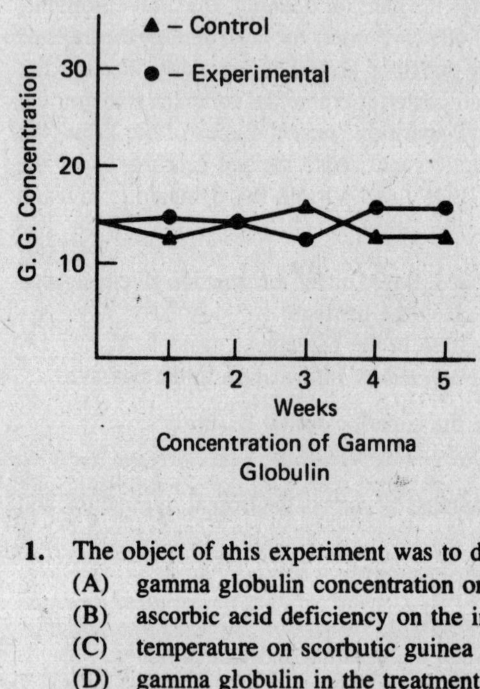

Concentration of Gamma Globulin

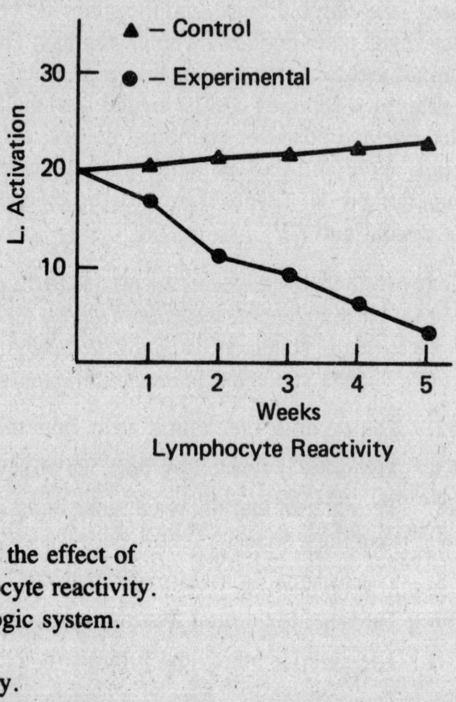

Lymphocyte Reactivity

1. The object of this experiment was to determine the effect of
   (A) gamma globulin concentration on lymphocyte reactivity.
   (B) ascorbic acid deficiency on the immunologic system.
   (C) temperature on scorbutic guinea pigs.
   (D) gamma globulin in the treatment of scurvy.

2. Another conclusion that can be reached from these data is
   (A) there are no sex differences in the response of guinea pigs to an ascorbic acid deficient diet.
   (B) temperature has a marked effect on gamma globulin concentration.
   (C) lymphocyte reactivity in the scorbutic guinea pig is independent of gamma globulin concentration.
   (D) gamma globulin concentration varies inversely with lymphocyte reactivity.

3. The experimenter may also conclude that
   (A) the scorbutic guinea pig probably has a partial immunologic deficiency.
   (B) lymphocyte reactivity varies widely in the normal guinea pig.
   (C) gamma globulin concentration is affected by biological rhythms.
   (D) there are no species differences in gamma globulin concentration.

A scientist sets up the following experiment. Ten male rats are placed in each of two cages. One cage is placed in a room regulated at a constant temperature of 37°C (group A) while the other cage is placed in a similar room kept at 45°C (group B). Food and water were provided *ad libitum* to both experimental sets. Food consumption, water consumption, ACTH blood level, and heart rate were determined for a period of ten days. The following bar graphs illustrated the results.

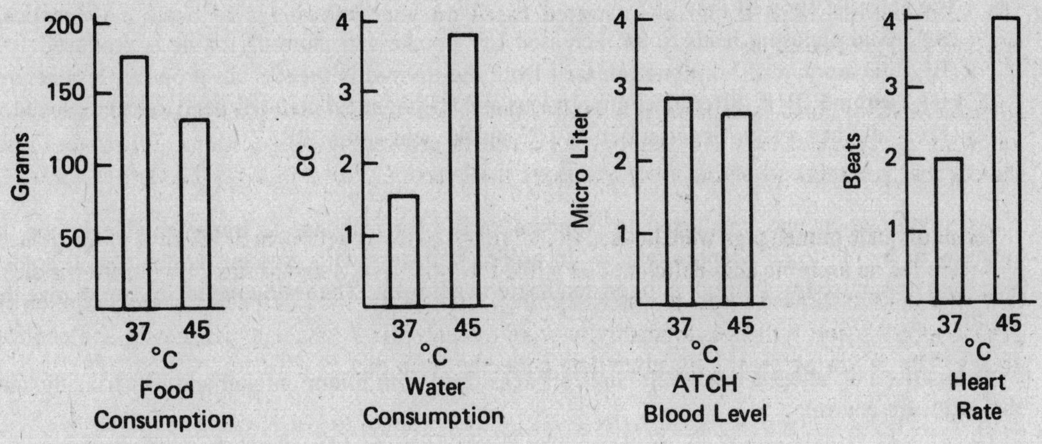

4. The objective of this experiment was to determine
   (A) food consumption in rats.
   (B) water consumption in rats.
   (C) heart rate in rats.
   (D) effect of temperature on rats.

5. The investigator after examining the four graphs can report that
   (A) at a higher temperature the rats were more active.
   (B) the rats maintained at 37°C developed a desire for water.
   (C) ACTH level is not markedly affected by the experimental conditions.
   (D) at higher temperatures more food is required.

Animals utilized in the following experiment were golden hamsters (*Mesocricetus auratus*). Normal diet consisted of Purina laboratory chow provided *ad libitum*. Animals were divided into 3 groups: group A—Control; group B—Cold exposed at 5°C ± 1°C for 5 days; group C—Cold exposed at 5°C ± 1°C for 30 days. Body weight (BW), Thyroid weight (TW), I^{131} uptake (I^{131}), and Serum Protein Bound Iodine^{127} (PBI^{127}) were measured.

Groups	BW grams	TW mg/100 gr BW	I^{131} Uptake 24 hours	Serum PBI µg/100 ml
A	97	5.89	5.88	4.09
B	79	5.55	15.37*	5.27*
C	110	6.25	11.06*	5.02*

*Fisher's "T" significant to .001

6. The scientist was interested to determine
   (A) whether hamsters can survive in the cold.
   (B) the basic metabolic rate of these animals.
   (C) the effect cold has on body weight.
   (D) the influence cold exposure has on several parameters used to assess thyroid function.

7. The data suggest that
   (A) the morphology of the thyroid gland was not altered since no significant weight change was recorded.
   (B) the thyroid gland is in a physiological state of hyperactivity in cold-exposed animals.
   (C) hamsters in the cold are in great distress.
   (D) the thyroid gland is in a physiological state of hypoactivity in cold-exposed animals.

8. The scientist showed that
   (A) cold exposure leads to an increased I^{131} uptake and more thyroxine is produced.
   (B) the amount of hormone released from the thyroid is greater but probably less active.
   (C) serum PBI^{127} differences are obvious and no statistical methods need to be employed.
   (D) cold has a significant effect on I^{131} uptake and serum PBI.

An investigation was conducted to compare early host response to transplantable tumor, as manifested by mast cell adenine release, in golden hamsters with growing tumor and in golden hamsters immunized with tumor antigen and bacteria adjuvant. The following tables summarize the results.

Comparison of adenine release in hamsters sensitized with tumor antigen and bacteria adjuvant and adjuvant controls.

TABLE 1

Groups	No. of Animals	% Release
Tumor antigen and bacteria adjuvant	40	66.51
Bacteria adjuvant	40	11.13

Comparison of adenine release in the golden hamster with growing tumor and untreated controls.

TABLE 2

Groups	No. of Animals	% Release
Tumor transplant	40	33.50
Normal controls	40	7.50

The following statements are related to the passage above. Based on the information given, select:
(A) if the statement is *supported by* the information in the passage.
(B) if the statement is *contradicted by* the information in the passage.
(C) if the statement is *neither supported nor contradicted by* information in the passage.

9. While adjuvant controls had more histamine release than untreated controls, their group average was significantly below that of the animals actively sensitized to tumor.

10. Animals that received transplants released half as much adenine as those given tumor antigen and bacteria adjuvant.

11. There is a significant difference between the tumor-bearing animals and their controls indicating some degree of enhanced cellular sensitization.

12. The experiments indicate that the immunological system of the golden hamster can respond with adenine release upon challenge with antigen prepared from that tumor.

13. Adenine release was a good parameter in the above study.

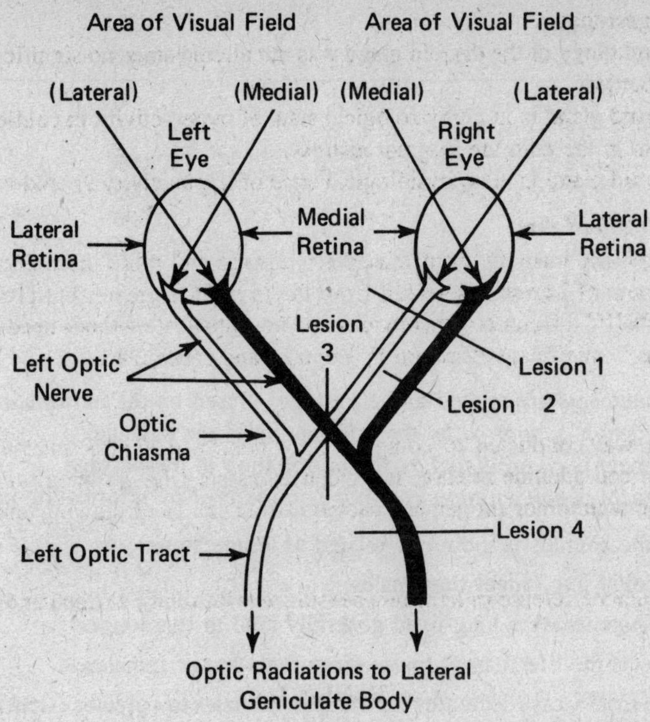

This diagram represents fiber pathways by which impulses from the retina are carried to the brain. Note components of each optic nerve and which retinal region, and corresponding visual field region, are carried by each optic nerve component.

Assume lesions 1-4 are functionally complete; that is, they result in complete sensory loss for a particular visual field region.

Based on location of the lesions in the preceding diagram, predict what the *visual field deficit* (black region) would be for each lesion.

14	15	16	17
Lesion 1	**Lesion 2**	**Lesion 3**	**Lesion 4**

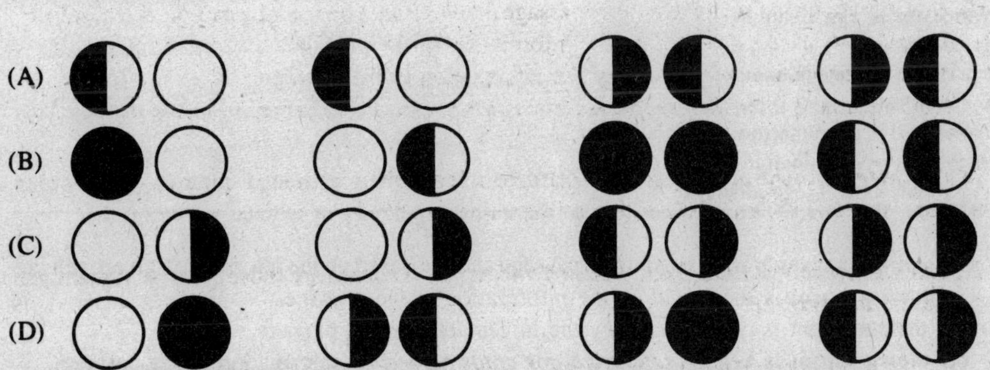

The life span of poikilotherms is related to the ambient temperature. In order to investigate the processes of aging in these animals one must keep meticulous records of the temperature. Various parameters, other than temperature, have been introduced into aging studies which alter the life span and one of these, Co^{60} γ rays, has been widely utilized with the following results.

No. of Animals	Temp. °C	Sex	Dose rads	Life Span days ± S.D.
100	18	M	0	55 ± 1
100	18	F	0	65 ± 2
100	18	M	10,000	40 ± 1
100	18	F	10,000	65 ± 2
100	20	M	10,000	55 ± 1
100	20	F	10,000	75 ± 2
100	20	M	0	65 ± 2
100	20	F	0	75 ± 2

The following statements are related to the passage. Based on the information, select:
(A) if the statement is *supported by* the information in the passage.
(B) if the statement is *contradicted by* the information in the passage.
(C) if the statement is *neither supported nor contradicted by* information in the passage.

18. Life span of the animals is indirectly related to temperature.

19. Females generally live longer than males.

20. Males whose parents were long-lived generally tend to live longer.

21. Radiation affects the life span of males more than that of females.

22. 10,000 rads of Co^{60} γ rays decreases the life span of males to a greater extent than a 2°C drop in temperature.

23. Males are less radiosensitive than females.

24. 10,000 rads of Co^{60} γ rays do not cause any chromosome damage.

25. Female life spans are not affected by 10,000 rads of Co^{60} γ rays.

The data below shows the result of an experiment concerning cell cooperation in the immune response. The experiment attempts to determine if thymus and bone marrow cells are required for antibody to be produced against egg albumin. Various donor cells (thymus or bone marrow) are injected into recipient mice whose immune system has been rendered nonresponsive by X-irradiation. Antibody levels were then determined in the serum of the recipient animals.

Donor Cells Injected	Antibody Production
1) Thymocytes + egg albumin	0
2) Thymocytes	0
3) Bone marrow + egg albumin	0
4) Bone marrow	0
5) Thymocytes + bone marrow + egg albumin	+++
6) Spleen cells + egg albumin	+++
7) Lymph node cells + egg albumin	+++

The following statements are related to the passage above. Based on the information given, select:
(A) if the statement is *supported by* the information in the passage.
(B) if the statement is *contradicted by* the information in the passage.
(C) if the statement is *neither supported nor contradicted by* information in the passage.

26. In this system, bone marrow and thymus cells are required for a mouse to make antibody to egg albumin.

27. Thymus cells or cells derived from the thymus are probably found in the spleen.

28. Thymus cells or bone marrow cells or both are capable of synthesizing antibody.

29. In the intact animal, the thymus would probably be important as a source of antibody.

A motor unit consists of the axon of a single motor neuron and all the skeletal muscle fibers it supplies. By the procedure of electromyography, membrane depolarization with resulting contraction of the muscle fibers can be detected. Briefly, electromyography involves positioning an electrode between muscle fibers and recording current flow on a suitable detection device such as an oscilloscope (CRO). Use this information and figures A and B to answer the next five questions.

Figure A

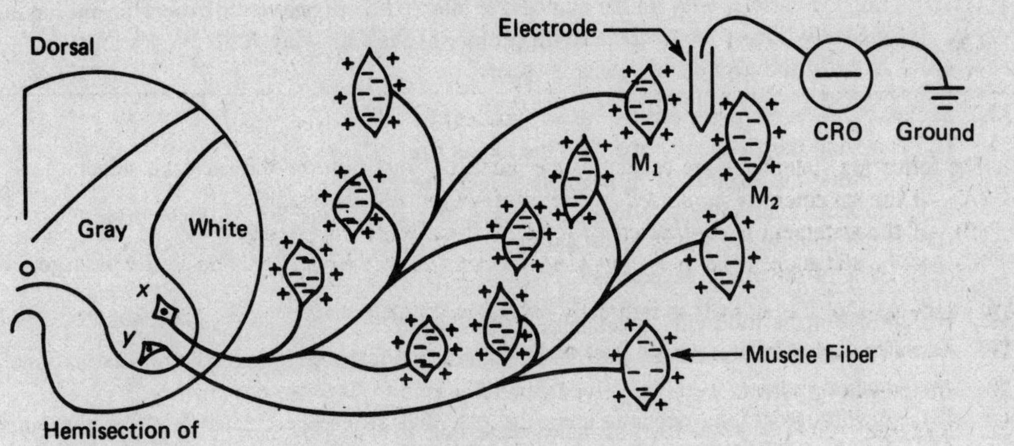

x and *y* represent cell bodies of motor neurons

Figure B

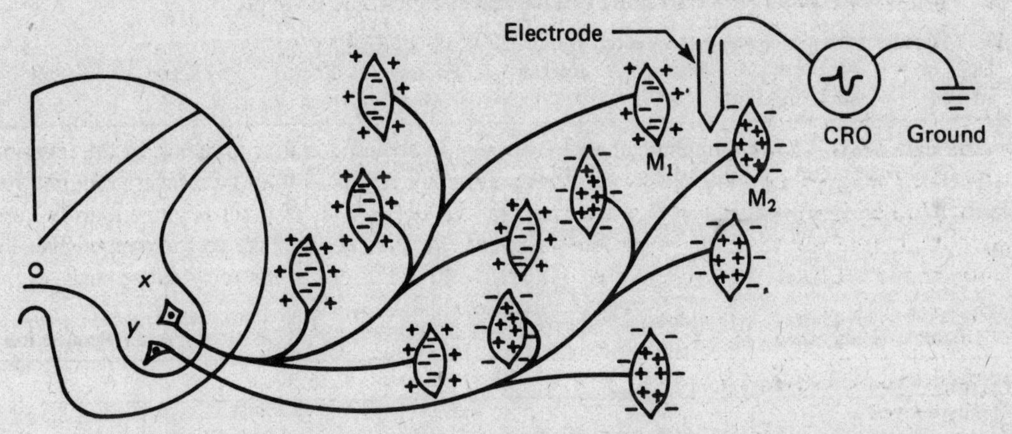

30. Which one of the following statements is correct?
(A) Cell bodies of motor neurons are anatomically located only in the dorsal gray matter of the spinal cord.
(B) Eleven (11) motor units are represented in figure A.
(C) All motor units represented in figure A are inactive (resting).
(D) A single axon supplies only a single muscle fiber.
(E) Motor units are unilaterally associated with the spinal cord.

31. Which one of the following statements is correct?
(A) Current will flow between muscle fibers m_1 and m_2 in figure A.
(B) Current will flow from muscle fiber m_1 toward fiber m_2 in figure B.
(C) All motor units shown in figure B are active.
(D) The axon of cell body *x* in figure B has fired.
(E) The cell membrane of muscle fiber m_1 in figure B has become permeable to sodium ions (Na^+).

32. Which one of the following statements is correct?
   (A) By inference from the given information, one would expect to find smaller motor units in an extraocular muscle (eye movements) than in the biceps muscle.
   (B) By inference from the given information, one would expect to find smaller motor units in the biceps muscle than in an extraocular muscle (eye movements).
   (C) The precision of movement permitted by a muscle is probably independent of the size of its motor units.
   (D) For two muscles with similar numbers of muscle fibers, one would expect the one having generally larger motor units to have more axons supplying it.
   (E) None of the above statements is correct.

33. Skeletal muscle response can be varied (graded) by
   (A) varying the frequency at which the axons fire.
   (B) varying the number of motor units which are active.
   (C) no means, because activity of the fibers of a given muscle is all or nothing.
   (D) both methods A and B given above.
   (E) none of the above responses.

34. Which one of the following statements is correct?
   (A) The electrode shown in figure A will record electrical activity directly from axons of cell bodies x and y.
   (B) Electromyography depends upon the potential difference created between the outer membranes of active and inactive skeletal muscle fibers.
   (C) Assuming fibers of equal size and equal mechanical advantage, firing of axon y in either figure A or figure B will produce the greatest contraction.
   (D) A lesion which destroys the cell body of axon x will cause the loss of six motor units.
   (E) None of the above statements is correct.

Days on Drug	Strength of Drug	Factor 1	Factor 2	Factor 3	Factor 4	Factor 5	Factor 6
0	0	12.5	33.0	26.5	9.3	6.2	71
6	0.05	10.7	17.0	47.0	9.6	5.0	73
6	0.10	3.0	9.8	64.0	7.0	4.8	80
6	0.20	4.8	8.9	49.2	2.4	4.6	62
6	0.50	12.0	7.9	55.8	10.7	6.6	73
12	0.05	12.5	9.8	23.1	12.9	11.0	45
12	0.10	4.4	7.9	40.7	8.3	9.1	49
12	0.20	6.8	7.2	43.0	5.9	16.7	54
12	0.50	3.9	5.7	34.2	5.3	23.0	43

The following statements are related to the table presented above. Based on the information given, select:
   (A) if the statement is *supported by* the information in the table.
   (B) if the statement is *contradicted by* the information in the table.
   (C) if the statement is *neither supported nor contradicted by* information in the table.

35. There is a significant difference in the analyzed factors between the 6-day and the 12-day treatment period.

36. The percentage of Factor 3 increased and that of Factor 2 decreased.

37. If there was an increase in Factor 3 and a decrease in Factor 2, there was a resultant rise in the Factor 3/Factor 2 ratio.

38. The proportion of isolated Factor 4 did not show any consistent trend.

39. The amount of Factor 6 did not demonstrate any obvious decline from the normal in the 6-day group; in the 12-day group, a decline is noted which could be due to decreased amounts of Factors 2 and 3.

40. The level of Factor 5 varied around control values in the 6-day treatment period but showed a definite rise in the 12-day group.

41. Results of the analysis of factors are dose dependent.

Graph 1

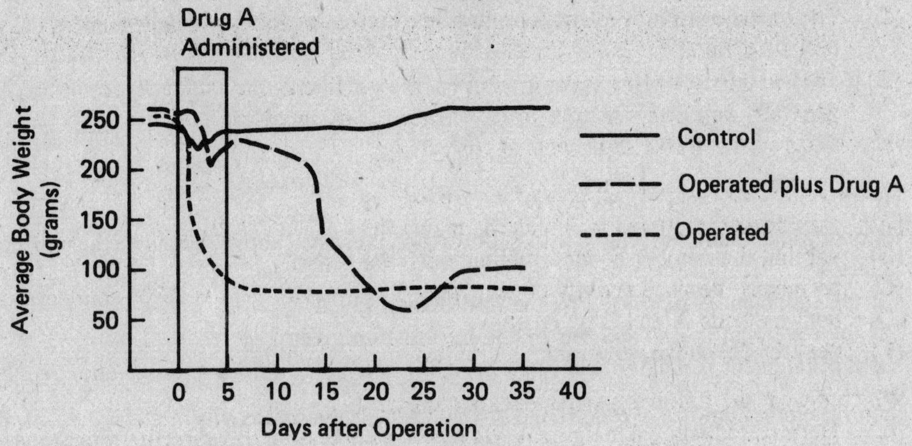

Graph 2

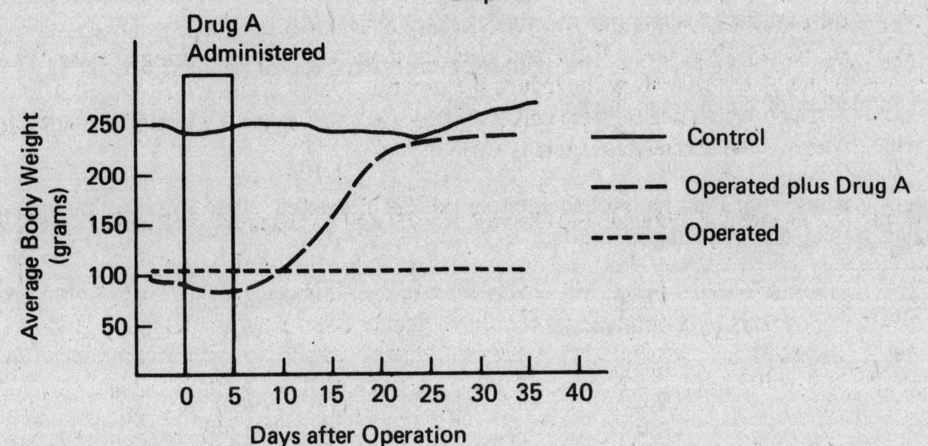

The following statements are related to the graphs presented above. Based on the information given, select:

(A) if the statement is *supported by* the information in the graph.
(B) if the statement is *contradicted by* the information in the graph.
(C) if the statement is *neither supported nor contradicted by* information in the graph.

42. In graph 1, the operated animals lacked a desire to eat for about 1 week, but then ate again to maintain their body weights at a reduced level.

43. In graph 1 the operated group that received drug A maintained their body weight while on the drug.

44. In graph 1, when the drug was discontinued, lack of desire to eat set in and remained until the animals' weights declined to the level of the animals that were operated on but did not receive the drug.

45. When we compare the results obtained in graph 1 to those obtained in graph 2, we note that reducing the body weight before the operation eliminated the lack of desire to eat.

46. Body weight was a significant factor in drug A action.

47. The experiments depicted were properly controlled.

The thickness of the human oral epithelium was measured in seven different areas of the oral cavity in thirty cadavers. The results are tabulated below.

Area	Average	Range
A	500μ	125-950μ
B	362μ	178-780μ
C	254μ	130-489μ
D	238μ	156-320μ
E	204μ	135-270μ
F	68μ	30-146μ
G	123μ	35-260μ

The following statements are related to the information presented above. Based on the information given, select:

(A) if the statement is *supported by* the information given.
(B) if the statement is *contradicted by* the information given.
(C) if the statement is *neither supported nor contradicted by* information given.

48. The oral epithelium has a wide range of thickness in the oral cavity.

49. The greatest range was observed in Area B.

50. The thinnest measurement was observed in Area G.

51. The results above are not valid since they were not attained from living subjects.

52. The range of thickness of the oral epithelium as observed was 30-950μ.

53. The median of the average thickness is 238μ.

Drug X is administered to a patient and a certain value is monitored. After 30 days of treatment the physician studies the following values:

% of Drug X Administered	Days	Mean Value of Y
0.000	0	6.51
0.025	3	6.61
0.05	3	7.39
0.10	3	7.90
0.20	3	8.00
0.025	15	9.02
0.05	15	9.07
0.10	15	9.27
0.20	15	9.53
0.025	30	10.80
0.05	30	11.80
0.10	30	12.00
0.20	30	12.51

The following statements are related to the information presented above. Based on the information given, select:

(A) if the statement is *supported by* the information given.
(B) if the statement is *contradicted by* the information given.
(C) if the statement is *neither supported nor contradicted by* information given.

54. The drug has an effect.

55. There is a dose relationship to the response.

56. The dose administered is of critical importance as can be deduced from the values.

57. The physician can expect the values of "Y" to continue to reflect dosage and period of treatment.

58. There were no side effects of this treatment.

59. The same values probably will be found if another patient were to be treated.

Distribution of relative amounts of radioiodinated amino acids in thyroid homogenates after administration of graded doses of PTU for three days.

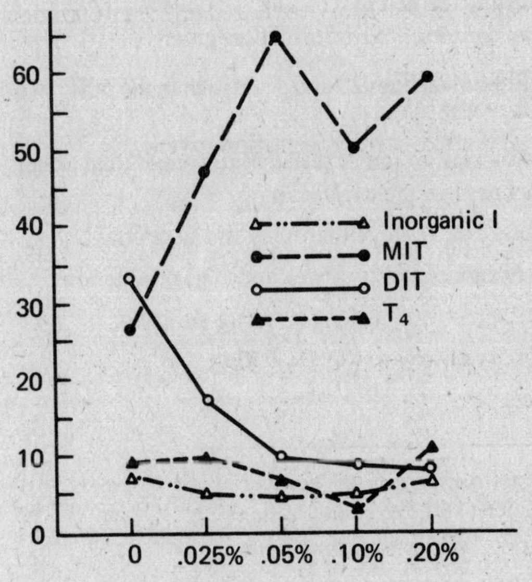

Distribution of relative amounts of radioiodinated amino acids in thyroid homogenates after administration of graded doses of PTU for six days.

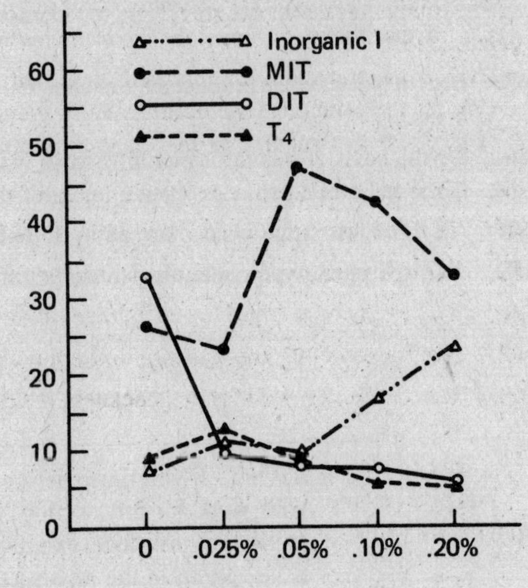

The following statements are related to the information presented above. Based on the information given, select:

(A) if the statement is *supported by* the information given.
(B) if the statement is *contradicted by* the information given.
(C) if the statement is *neither supported nor contradicted by* information given.

60. The percentage of labeled MIT increased and that of labeled DIT decreased; in the 6-day treated group there is a rise and then a decline in the MIT detected.

61. The amount of MIT rose from 26% in the controls to 64% in the 3-day experimentally treated animals.

62. A rise in the MIT/DIT ratio is observed.

63. The level of inorganic iodide varied around control values in the 3-day group but showed a definite rise in the 6-day group.

64. The enzymatic digest yields information on the distribution of radioactive iodide among the various iodinated amino acids studied.

Maloney sarcoma tumors were implanted in Brown Norway (BN), Lewis (Le), and Lewis-Brown Norway (LBN) rats. Studies were then done to determine the types and amounts of host serum antibodies produced against the protein components of the virus contained in the tumor cells. The following data are from one such experiment.

ANTIPROTEIN 30 ACTIVITY IN SERA OF TUMOR BEARING BN, Le, AND LBN RATS

Host	AgB Phenotype	Mg Equivalent Day 25 Post Implant	Anti-p30 Antibody Day 31 Post Implant
BN	3/3	3.5 ± 0.8	5.3 ± 1.7
LBN	1/3	2.4 ± 0.4	4.5 ± 1.4
Le	1/1	0.4 ± 0.1	0.4 ± 0.2

The following statements are related to the information presented. Based on the information given, select:

(A) if the statement is *supported by* the information given.
(B) if the statement is *contradicted by* the information given.
(C) if the statement is *neither contradicted nor supported by* information given.

65. Brown Norway rats produced more anti-p30 antibody at both 25 and 31 days than the other two hosts.

66. On the basis of this information, Brown Norway rats are more resistant to cancer than either LBN or Le rats.

67. All three hosts produced more anti-p30 antibody at 31 days than they did at 25 days.

68. An AgB phenotype containing threes seems to be related to lower anti-p30 production.

STOP. If you finish before the time limit is up, go over your work for this section. DO NOT look at any other sections of the model examination. When your time limit is up, go on to the next section.

Model Test B Answers*

SCIENCE KNOWLEDGE

Biology

1. C
2. C
3. D
4. C
5. E
6. C
7. C
8. A
9. D
10. C
11. D
12. D
13. A
14. E
15. D
16. B
17. D
18. E
19. C
20. B
21. C
22. D
23. B
24. A
25. A
26. D
27. C
28. B
29. B
30. A
31. E
32. B
33. D
34. B
35. B
36. B
37. C
38. D

Chemistry

1. D
2. A
3. D
4. C
5. B
6. C
7. C
8. A
9. D
10. E
11. B
12. B
13. D
14. C
15. B
16. C
17. C
18. A
19. B
20. E
21. D
22. B
23. D
24. B
25. D
26. A
27. B
28. C
29. A
30. C
31. B
32. A
33. D
34. A
35. E
36. C
37. E
38. D
39. B
40. B
41. C
42. B
43. D
44. B
45. C
46. C
47. D
48. B
49. D

Physics

1. C
2. A
3. B
4. B
5. E
6. E
7. A
8. C
9. E
10. D
11. C
12. C
13. C
14. B
15. A
16. A
17. C
18. D
19. A
20. D
21. B
22. A
23. A
24. C
25. E
26. B
27. A
28. C
29. C
30. A
31. E
32. B
33. D
34. D
35. C
36. C
37. A
38. B

*Explanations for science answers can be found on p. 193.

SCIENCE PROBLEMS

1. B
2. A
3. E
4. E
5. B
6. E
7. B
8. A
9. E
10. D
11. B
12. B
13. A
14. A
15. B
16. C
17. A
18. D
19. C
20. A
21. B
22. E
23. A
24. B
25. A
26. A
27. B
28. A
29. C
30. B
31. C
32. D
33. E
34. C
35. B
36. B
37. D
38. B
39. A
40. A
41. E
42. A
43. A
44. C
45. B
46. C
47. C
48. E
49. A
50. B
51. B
52. E
53. E
54. A
55. D
56. E
57. C
58. E
59. E
60. B
61. C
62. B
63. E
64. A
65. D
66. A

SKILLS ANALYSIS: READING

1. A
2. B
3. A
4. A
5. C
6. A
7. B
8. A
9. B
10. A
11. B
12. A
13. D
14. B
15. C
16. C
17. B
18. A
19. A
20. C
21. A
22. C
23. A
24. A
25. A
26. C
27. B
28. A
29. C
30. B
31. C
32. A
33. C
34. C
35. B
36. C
37. A
38. C
39. A
40. B
41. C
42. A
43. A
44. A
45. C
46. A
47. B
48. B
49. C
50. B
51. A
52. C
53. A
54. A
55. C
56. C
57. A
58. C
59. B
60. C
61. C
62. C
63. A
64. A
65. B
66. B
67. C
68. C

SKILLS ANALYSIS: QUANTITATIVE

1. B
2. C
3. A
4. D
5. C
6. D
7. B
8. D
9. A
10. A
11. C
12. A
13. A
14. D
15. B
16. C
17. B
18. A
19. A
20. C
21. A
22. A
23. B
24. C
25. A
26. A
27. A
28. C
29. B
30. C
31. B
32. A
33. D
34. B
35. B
36. A
37. A
38. A
39. A
40. A
41. B
42. A
43. A
44. A
45. A
46. A
47. B
48. A
49. B
50. B
51. C
52. A
53. A
54. A
55. A
56. B
57. C
58. C
59. C
60. A
61. A
62. A
63. A
64. A
65. A
66. C
67. B
68. B

Explanation of Answers for Science Questions-Model Test B

SCIENCE KNOWLEDGE

Biology

1. (C) The gastric mucosa secretes hydrochloric acid; mucin, and the enzymes rennin, pepsin, and lipase. An average of 2 to 3 liters is secreted within a 24 hour time period. The pH of gastric juice usually varies from 0.9 to 1.5. This acidity allows pepsin to act while it inhibits ptyalin (salivary amylase). Food usually remains in the stomach for 3 to 4 hours.

2. (C) Multiple alleles determine the human blood types. The common blood types are: A, B, AB, and O. Red blood cells of a person classified as "Type A" contain "Agglutinogen A" and their serum contains "Agglutinin b." Type AB contains agglutinogens A and B but no agglutinins. Type O possesses no agglutinogens but the serum carries a + b agglutinins. Rhesus (Rh) agglutinogen is present in humans and is represented by a dominant gene R. The agglutinogen of an Rh positive fetus passes across the placenta, enters the maternal blood stream and elicits the production of an agglutinin (antibody) by the mother. The agglutinin passes into the circulation of the fetus and if present in sufficient concentration can produce agglutination, at times fatal to the developing fetus.

3. (D) Light must penetrate the retina to reach the rods and cones. The fovea centralis is the central portion of the macula lutea; it is the region of sharpest vision. It is thinner than the rest of the retina and only cones are present. Rods are absent from this area. Cones are regarded as color receptors, while rods are achromatic receptors of low intensity light.

4. (C) In a parfocal optical microscope the objective lenses are so constructed or mounted that one may change from one to another and the image remains focused; the lenses have focal points in the same plane.

5. (E) The reproductive cycle is under hormonal regulation; gonadotropic hormones of the pituitary (anterior lobe) stimulate the ovaries to produce a mature egg. The pituitary and ovaries have a reciprocal effect upon each other. FSH (follicle stimulating hormone) from the pituitary elicits estrogen production from the developing follicle. When estrogen concentration reaches a certain blood level, it inhibits FSH production. At that time the egg is discharged and the cells lining the follicle come under the influence of another gonadotropin LH (luteinizing hormone) which influences the development of the corpus luteum. The corpus luteum produces the hormone progesterone which influences the wall of the uterus in preparation for implantation. As the concentration of progesterone rises, LH production is checked. If fertilization has occurred, the production of FSH is curtailed throughout the period of gestation through the production of estrogen by the placenta and ovary. If fertilization does not occur, the cycle begins anew.

6. (C) Langerhans described the beta cells (within the islets of Langerhans) of the pancreas which produce insulin that affects the metabolism of glucose directly. Fat and protein are indirectly affected. After a meal the level of blood sugar rises eliciting the production of insulin which stimulates the absorption of glucose by the cells and helps in its conversion to glycogen. Insulin deficiency leads to high blood sugar levels and the disease called diabetes mellitus.

7. (C) Anterior-posterior diameters of eyeballs vary. A long eye is considered near-sighted or myopic; light rays come to focus before they reach the retina; therefore, a concave lens if needed for correction. A short eye results in far-sightness or hypermetropia; light rays would come to focus in back of the retina and, therefore, a convex lens is needed for correction.

8. (A) Development in animals results from the cleavage divisions of the zygote. The zygote divides first into two cells, then these divide into four, and so on, until it becomes a cell mass called the morula. Through more divisions the morula becomes a hollow ball of cells which is called the blastula.

9. (D) The mystery of the origin of life still eludes

us. Two basic concepts are proposed: 1. Vitalistic—a vital force created life; 2. Mechanistic—forces of nature were instrumental. Oparin suggested that the primitive atmosphere was made up of gases like methane, ammonia, hydrogen, and water vapor. Miller discharged electricity through the above environment and found after a week, a variety of organic compounds, including amino acids were produced. Combinations of these then could theoretically have led to the build-up of complex molecules and eventually protoplasm.

10. (C) This is the general body plan, a slight modification as found in the annelids.

11. (D) This is a disease which results from eating poorly cooked pork which contains *Trichinella spiralis*. Eosinophilia, nausea, fever, diarrhea, stiffness, and painful swelling of muscles are characteristic.

12. (D) Epithelium is a group of cells forming a tissue. Epithelium lines the gut, the respiratory system, the genito-urinary system and forms the epidermis. It, therefore, can protect, secrete, and absorb.

13. (A) Symbiosis is defined as association of organisms from which each member derives some advantage. Commensalism is defined as association of organisms which share the same food, etc. (one utilizing the leftovers from the other). Saprophytism is defined as organisms living on dead organisms or products of living ones; they bring about putrefaction or decay. Parasitism is defined as organisms that live in or on their hosts and feed on their tissues or their products.

14. (E) A contractile vacuole is found in fresh-water protozoa; it periodically expels water to the outside. In this manner excess water leaves the cell. Due to its osmotic relationship with its environment, water is entering and the cell must maintain the water level of its protoplasm.

15. (D) A backcross consists of crossing a dominant phenotype with a pure homozygous recessive. In this manner the breeder determines if the phenotype is heterozygous or homozygous.

16. (B) Tonus refers to muscular activity in which a shortened condition is maintained for a prolonged period. Visceral muscle is the outstanding example. The word tonus can be applied to any sustained process which is the result of probable regularly repeated excitation.

17. (D) The gray matter of the spinal cord is divided into two (2) components: motor and receptor. The motor part is comprised of the ventral and intermediolateral columns and gives rise to the ventral roots. Ventral horn cells supply voluntary muscles; intermediolateral cells give rise to preganglionic sympathetic fibers of the thoraco-lumbar system. The receptor portion is located in the dorsal horn. The white matter of the spinal cord is composed of nerve fibers in a network of connective tissue.

18. (E) Many activities are attributed to the hypothalamus. Lesions of this area may produce diabetes insipidus, obesity, sexual dystrophy, and loss of temperature control.

19. (C) Blood pressure is usually measured by placing the sphygmomanometer cuff around the arm compressing the brachial artery and vein. Maximum blood pressure is obtained during ventricular contraction (systole); in our case 160. Minimum blood pressure indicates ventricular rest (diastole); in our case 90.

20. (B) Mesoderm is the middle layer of the three primary germ layers. The following are considered to be of mesodermal origin:
   1. connective tissue, cartilage, and bone
   2. striated and smooth muscle
   3. blood and lymph cells
   4. walls of the circulatory system
   5. genito-urinary system
   6. spleen

21. (C) The cause of muscle fatigue is said to be the accumulated anaerobically produced lactic acid. Lactic acid may later be broken down into carbon dioxide and water for elimination, or it may be converted into glycogen and stored for future use.

22. (D) The autonomic nervous system innervates all smooth muscle, and glands. The autonomic nervous system is divided into a sympathetic (flight and fight) component and parasympathetic (maintains homeostasis) component. It exerts important influences on the intrinsic eye musculature; skin glands; and the cardiovascular, respiratory, endocrine, and reproductive systems. Fear, rage, pain, etc., evoke sympathetic activity which mobilizes the resources of the body. Gastrointestinal activity is curtailed; heart rate and blood pressure increase; and coronary arteries and bronchioles dilate.

23. (B) Alternating periods of light and darkness and the proportion thereof are extremely important to the functioning (cycles) of plant and animal life observed.

24. (A) See also question 5. FSH stimulates the production of estrogen by the developing follicle. LH

stimulates the production of progesterone by the corpus luteum.

25. (A) Directly underlying epithelium is found a homogeneous, noncellular material, composed of reticular fibers and protein polysaccharides which serves to bind down the tissue; this structure is the basement membrane.

26. (D) An anticoagulant is a substance that prevents or retards coagulation of blood. Heparin is an acid mucopolysaccharide; it occurs most abundantly in the liver. Aspirin (acetylsalicylic acid) is an analgesic, antipyretic, antirheumatic compound that possesses anticoagulant properties. Dicumarol is a trademark for bishydroxycoumarin, an excellent anticoagulant.

27. (C) A niche is defined as the position or status that an organism occupies with respect to the other organisms with which it associates.

28. (B) At the time of puberty usually an increase in sex drive, beard growth, and development of a deeper voice are experienced. The external genitalia are part of the organism and will develop and grow as the organism does. They are genetically determined and are a primary characteristic of the male.

29. (B) The cell bodies of the motor (efferent) system are located in the ventral horns (gray matter) of the spinal cord and their fibers leave the cord via ventral (anterior) roots which join with the dorsal (sensory) roots to form a spinal nerve. If a spinal nerve were sectioned, loss of both sensation and motor activity would be experienced. In this case only motor functions were interrupted.

30. (A) Reception via afferent (sensory) receptors, conduction via sensory fibers to the central nervous system (spinal cord), and propagation of the impulses to the efferent (motor) system will then result in appropriate action. Usually most reflex arcs include one association neuron in the spinal cord between their afferent and efferent fibers. The medulla is not a part of the spinal cord; it is a part of the brain, and usually reflex arcs do not utilize higher centers.

31. (E) This is a definition and should be memorized.

32. (B) The medulla is a part of the brain stem and connects to the spinal cord at the foramen magnum. The following cranial nerves are associated with the medulla: a, XII—hypoglossal nerve; b, XI—spinal accessory nerve; c, X—vagus nerve; d, IX—glossopharyngeal nerve; e, VIII—stato-acoustic nerve; and f, portions of the facial nerve (VII). The vagus nerve (X) is the most important parasympathetic nerve. Stimulation of vagal fibers slows the heart rate; constricts the smooth muscles of the bronchial tree; stimulates secretion by the bronchial mucosa; and promotes peristalsis, gastric, and pancreatic secretions. Blood pressure control also involves aortic body, carotid sinus, and carotid body receptor modulation by the glossopharyngeal (IX) and vagus (X) nerves.

33. (D) The percentage of white blood cells varies as listed:

Agranular cells:	
1. lymphocytes	20-25%
2. monocytes	3-8%
Granular cells:	
1. neutrophils	65-75%
2. eosinophils	2-5%
3. basophils	0.5% or less

34. (B) Bile is secreted by the liver, stored and concentrated in the gall bladder and poured into the duodenum. It contains bile salts, cholesterol, lecithin, fat, pigments, and mucin. It aids in the emulsification, digestion, and absorption of fat. It contributes to the alkalinization of the intestines.

35. (B) The class Cyclostomata of the phylum Chordata and sub-phylum Craniata are jawless, finless, without scales or bony plates, have a sucking mouth and possess 6-14 gill slits in the adult. The cyclostomes are the lampreys and hag-fishes.

36. (B) The cell membrane is semipermeable, can be resolved by the electron microscope, is about 75 Å wide and appears on electron micrographs as two (2) dark lines with a light space between them. Evidence indicates that the two bordering dark lines are composed of proteins while the middle (light) layer contains lipids.

37. (C) If more than two stimuli are given to a muscle in rapid succession, a partial fusion of all contractions results. The contractions occur before relaxation can take place or is completed. If a contraction is steadily maintained and no relaxation occurs between separate stimuli, the contraction is known as tetanus.

38. (D) Use your basic genetic knowledge.
1. 100% aa
2. 25% AA, 50% Aa, 25% aa
3. 100 Aa
4. 50% Aa, 50% aa

Chemistry

1. **(D)** Fatty acids are esterified with glycerol to form triglycerides (commonly known as fat). Fatty acid is thus a component of the larger triglyceride molecule (fat) as glucose is a component of the polysaccharides listed here (starch, glycogen and cellulose).

2. **(A)** The reaction of sodium alkoxide with alkyl halide is often used in the synthesis of ethers. This is known as the Williamson synthesis.

3. **(D)** Alcohols are not appreciably acidic. Methanol (answer A) and cyclohexanol (B) are alcohols. Phenols (C,D) are acidic as a result of resonance of the ring. Nitro substituents increase the acidity of phenols through inductive and resonance effects.

4. **(C)** Ethers are generally unreactive and for this reason often serve as the solvent in various reactions. They may, however, be cleaved with strong halogen acids (hydrogen iodide being most reactive).

5. **(B)** This reaction utilizes the activating effect of the carbonyl replacement of an alpha-hydrogen by halogen. This is a useful reaction which allows the introduction of a functional group on the alpha-carbon.

6. **(C)** Glucose is an aldohexose, a reducing sugar, and a monosaccharide. It has a number of asymmetric centers and possesses optical activity. It is *not* a disaccharide.

7. **(C)** Ammoniacal silver nitrate is reduced and produces a silver mirror in the presence of aldehydes but not ketones.

8. **(A)** Periodate (HIO_4) will oxidize only vicinal hydroxyls (i.e., on adjacent carbon atoms).

9. **(D)** Hydrogen bonding occurs between alcohol molecules as between water molecules to produce the comparatively high boiling points of alcohols.

10. **(E)** A catalyst is a substance which increases the velocity of a chemical reaction. The substance remains chemically unaltered and its concentration remains the same throughout the reaction.

11. **(B)** Note that the question asks for *nitrogenous* metabolic waste products. The compounds in answer A are *not* nitrogenous. Amino acids, glucosamine, and nucleic acids (DNA or RNA) are not ordinarily metabolic waste products.

12. **(B)** The double bonds in the unsaturated fatty acids of margarine and shortening are susceptible to oxidative rancidity. Hydrogenation decreases the rancidity by decreasing the number of double bonds.

13. **(D)** Since more saturated fatty acids (and fats) have a higher melting point, hydrogenation raises the melting point.

14. **(C)** Under the stated conditions aldehyde (except formaldehyde) $\rightarrow$ secondary alcohol; carboxylic acid $\rightarrow$ methane + carboxylic acid; ester $\rightarrow$ ketone; ketone $\rightarrow$ tertiary alcohol.

15. **(B)** *Hypertonic:* the solution has a higher osmotic pressure than the solution with which it is compared. There is a higher concentration of solute and a lower concentration of solvent. *Hypotonic:* a lower concentration of solute and a higher concentration of solvent are present. *Isotonic:* both solutions have the same osmotic pressure.

16. **(C)** One mole of any compound contains 6.02×10^{23} molecules. Two moles of carbon dioxide would contain one mole of molecules more than that contained by one mole of oxygen.

17. **(C)** Fatty acids are the long chain monocarboxylic acids found in fats. Ordinarily they contain an even number of carbon atoms such as $CH_3(CH_2)_{12}COOH$

18. **(A)** Acid salts are formed by di- and tribasic acids. For example, H_2CO_3 can form the acid salt ($NaHCO_3$) known as sodium hydrogen carbonate or sodium bicarbonate.

19. **(B)** Acetals are formed from the reaction of two moles of alcohol with one mole of aldehyde. The reaction of equimolar quantities of alcohol and aldehyde produces a hemiacetal.

20. **(E)** The capture of a neutron by the nucleus increases the atomic weight by one and has no effect on the atomic number. Negatron decay (loss of a negative electron from the nucleus) increases the atomic number by one without appreciable effect on the atomic weight. The net effect of the two events is to increase both the atomic weight and the atomic number by one.

21. **(D)** NaOH may be called a base because it produces OH^- ions, but it is more properly called a base because it consumes H^+ ions.

22. **(B)** Cholesterol is an intermediate in the biosynthesis of steroid hormones, bile acids, and vitamin D_3. Essential fatty acids and essential amino acids must be consumed by the organism in the diet.

23. **(D)** Prostaglandins are potent compounds; they are structurally unique in the respect that they contain 20 carbon atoms and are formed from essential fatty acids. They affect the nervous system, circulation, reproductive organs, and metabolism.

24. **(B)** 2-Butyne (or dimethylacetylene) contains a triple bond between C_2 and C_3. Catalytic hydrogenation may be utilized to add hydrogen across the triple bond, creating a cis-double bond.

25. **(D)** Concentrated sulfuric acid protonates double or triple bonds to produce the polar carbonium ion. This will aid in solubilizing these unsaturated compounds (further reactions, however, may preclude simple recovery of the alkenes and alkynes). Saturated hydrocarbons do not react and are essentially insoluble.

26. **(A)** Dehydrohalogenation of an alkyl halide is a good reaction for the production of an alkene. In choosing between a primary halide and a secondary halide, remember that the adjacent carbon having the smaller number of hydrogen atoms will lose hydrogen. (That is, answer B would produce 2-butene.) Sulfuric acid dehydration of the primary alcohol produces the ether as a major product depending on conditions. Hydrogenation of the alkyne with Pt catalyst would probably not stop at the alkene, but the unsaturation is not in the right position anyway.

27. **(B)** Remember that the nitro group withdraws electrons from the ring and thus deactivates the ring to electrophilic substitution reactions. Although the ring has been deactivated, the highest electron density is in the meta-position.

28. **(C)** See explanation for question 27.

29. **(A)** Beta decay (negatron loss) converts a neutron to a proton plus a negatron. Retention of the proton by the nucleus results in an increase in atomic number (i.e., number of protons) and only a negligible decrease in atomic weight.

30. **(C)** The thermal decomposition of $KClO_3$ to produce oxygen will occur if the temperature is sufficiently high. The addition of a catalyst MnO_2 will decrease the activation energy and increase the rate at a lower temperature.

31. **(B)** See explanation for question 30.

32. **(A)** Long hydrocarbon chains have substantial flexibility. The major problem in preparing large ring compounds is that of bringing the reactive groups close enough to each other to effect ring closure. Once formed, these compounds possess a high degree of stability.

33. **(D)** In the bromination of benzene, Br^+ is the electrophile and benzene is the nucleophile.

34. **(A)** As with any reaction, the equilibrium constant is equal to the arithmetic product of the concentration of the species produced divided by the concentration of the unreacted species.

35. **(E)** Iso-octane is assigned an octane rating of 100, and n-heptane has an octane rating of zero. In the case of a simple mixture of the two compounds, the percentage of iso-octane will be equal to the octane rating.

36. **(C)** Compound 3 has two asymmetric centers (carbons 2 and 3), but there is a plane of symmetry between carbons 2 and 3. This is called a meso compound and is devoid of optical activity. Compound 1 is not a meso compound since the functional groups on carbons 1 and 4 are different and there is no plane of symmetry.

37. **(E)** A racemic mixture contains equal proportions of levorotatory and dextrorotatory isomers.

38. **(D)** A stronger acid will be more highly ionized, will have a larger ionization constant (i.e., K_a) and will produce a lower pH for a given acid concentration. But $pK_a = \log(1/K_a)$. Therefore a larger K_a will correspond to a smaller pK_a. For this reason a stronger acid has a smaller pK_a.

39. **(B)** Ammoniacal silver nitrate (Tollens' reagent) is commonly used to differentiate between aldehydes and ketones. The formation of the silver mirror indicates the presence of an aldehyde, but 2-butanone is a ketone.

40. **(B)** The reaction of a nonmetal and oxygen does not produce a salt.

41. **(C)** The strongest, most polar bond of those listed is the C-F bond.

42. **(B)** In the passage of a gas through a pinhole, the rate of exiting is inversely proportional to the square root of molecular weight.
MW C_2H_4 is approximately 28.
MW CO_2 is approximately 44.
Since there is an inverse relationship, C_2H_4 will exit more rapidly and more CO_2 will remain behind.

43. **(D)** The base simply reacts with each of the available hydrogens to produce the trisodium salt.

44. **(B)** The hydrogen content of fat is highest, and its oxidation produces the most water for a given weight.

45. **(C)** The definition of an ion is an atom or group of atoms that have either lost or gained one or more electrons.

46. **(C)** The atomic number is equal to the number of protons, all of which are in the nucleus.

47. **(D)** The statements refer to common sense general characteristics of fats.

48. **(B)** Brownian movement is a constant and spontaneous movement due to the kinetic energy of matter. It is physical due to molecular bombardment of suspended particles. If a particle is hit in one place, then another, etc., it will be displaced first in one direction and then in another, etc., and the particles will oscillate in all planes.

49. **(D)** A Grignard reagent (RMgX) reacts with reactive hydrogen to produce RH; a carboxylic acid, acetylene, or an alcohol has sufficiently reactive hydrogen. A Grignard reagent will react with an aldehyde (R′ — CHO) to produce an organometallic compound which may be hydrolyzed to a secondary alcohol.

Physics

1. **(C)** Work is equal to force times distance. A mass of 200 lb. exerts a force of 200 lb. with our gravitational acceleration. 200 lb. × 60 ft. = 12,000 ft.-lb.

2. **(C)** $\frac{P_1V_1}{T_1} = \frac{P_2V_2}{T_2}$ where P is pressure, V is volume, and T is temperature in °K. STP (standard temperature and pressure) is 273°K and 1 atm pressure.

$$\frac{1 \times 4}{273} = \frac{2V_2}{819°K}$$

$$V_2 = 6$$

3. **(B)** Boyle's law states that the product of volume and pressure of a gas is a constant at constant temperature.

$$P_1V_1 = P_2V_2$$

$$V_2 = \frac{P_1}{P_2}V_1$$

If pressure is doubled $\frac{P_1}{P_2} = \frac{1}{2}$. Thus $V_2 = \frac{1}{2}V_1$

4. **(B)** $S = V_it - \frac{gt^2}{2}$. S, the distance, equals zero when the object has returned. V_i, the initial velocity, equals 64 ft/sec. g, the acceleration of gravity equals 32 ft/sec.²

$$0 = 64t - \frac{32t^2}{2} = 64t - 16t^2$$

$$16t^2 - 64t = 0$$

Factoring, $t(16t - 64) = 0$. When the product equals zero, one of the factors must equal zero.

Either $t = 0$ (not valid)

or $16t - 64 = 0$

and $t = \frac{64}{16} = 4$ sec.

5. **(E)** The boiling point of a liquid is the temperature at which the vapor pressure of the liquid equals the external pressure to which the system is subjected.

6. **(E)** The kinetic molecular theory (or the kinetic theory of gases) tells us that the temperature (°K) is a measure of the average kinetic energy of a gas without respect to the identity of the gas.

7. **(A)** The volume of the particles is equal to the increase in liquid level (i.e., 45 − 30 = 15) $\frac{90\text{ g}}{15\text{ ml}} = 6$ g/ml.

8. **(C)** In the absence of friction the horizontal component requires no work. Thus the same work is required to raise the mass the same height whether directly or on an inclined plane.

9. **(E)** Neither the wave theory nor particle theory alone satisfactorily explains the nature of light; its properties are best explained by a combination of the two theories.

10. **(D)** $S = V_0t + \frac{1}{2}gt^2$

$$S = (0)t + \tfrac{1}{2}(32)(4)^2$$

$$S = 0 + 16(16) = 256 \text{ ft.}$$

11. **(C)** Only 2 factors play a role; the coin has 2 sides, 1 head and 1 tail, and the gambler's chance is 50%. No previous experience or odds apply.

12. **(C)** $V = at$; $t = 30$ sec. $= \frac{30}{3600}$ hr.

$$600 = a\frac{30}{3600} = \frac{a}{120}$$

$a = 72{,}000$ mi./hr.².

In a problem like this, be sure that you convert all your units to agree (as we converted sec. to hrs. in this problem in order that all time would be in hrs.).

13. **(C)** Since the resultant force is the difference between the two forces, the two forces must be directly opposing each other (i.e., at 180°).

14. **(B)** The gravitational acceleration on a body is unaffected by the horizontal velocity. Thus the two cannonballs will strike the ground simultaneously.

15. **(A)** Momentum = mv = $m_1v_1 + m_2v_2$ = (50)(0.2) + (10)(0) = 10 gm-m/sec.

16. **(A)** Momentum is conserved.

17. **(C)** Momentum is conserved. 10 gm-m/sec. = (50 + 10)V. $V = \frac{10}{60} = 0.17$ m/sec.

18. **(D)** Kinetic energy = $\frac{1}{2}mv^2 = \frac{60}{2}(0.17)^2$
$= 30(0.0289)$
$= 0.867$ gm gm-m²/sec.².

19. **(A)** If the half-life is 7.5 days, then 15 days would represent two half-lives. In the first half-life 50% will be lost, and in the second half-life 50% of the remainder will be lost.
Remainder = 0.5^n and n = number of half-lives.
Remainder = $(0.5)^2 = 0.25$ or 25%

20. **(D)** There is no sound in a vacuum.

21. **(B)** Surface tension is the explanation for the fact that a steel needle may be floated on water in spite of the fact that steel is denser. The addition of detergent decreases surface tension, and the needle will sink.

22. **(A)** This question is related to the Doppler effect. Since the point of generation of the sound is approaching, the frequency of the tone as perceived by the stationary listener will be higher. After the locomotive has passed and is moving away, the frequency perceived is lower.

23. **(A)** $F = \frac{mv^2}{r} = \frac{(0.5)(2)^2}{10} = 0.2$ Since mass is in kg, velocity in m/sec.², and distance in meters, the unit of force will be the newton. Note that the diameter of the circle was given, but the radius is required in the equation.

24. **(C)** The heat produced by a nuclear reactor is utilized in the production of steam. The steam is used to run steam turbines for the production of electricity.

25. **(E)** The magnification of a compound microscope may be calculated by multiplying the magnifications of the component lenses. In this case 10 × 97 = 970.

26. **(B)** The critical temperature of a compound is the highest at which its gas may be liquefied no matter what pressure is applied.

27. **(A)** In series, the equivalent resistance is equal to the sum of the individual resistances. 3 + 6 + 2 = 11 ohms.

28. **(C)** In parallel, the equivalent resistance may be calculated as follows:

$$\frac{1}{R_{eq}} = \frac{1}{R_1} + \frac{1}{R_2} + \frac{1}{R_2}$$

$$\frac{1}{R_{eq}} = \frac{1}{3} + \frac{1}{6} + \frac{1}{2} = \frac{2}{6} + \frac{1}{6} + \frac{3}{6} = \frac{6}{6} = 1$$
$$R_{eq} = 1$$

29. **(C)** The colors in the visible spectrum are usually listed in order as red, orange, yellow, green, blue, indigo, and violet.

30. **(A)** The equivalent resistance of series resistances is the sum of their single resistances. (In this case 2 + 3 + 5 = 10 ohms.)
$I = \frac{E}{R} = \frac{20 \text{ volts}}{10 \text{ ohms}} = 2$ amps

31. **(E)** The oldest rocks are said to be about 3,500,000,000 years old. Utilizing half-life information man has been able to quite accurately date many phenomena.
Rubidium-87: half-life around 50 billion years
Potassium-40: half-life around 1.3 billion years
Carbon-14: half-life around 5565 years
Uranium-238: half-life around 4.5 billion years

32. **(B)** The laboratory bench measures 78 cm; 1 inch = 2.54 cm; therefore, we divide 78 by 2.54 to find the number of inches. The answer is 30.7 inches.

33. **(D)** We can increase the strength of an electromagnet also by concentrating the lines of force into a smaller area; increasing current, adding more coiled wire, and increasing the size of the iron core are the other modes.

34. **(D)** The calorie is the unit of heat used in measuring the value of foods for producing heat and energy in the human body. It is equivalent to the amount of heat that is required to raise the temperature of one kilogram of water one degree Celsius.

35. **(C)** We know the conversion factors:
$°F = \frac{9}{5}C° + 32$
$°C = \frac{5}{9}(F° - 32)$
$°F = \frac{9}{5}(45) + 32$
$°F = 81 + 32$
$°F = 113$

36. **(C)** Gravitational pull will cause an object to be accelerated at 32 ft./sec.². This fact varies somewhat depending on location on the earth since the earth is not an absolutely perfect sphere.
$v_f = at = (32) \times (1) = 32$ ft./sec.

37. **(A)** $S = v_0t + \frac{at^2}{2}$
$S = (0)(1) + \frac{32(1)^2}{2} = 16$ ft.

38. **(B)** Galileo in the 16th century pointed out that all objects will fall at the same rate if the resistance of air is nullified. In a vacuum all objects will fall at the same rate.

SCIENCE PROBLEMS

1-3. **(1-B) (2-A) (3-E)** The experimental design illustrates the process of respiration during which oxygen is used up and carbon dioxide is produced. Lime water is commonly used to test for carbon dioxide. Only the O_2 is used up and, therefore, the mercury manometer reading will be about 15 cm since O_2 comprises about 20% of air with nitrogen contributing about 80% to the system. If all the air could be used in the above experiment the manometer reading would be 76 cm, also known as standard atmospheric pressure.

4. **(E)** The distillate would be only 95.6% ethanol. When all the ethanol had been distilled (as the major component of the 95.6% purity product), the remaining material in the distillation flask would be pure water. This could be distilled at 100°C.

5. **(B)** Since the binary azeotrope of 95.6% ethanol has the lowest boiling point, this product must be removed first. The remainder is pure water that may be recovered from the distillation flask or collected as the second fraction in distillation (100°C).

$$(0.956)X = 500 \text{ g}$$
$$X = \frac{500}{0.956}$$
$$X = 523 \text{ g of the 95.6\% mixture}$$
$$1000 \text{ g} - 523 \text{ g} = 477 \text{ g of water}$$

6. **(E)** The binary azeotrope (95.6% ethanol, 4.4% water) boils below the boiling point of pure ethanol. The binary azeotrope will be the only product until all the ethanol has been removed from the distillation flask if the beginning mixture contains at least 4.4% water. Redistillation of the 95.6% ethanol would not improve the purity but the addition of the proper amount of benzene will allow the water to be removed as the lower boiling binary azeotrope (benzene/ethanol/water), and the remaining pure ethanol may then be collected.

7. **(B)** Given $v = v_0 + at; x = v_0t + ½at^2, v_0 = 0$ and $a = 9.8$ m/sec.^{2}, calculate v at the end of 1 second:

$$v = 0 + (9.8)(1)$$
$$v_{1sec.} = 9.8 \text{ m/sec.}$$

8. **(A)** How far has the ball dropped?

$$x = vt + ½at^2$$
$$x = 0 + (½)(9.8)(1)$$
$$x_{1sec.} = 4.9 \text{ m}$$

9. **(E)** When will the ball strike the ground if $x = 19.6$ m?

$$x = vt + ½at^2$$
$$19.6 = 0 + (½)(9.8)(t^2)$$
$$19.6 = 4.9t^2$$
$$t = 2 \text{ sec.}$$

10. **(D)** Since $\text{pH} = pK_a + \log \frac{\text{salt}}{\text{weak acid}}$, then $\text{pH} = pK_a + \log \frac{10}{1}$ and the log 10 is 1, so $\text{pH} = pK_a + 1$.

11. **(B)** With the Henderson-Hasselbalch equation $\text{pH} = pK + \log \frac{\text{salt}}{\text{weak acid}}$. The $\log \frac{\text{salt}}{\text{weak acid}}$ is zero which happens when the ratio of salt to weak acid is one.

12. **(B)** $\text{pH} = 5 + \log \frac{0.1}{0.1}$. Since $\frac{0.1}{0.1}$ is 1 and the log 1 is 0, the pH is 5.

13. **(A)** Ninhydrin will react with free amino groups. In a polypeptide the free amino groups are the alpha group at the amino terminal end of the chain as well as epsilon amino groups (e.g., lysine) within the polypeptide. The number of free amino groups will be increased by any reaction that hydrolyzes peptide bonds. Hydrolysis of peptide bonds may be accomplished by acid hydrolysis or by a peptidase enzyme.

14. **(A)** See answer to question 13.

15. **(B)** See previous answer. The inhibitor will decrease the activity of the peptidase enzyme. Thus the sample with enzyme and inhibitor will have fewer free amino groups than the sample with enzyme and no inhibitor.

16. **(C)** Absorption at 10.3 microns is characteristic of *trans* double bonds.

17. **(A)** Catalytic hydrogenation will convert both *cis* and *trans* unsaturated fatty acids to saturated ones.

18. **(D)** Animals and higher plants have almost exclusively *cis* double bonds in their unsaturated fatty acids. *Trans* fatty acids are more common in certain bacteria.

19. **(C)** In calculating the mass, recall that density = m/v. m = ?. $v = 30$ cm^3. ρHg = 13.6 gm/cm^3.

$$m = \rho v = (13.6)(30)$$
$$m = 408 \text{ gm (convert to kg)}$$
$$m = 408 \times 10^{-3} \text{ kg} = 0.408 \text{ kg}$$

20. **(A)** What is the mass of the same volume of water? Repeat the above calculation for water which tells us that: $m = 30$ gm or 0.030 kg. Or recall that mercury is 13.6 times denser than the water and therefore the mass of an equal volume = $\frac{0.408}{13.6} = 0.030$ kg.

21. **(B)** Specific gravity = 13.6 by definition.

22. **(E)** $\frac{0.5 \text{ mg}}{0.1 \text{ ml}} = \frac{X}{10 \text{ ml}}$

$$X = \frac{(0.5)(10)}{0.1} = 50 \text{ mg}$$

This 50 mg represents the total amount in the entire 3 ml of plasma that was extracted.

$\frac{50 \text{ mg}}{3 \text{ ml}} = \frac{X}{100 \text{ ml}}$

$$X = \frac{(50)(100)}{3} = 1667 \text{ mg/100 ml}$$

23. **(A)** See the above answer. The calculation is based on 100 ml plasma rather than on whole blood.

24. **(B)** Exceeding the linear range would ordinarily lead to a lower absorbance than expected. An error in weighing to prepare the standard solution would introduce a constant error. The remaining possibility, a pipetting error, is most likely. Pipetting errors may be positive or negative.

25. **(A)** The velocity of a wave (C) is directly related to its wavelength and inversely related to its period. The frequency of a wave is inversely proportional to its period, so that in this case the period is 10 seconds and consequently the frequency is $\frac{1}{10}$.

26. **(A)** The velocity is simply $C = L/T$ where $L = 50$ meters and $T = 10$ seconds. $C = 5$ m/sec.

27. **(B)** Wave refraction tends to make wave trains parallel to shore.

28-30. **(28-A) (29-C) (30-B)** The staircase phenomenon or treppe is due to a gradual increase in the extent of muscle contraction; a limit will be reached after rapid repeated stimuli. Fatigue is the decreased response of the nerve to stimulation.

31. **(C)** The activity of lactic dehydrogenase may be expressed as the rate of reduction of NAD^+. The significance of a reduced activity of lactic dehydrogenase is not discussed here.

32. **(D)** The way the question is stated it appears that total activity is being compared between patients B and E. If 0.1 ml of serum from B has 4 times the enzymatic activity of 0.2 ml of serum from E, then the unit activity of B is 8 times that of E. $8 \times 40 = 320$ units/ml.

33. **(E)** The rate of appearance of NADH + H^+ must be equal to the rate of disappearance of NAD^+ in enzymatic reactions such as this. The only time this will not be true is when another reaction is destroying one of the forms of the coenzyme.

34. **(C)** $n = C/S_m$. $C = 3 \times 10^8$. $S_m = 2.25 \times 10^8$. n_m = index of refraction of water = 1.333

35. **(B)** The index of refraction for a vacuum = 1 because $Sm = C = 3 \times 10^8$ m/sec. Therefore, $n = 1$. Snell's Law states that $\sin\theta_i/\sin\theta_r = n_r/n_i$ and so $n_r/n_i > 1$ because $n_r = 1.33$

36. **(B)** In this case n_r = vacuum = 1.0; n_i = water = 1.33. Therefore, $n_r/n_i = 1.00/1.33 = 0.75 < 1$ and the beam would bend *away* from the normal.

37-39. **(37-D) (38-B) (39-A)** The answers to questions 37-39 are self-explanatory.

40. **(A)** $K_i = \frac{[H^+][F^-]}{[HF]}$

$[H^+][F^-] = K_i\,[HF]$

Since $[H^+]$ and $[F^-]$ should be equal,

$[H^+] = \sqrt{K_i\,[HF]} = \sqrt{(2 \times 10^{-4})(0.5)}$

$[H^+] = \sqrt{1 \times 10^{-4}} = 1 \times 10^{-2}$

$pH = -\log\,[H^+] = 2$

41. **(E)** $[H^+][OH^-] = 1 \times 10^{-14}$

$[H^+] = 1 \times 10^{-7}$

$(1 \times 10^{-2}) + (1 \times 10^{-7}) = 1.00001 \times 10^{-2}$

The logarithm of the above number is not significantly different from that in the previous question. Thus failure to include the ionization of water leads to an "error" which is substantially less than 0.001 pH units. This "error" is less than that introduced by other assumptions and simplifications.

42. **(A)** For a monoprotic acid normality and molarity are equal. See the two answers above.

43. **(A)** $4H + O_2 \rightarrow 2H_2O$

$\frac{X}{4} = \frac{0.138}{36}$

$X = 0.0153$ gal hydrogen in 0.100 g of compound

$\frac{0.0153}{1} = 0.0153$ g atoms hydrogen in 0.100 g of compound

$C + O_2 \rightarrow CO_2$

$\frac{X}{12} = \frac{0.677}{44}$

$X = 0.185$ g of carbon in 0.100 g of compound

$\frac{0.185}{12} = 0.0154$ g atoms carbon in 0.100 g of compound. Obviously carbon and hydrogen appear in equal atomic amounts, and the empirical formula is CH.

44. (C) The molecular formula will be a multiple of the empirical formula. Since the empirical formula is CH, the molecular formula must be a multiple such as C_2H_2, C_3H_3, C_4H_4, etc.

45. (B) Colligative properties are those that depend on the number of particles in solution. Freezing point depression is a colligative property and could be used to determine the number of particles in a given weight (and thus determine the molecular weight). With this information the multiple to be used in converting empirical formula to molecular formula is known. In this particular problem dissolving the necessary amount of the compound (i.e., C_2H_2) in water may be difficult, but the principle is sound for use with a variety of compounds.

46. (C) $[Ag^{+\,2}][SO_4^{=}] = 6.4 \times 10^{-5}$

$$[SO_4^{=}] = \frac{6.4 \times 10^{-5}}{[Ag^{+\,2}]} = \frac{6.4 \times 10^{-5}}{(0.1)^2} = 6.4 \times 10^{-3}$$

47. (C) Na_2SO_4 is a strongly ionized salt. If it were weakly ionized (as the question supposes), the additional Na^+ ions introduced by $NaNO_3$ would depress the ionization of Na_2SO_4 and decrease the $SO_4^{=}$ concentration. If Na_2SO_4 were weakly ionized, however, the $SO_4^{=}$ concentration would already be less than what is assumed in the previous question for a strongly ionized salt.

48. (E) AgCl is even less soluble than Ag_2SO_4. (K_{sp} of AgCl is 2.4×10^{-10} as compared to 6.4×10^{-5} for Ag_2SO_4.)

49. (A) The total resistance is composed of R_1 and the resistance from the parallel resistors in the branch composed of R_2, R_3, and R_4. For resistors connected in parallel, the following statement holds: $\frac{1}{R} = \frac{1}{Ra} + \frac{1}{Rb} + \frac{1}{Rc} \ldots$ in our case:

$$\frac{1}{R} = \frac{1}{5} + \frac{1}{10} + \frac{1}{15}$$

$$\frac{1}{R} = \frac{12 + 6 + 4}{60} = \frac{22}{60}$$

$$22R = 60$$

$$Rp = 2.7 \text{ ohms}$$

50. (B) $R_{tot} = R_1 + R_P = 20 + 22.7$ ohms

51. (B) $I = V/R$ where I = current in amps, V = potential difference (volts), and R = resistance (ohms).

$V = RI$

$V = (5)(22.7)$

$V = 114$ volts

52. (E) Using $\alpha = \Delta L/L_0\, \Delta T$; $\alpha = 9 \times 10^{-6}$ per °C, $\Delta T = 10$°C, $\Delta L = 1 \times 10^{-2}$ cm, and L_0 = desired.

$$L_0 = \frac{\Delta L}{\alpha\, \Delta T} = 1 \times \frac{10^{-2}}{9} \times 10^{-6} \times 10$$

$$L_0 = 0.11 \times 10^3 \text{ cm} = 110 \text{ cm}$$

53. (E) Length L_0 = 110 cm at 10°C, therefore to find the length of the bar at 0°C:

$\Delta L = (\alpha)(L_0)(\Delta T)$

$\Delta L = (9 \times 10^{-6})(110)(10)$

$\Delta L = 9 \times 110 \times 10^{-5}$

$\Delta L = 990 \times 10^{-5}$ cm

$L_0 = 110$ cm

(new) $L = [110 - (990 \times 10^{-5})]$ cm

$L = 110 - 0.01$

$L_{\text{at } 0°C} = 109.00$ cm

54. (A) The answer to this question is self-explanatory.

55. (D) To produce all black cows (BB or Bb, 3 out of 4) we must multiply $\frac{3}{4} \times \frac{3}{4} \times \frac{3}{4} \times \frac{3}{4} = \frac{81}{256}$.

56. (E) To produce all gray cows (bb, 1 out of 4) we must multiply $\frac{1}{4} \times \frac{1}{4} \times \frac{1}{4} \times \frac{1}{4} = \frac{1}{256}$.

57. (C) In order for the breeder to determine if a line is genotypically pure a backcross is used. A backcross consists of crossing a dominant phenotype with a pure homozygous recessive (in our case bb).

58. (E) Although the solution is at the equivalence point of acid and base, we are unable to predict the pH.

59. (E) See the above answer. Since we are dealing with normality rather than molarity, the formula has no effect on our predictions.

60. (B) The salt is that of a weak base and a strong acid. $CaCl_2 + 2H_2O \rightleftharpoons Ca(OH_2)_2 + 2HCl$. Since $Ca(OH)_2$ is less weakly ionized than HCl, the solution will be somewhat acidic.

61-63. (61-C) (62-B) (63-E) The answers to questions 61-63 are self-explanatory.

64. (A) 284.47 − 282.45 = 2.02
A difference of 2.02 between the molecular weights represents two hydrogen atoms; thus, there is one double bond per molecule.

65. (D) There is no way to determine whether the double bonds are *cis*, *trans*, or a mixture of the two based on the information given.

66. (A) 282.45 − 2.02 = 280.43

Answer Sheet–Model Test C

SCIENCE KNOWLEDGE

Biology

1. Ⓐ Ⓑ Ⓒ Ⓓ Ⓔ
2. Ⓐ Ⓑ Ⓒ Ⓓ Ⓔ
3. Ⓐ Ⓑ Ⓒ Ⓓ Ⓔ
4. Ⓐ Ⓑ Ⓒ Ⓓ Ⓔ
5. Ⓐ Ⓑ Ⓒ Ⓓ Ⓔ
6. Ⓐ Ⓑ Ⓒ Ⓓ Ⓔ
7. Ⓐ Ⓑ Ⓒ Ⓓ Ⓔ
8. Ⓐ Ⓑ Ⓒ Ⓓ Ⓔ
9. Ⓐ Ⓑ Ⓒ Ⓓ Ⓔ
10. Ⓐ Ⓑ Ⓒ Ⓓ Ⓔ
11. Ⓐ Ⓑ Ⓒ Ⓓ Ⓔ
12. Ⓐ Ⓑ Ⓒ Ⓓ Ⓔ
13. Ⓐ Ⓑ Ⓒ Ⓓ Ⓔ
14. Ⓐ Ⓑ Ⓒ Ⓓ Ⓔ
15. Ⓐ Ⓑ Ⓒ Ⓓ Ⓔ
16. Ⓐ Ⓑ Ⓒ Ⓓ Ⓔ
17. Ⓐ Ⓑ Ⓒ Ⓓ Ⓔ
18. Ⓐ Ⓑ Ⓒ Ⓓ Ⓔ
19. Ⓐ Ⓑ Ⓒ Ⓓ Ⓔ
20. Ⓐ Ⓑ Ⓒ Ⓓ Ⓔ
21. Ⓐ Ⓑ Ⓒ Ⓓ Ⓔ
22. Ⓐ Ⓑ Ⓒ Ⓓ Ⓔ
23. Ⓐ Ⓑ Ⓒ Ⓓ Ⓔ
24. Ⓐ Ⓑ Ⓒ Ⓓ Ⓔ
25. Ⓐ Ⓑ Ⓒ Ⓓ Ⓔ
26. Ⓐ Ⓑ Ⓒ Ⓓ Ⓔ
27. Ⓐ Ⓑ Ⓒ Ⓓ Ⓔ
28. Ⓐ Ⓑ Ⓒ Ⓓ Ⓔ
29. Ⓐ Ⓑ Ⓒ Ⓓ Ⓔ
30. Ⓐ Ⓑ Ⓒ Ⓓ Ⓔ
31. Ⓐ Ⓑ Ⓒ Ⓓ Ⓔ
32. Ⓐ Ⓑ Ⓒ Ⓓ Ⓔ
33. Ⓐ Ⓑ Ⓒ Ⓓ Ⓔ
34. Ⓐ Ⓑ Ⓒ Ⓓ Ⓔ
35. Ⓐ Ⓑ Ⓒ Ⓓ Ⓔ
36. Ⓐ Ⓑ Ⓒ Ⓓ Ⓔ
37. Ⓐ Ⓑ Ⓒ Ⓓ Ⓔ
38. Ⓐ Ⓑ Ⓒ Ⓓ Ⓔ

Chemistry

1. Ⓐ Ⓑ Ⓒ Ⓓ Ⓔ
2. Ⓐ Ⓑ Ⓒ Ⓓ Ⓔ
3. Ⓐ Ⓑ Ⓒ Ⓓ Ⓔ
4. Ⓐ Ⓑ Ⓒ Ⓓ Ⓔ
5. Ⓐ Ⓑ Ⓒ Ⓓ Ⓔ
6. Ⓐ Ⓑ Ⓒ Ⓓ Ⓔ
7. Ⓐ Ⓑ Ⓒ Ⓓ Ⓔ
8. Ⓐ Ⓑ Ⓒ Ⓓ Ⓔ
9. Ⓐ Ⓑ Ⓒ Ⓓ Ⓔ
10. Ⓐ Ⓑ Ⓒ Ⓓ Ⓔ
11. Ⓐ Ⓑ Ⓒ Ⓓ Ⓔ
12. Ⓐ Ⓑ Ⓒ Ⓓ Ⓔ
13. Ⓐ Ⓑ Ⓒ Ⓓ Ⓔ
14. Ⓐ Ⓑ Ⓒ Ⓓ Ⓔ
15. Ⓐ Ⓑ Ⓒ Ⓓ Ⓔ
16. Ⓐ Ⓑ Ⓒ Ⓓ Ⓔ
17. Ⓐ Ⓑ Ⓒ Ⓓ Ⓔ
18. Ⓐ Ⓑ Ⓒ Ⓓ Ⓔ
19. Ⓐ Ⓑ Ⓒ Ⓓ Ⓔ
20. Ⓐ Ⓑ Ⓒ Ⓓ Ⓔ
21. Ⓐ Ⓑ Ⓒ Ⓓ Ⓔ
22. Ⓐ Ⓑ Ⓒ Ⓓ Ⓔ
23. Ⓐ Ⓑ Ⓒ Ⓓ Ⓔ
24. Ⓐ Ⓑ Ⓒ Ⓓ Ⓔ
25. Ⓐ Ⓑ Ⓒ Ⓓ Ⓔ
26. Ⓐ Ⓑ Ⓒ Ⓓ Ⓔ
27. Ⓐ Ⓑ Ⓒ Ⓓ Ⓔ
28. Ⓐ Ⓑ Ⓒ Ⓓ Ⓔ
29. Ⓐ Ⓑ Ⓒ Ⓓ Ⓔ
30. Ⓐ Ⓑ Ⓒ Ⓓ Ⓔ
31. Ⓐ Ⓑ Ⓒ Ⓓ Ⓔ
32. Ⓐ Ⓑ Ⓒ Ⓓ Ⓔ
33. Ⓐ Ⓑ Ⓒ Ⓓ Ⓔ
34. Ⓐ Ⓑ Ⓒ Ⓓ Ⓔ
35. Ⓐ Ⓑ Ⓒ Ⓓ Ⓔ
36. Ⓐ Ⓑ Ⓒ Ⓓ Ⓔ
37. Ⓐ Ⓑ Ⓒ Ⓓ Ⓔ
38. Ⓐ Ⓑ Ⓒ Ⓓ Ⓔ
39. Ⓐ Ⓑ Ⓒ Ⓓ Ⓔ
40. Ⓐ Ⓑ Ⓒ Ⓓ Ⓔ
41. Ⓐ Ⓑ Ⓒ Ⓓ Ⓔ
42. Ⓐ Ⓑ Ⓒ Ⓓ Ⓔ
43. Ⓐ Ⓑ Ⓒ Ⓓ Ⓔ
44. Ⓐ Ⓑ Ⓒ Ⓓ Ⓔ
45. Ⓐ Ⓑ Ⓒ Ⓓ Ⓔ
46. Ⓐ Ⓑ Ⓒ Ⓓ Ⓔ
47. Ⓐ Ⓑ Ⓒ Ⓓ Ⓔ
48. Ⓐ Ⓑ Ⓒ Ⓓ Ⓔ
49. Ⓐ Ⓑ Ⓒ Ⓓ Ⓔ

Physics

1. Ⓐ Ⓑ Ⓒ Ⓓ Ⓔ
2. Ⓐ Ⓑ Ⓒ Ⓓ Ⓔ
3. Ⓐ Ⓑ Ⓒ Ⓓ Ⓔ
4. Ⓐ Ⓑ Ⓒ Ⓓ Ⓔ
5. Ⓐ Ⓑ Ⓒ Ⓓ Ⓔ
6. Ⓐ Ⓑ Ⓒ Ⓓ Ⓔ
7. Ⓐ Ⓑ Ⓒ Ⓓ Ⓔ
8. Ⓐ Ⓑ Ⓒ Ⓓ Ⓔ
9. Ⓐ Ⓑ Ⓒ Ⓓ Ⓔ
10. Ⓐ Ⓑ Ⓒ Ⓓ Ⓔ
11. Ⓐ Ⓑ Ⓒ Ⓓ Ⓔ
12. Ⓐ Ⓑ Ⓒ Ⓓ Ⓔ
13. Ⓐ Ⓑ Ⓒ Ⓓ Ⓔ
14. Ⓐ Ⓑ Ⓒ Ⓓ Ⓔ
15. Ⓐ Ⓑ Ⓒ Ⓓ Ⓔ
16. Ⓐ Ⓑ Ⓒ Ⓓ Ⓔ
17. Ⓐ Ⓑ Ⓒ Ⓓ Ⓔ
18. Ⓐ Ⓑ Ⓒ Ⓓ Ⓔ
19. Ⓐ Ⓑ Ⓒ Ⓓ Ⓔ
20. Ⓐ Ⓑ Ⓒ Ⓓ Ⓔ
21. Ⓐ Ⓑ Ⓒ Ⓓ Ⓔ
22. Ⓐ Ⓑ Ⓒ Ⓓ Ⓔ
23. Ⓐ Ⓑ Ⓒ Ⓓ Ⓔ
24. Ⓐ Ⓑ Ⓒ Ⓓ Ⓔ
25. Ⓐ Ⓑ Ⓒ Ⓓ Ⓔ
26. Ⓐ Ⓑ Ⓒ Ⓓ Ⓔ
27. Ⓐ Ⓑ Ⓒ Ⓓ Ⓔ
28. Ⓐ Ⓑ Ⓒ Ⓓ Ⓔ
29. Ⓐ Ⓑ Ⓒ Ⓓ Ⓔ
30. Ⓐ Ⓑ Ⓒ Ⓓ Ⓔ
31. Ⓐ Ⓑ Ⓒ Ⓓ Ⓔ
32. Ⓐ Ⓑ Ⓒ Ⓓ Ⓔ
33. Ⓐ Ⓑ Ⓒ Ⓓ Ⓔ
34. Ⓐ Ⓑ Ⓒ Ⓓ Ⓔ
35. Ⓐ Ⓑ Ⓒ Ⓓ Ⓔ
36. Ⓐ Ⓑ Ⓒ Ⓓ Ⓔ
37. Ⓐ Ⓑ Ⓒ Ⓓ Ⓔ
38. Ⓐ Ⓑ Ⓒ Ⓓ Ⓔ

SCIENCE PROBLEMS

1. Ⓐ Ⓑ Ⓒ Ⓓ Ⓔ
2. Ⓐ Ⓑ Ⓒ Ⓓ Ⓔ
3. Ⓐ Ⓑ Ⓒ Ⓓ Ⓔ
4. Ⓐ Ⓑ Ⓒ Ⓓ Ⓔ
5. Ⓐ Ⓑ Ⓒ Ⓓ Ⓔ
6. Ⓐ Ⓑ Ⓒ Ⓓ Ⓔ
7. Ⓐ Ⓑ Ⓒ Ⓓ Ⓔ
8. Ⓐ Ⓑ Ⓒ Ⓓ Ⓔ
9. Ⓐ Ⓑ Ⓒ Ⓓ Ⓔ
10. Ⓐ Ⓑ Ⓒ Ⓓ Ⓔ
11. Ⓐ Ⓑ Ⓒ Ⓓ Ⓔ
12. Ⓐ Ⓑ Ⓒ Ⓓ Ⓔ
13. Ⓐ Ⓑ Ⓒ Ⓓ Ⓔ
14. Ⓐ Ⓑ Ⓒ Ⓓ Ⓔ
15. Ⓐ Ⓑ Ⓒ Ⓓ Ⓔ
16. Ⓐ Ⓑ Ⓒ Ⓓ Ⓔ
17. Ⓐ Ⓑ Ⓒ Ⓓ Ⓔ
18. Ⓐ Ⓑ Ⓒ Ⓓ Ⓔ
19. Ⓐ Ⓑ Ⓒ Ⓓ Ⓔ
20. Ⓐ Ⓑ Ⓒ Ⓓ Ⓔ
21. Ⓐ Ⓑ Ⓒ Ⓓ Ⓔ
22. Ⓐ Ⓑ Ⓒ Ⓓ Ⓔ
23. Ⓐ Ⓑ Ⓒ Ⓓ Ⓔ
24. Ⓐ Ⓑ Ⓒ Ⓓ Ⓔ
25. Ⓐ Ⓑ Ⓒ Ⓓ Ⓔ
26. Ⓐ Ⓑ Ⓒ Ⓓ Ⓔ
27. Ⓐ Ⓑ Ⓒ Ⓓ Ⓔ
28. Ⓐ Ⓑ Ⓒ Ⓓ Ⓔ
29. Ⓐ Ⓑ Ⓒ Ⓓ Ⓔ
30. Ⓐ Ⓑ Ⓒ Ⓓ Ⓔ
31. Ⓐ Ⓑ Ⓒ Ⓓ Ⓔ
32. Ⓐ Ⓑ Ⓒ Ⓓ Ⓔ
33. Ⓐ Ⓑ Ⓒ Ⓓ Ⓔ
34. Ⓐ Ⓑ Ⓒ Ⓓ Ⓔ
35. Ⓐ Ⓑ Ⓒ Ⓓ Ⓔ
36. Ⓐ Ⓑ Ⓒ Ⓓ Ⓔ
37. Ⓐ Ⓑ Ⓒ Ⓓ Ⓔ
38. Ⓐ Ⓑ Ⓒ Ⓓ Ⓔ
39. Ⓐ Ⓑ Ⓒ Ⓓ Ⓔ
40. Ⓐ Ⓑ Ⓒ Ⓓ Ⓔ
41. Ⓐ Ⓑ Ⓒ Ⓓ Ⓔ
42. Ⓐ Ⓑ Ⓒ Ⓓ Ⓔ
43. Ⓐ Ⓑ Ⓒ Ⓓ Ⓔ
44. Ⓐ Ⓑ Ⓒ Ⓓ Ⓔ
45. Ⓐ Ⓑ Ⓒ Ⓓ Ⓔ
46. Ⓐ Ⓑ Ⓒ Ⓓ Ⓔ
47. Ⓐ Ⓑ Ⓒ Ⓓ Ⓔ
48. Ⓐ Ⓑ Ⓒ Ⓓ Ⓔ
49. Ⓐ Ⓑ Ⓒ Ⓓ Ⓔ
50. Ⓐ Ⓑ Ⓒ Ⓓ Ⓔ
51. Ⓐ Ⓑ Ⓒ Ⓓ Ⓔ
52. Ⓐ Ⓑ Ⓒ Ⓓ Ⓔ
53. Ⓐ Ⓑ Ⓒ Ⓓ Ⓔ
54. Ⓐ Ⓑ Ⓒ Ⓓ Ⓔ
55. Ⓐ Ⓑ Ⓒ Ⓓ Ⓔ
56. Ⓐ Ⓑ Ⓒ Ⓓ Ⓔ
57. Ⓐ Ⓑ Ⓒ Ⓓ Ⓔ
58. Ⓐ Ⓑ Ⓒ Ⓓ Ⓔ
59. Ⓐ Ⓑ Ⓒ Ⓓ Ⓔ
60. Ⓐ Ⓑ Ⓒ Ⓓ Ⓔ
61. Ⓐ Ⓑ Ⓒ Ⓓ Ⓔ
62. Ⓐ Ⓑ Ⓒ Ⓓ Ⓔ
63. Ⓐ Ⓑ Ⓒ Ⓓ Ⓔ
64. Ⓐ Ⓑ Ⓒ Ⓓ Ⓔ
65. Ⓐ Ⓑ Ⓒ Ⓓ Ⓔ
66. Ⓐ Ⓑ Ⓒ Ⓓ Ⓔ

SKILLS ANALYSIS: READING

1. Ⓐ Ⓑ Ⓒ
2. Ⓐ Ⓑ Ⓒ
3. Ⓐ Ⓑ Ⓒ
4. Ⓐ Ⓑ Ⓒ
5. Ⓐ Ⓑ Ⓒ
6. Ⓐ Ⓑ Ⓒ
7. Ⓐ Ⓑ Ⓒ
8. Ⓐ Ⓑ Ⓒ
9. Ⓐ Ⓑ Ⓒ
10. Ⓐ Ⓑ Ⓒ
11. Ⓐ Ⓑ Ⓒ
12. Ⓐ Ⓑ Ⓒ
13. Ⓐ Ⓑ Ⓒ
14. Ⓐ Ⓑ Ⓒ
15. Ⓐ Ⓑ Ⓒ
16. Ⓐ Ⓑ Ⓒ
17. Ⓐ Ⓑ Ⓒ
18. Ⓐ Ⓑ Ⓒ
19. Ⓐ Ⓑ Ⓒ
20. Ⓐ Ⓑ Ⓒ
21. Ⓐ Ⓑ Ⓒ
22. Ⓐ Ⓑ Ⓒ
23. Ⓐ Ⓑ Ⓒ
24. Ⓐ Ⓑ Ⓒ
25. Ⓐ Ⓑ Ⓒ
26. Ⓐ Ⓑ Ⓒ
27. Ⓐ Ⓑ Ⓒ
28. Ⓐ Ⓑ Ⓒ
29. Ⓐ Ⓑ Ⓒ
30. Ⓐ Ⓑ Ⓒ
31. Ⓐ Ⓑ Ⓒ
32. Ⓐ Ⓑ Ⓒ
33. Ⓐ Ⓑ Ⓒ
34. Ⓐ Ⓑ Ⓒ
35. Ⓐ Ⓑ Ⓒ
36. Ⓐ Ⓑ Ⓒ
37. Ⓐ Ⓑ Ⓒ
38. Ⓐ Ⓑ Ⓒ
39. Ⓐ Ⓑ Ⓒ
40. Ⓐ Ⓑ Ⓒ
41. Ⓐ Ⓑ Ⓒ
42. Ⓐ Ⓑ Ⓒ
43. Ⓐ Ⓑ Ⓒ
44. Ⓐ Ⓑ Ⓒ
45. Ⓐ Ⓑ Ⓒ
46. Ⓐ Ⓑ Ⓒ
47. Ⓐ Ⓑ Ⓒ
48. Ⓐ Ⓑ Ⓒ
49. Ⓐ Ⓑ Ⓒ
50. Ⓐ Ⓑ Ⓒ
51. Ⓐ Ⓑ Ⓒ Ⓓ Ⓔ
52. Ⓐ Ⓑ Ⓒ Ⓓ Ⓔ
53. Ⓐ Ⓑ Ⓒ Ⓓ Ⓔ
54. Ⓐ Ⓑ Ⓒ Ⓓ Ⓔ
55. Ⓐ Ⓑ Ⓒ Ⓓ Ⓔ
56. Ⓐ Ⓑ Ⓒ Ⓓ Ⓔ
57. Ⓐ Ⓑ Ⓒ Ⓓ Ⓔ
58. Ⓐ Ⓑ Ⓒ Ⓓ Ⓔ
59. Ⓐ Ⓑ Ⓒ Ⓓ Ⓔ
60. Ⓐ Ⓑ Ⓒ Ⓓ Ⓔ
61. Ⓐ Ⓑ Ⓒ Ⓓ Ⓔ
62. Ⓐ Ⓑ Ⓒ Ⓓ Ⓔ
63. Ⓐ Ⓑ Ⓒ
64. Ⓐ Ⓑ Ⓒ
65. Ⓐ Ⓑ Ⓒ
66. Ⓐ Ⓑ Ⓒ
67. Ⓐ Ⓑ Ⓒ
68. Ⓐ Ⓑ Ⓒ

SKILLS ANALYSIS: QUANTITATIVE

1. Ⓐ Ⓑ Ⓒ Ⓓ
2. Ⓐ Ⓑ Ⓒ Ⓓ
3. Ⓐ Ⓑ Ⓒ Ⓓ
4. Ⓐ Ⓑ Ⓒ Ⓓ
5. Ⓐ Ⓑ Ⓒ Ⓓ
6. Ⓐ Ⓑ Ⓒ Ⓓ
7. Ⓐ Ⓑ Ⓒ Ⓓ
8. Ⓐ Ⓑ Ⓒ Ⓓ
9. Ⓐ Ⓑ Ⓒ Ⓓ
10. Ⓐ Ⓑ Ⓒ Ⓓ
11, Ⓐ Ⓑ Ⓒ Ⓓ
12. Ⓐ Ⓑ Ⓒ Ⓓ
13. Ⓐ Ⓑ Ⓒ Ⓓ
14. Ⓐ Ⓑ Ⓒ Ⓓ
15. Ⓐ Ⓑ Ⓒ Ⓓ
16. Ⓐ Ⓑ Ⓒ Ⓓ
17. Ⓐ Ⓑ Ⓒ Ⓓ
18. Ⓐ Ⓑ Ⓒ Ⓓ
19. Ⓐ Ⓑ Ⓒ
20. Ⓐ Ⓑ Ⓒ
21. Ⓐ Ⓑ Ⓒ
22. Ⓐ Ⓑ Ⓒ
23. Ⓐ Ⓑ Ⓒ
24. Ⓐ Ⓑ Ⓒ
25. Ⓐ Ⓑ Ⓒ
26. Ⓐ Ⓑ Ⓒ
27. Ⓐ Ⓑ Ⓒ
28. Ⓐ Ⓑ Ⓒ
29. Ⓐ Ⓑ Ⓒ Ⓓ
30. Ⓐ Ⓑ Ⓒ Ⓓ Ⓔ
31. Ⓐ Ⓑ Ⓒ Ⓓ Ⓔ
32. Ⓐ Ⓑ Ⓒ Ⓓ Ⓔ
33. Ⓐ Ⓑ Ⓒ Ⓓ Ⓔ
34. Ⓐ Ⓑ Ⓒ Ⓓ
35. Ⓐ Ⓑ Ⓒ Ⓓ
36. Ⓐ Ⓑ Ⓒ Ⓓ
37. Ⓐ Ⓑ Ⓒ Ⓓ
38. Ⓐ Ⓑ Ⓒ Ⓓ
39. Ⓐ Ⓑ Ⓒ Ⓓ
40. Ⓐ Ⓑ Ⓒ Ⓓ
41. Ⓐ Ⓑ Ⓒ Ⓓ
42. Ⓐ Ⓑ Ⓒ Ⓓ
43. Ⓐ Ⓑ Ⓒ Ⓓ
44. Ⓐ Ⓑ Ⓒ Ⓓ
45. Ⓐ Ⓑ Ⓒ Ⓓ
46. Ⓐ Ⓑ Ⓒ
47. Ⓐ Ⓑ Ⓒ
48. Ⓐ Ⓑ Ⓒ
49. Ⓐ Ⓑ Ⓒ
50. Ⓐ Ⓑ Ⓒ
51. Ⓐ Ⓑ Ⓒ
52. Ⓐ Ⓑ Ⓒ
53. Ⓐ Ⓑ Ⓒ
54. Ⓐ Ⓑ Ⓒ
55. Ⓐ Ⓑ Ⓒ
56. Ⓐ Ⓑ Ⓒ
57. Ⓐ Ⓑ Ⓒ
58. Ⓐ Ⓑ Ⓒ
59. Ⓐ Ⓑ Ⓒ
60. Ⓐ Ⓑ Ⓒ
61. Ⓐ Ⓑ Ⓒ
62. Ⓐ Ⓑ Ⓒ
63. Ⓐ Ⓑ Ⓒ
64. Ⓐ Ⓑ Ⓒ
65. Ⓐ Ⓑ Ⓒ
66. Ⓐ Ⓑ Ⓒ
67. Ⓐ Ⓑ Ⓒ
68. Ⓐ Ⓑ Ⓒ

The New MCAT Model Examination C*

SCIENCE KNOWLEDGE

135 MINUTES
125 QUESTIONS

The following questions are based on your knowledge of science. The questions are varied; therefore, you are advised to pay careful attention to the instructions for each portion.

Biology

DIRECTIONS: In the following questions, four words or phrases are presented that have been labeled A-D. For each question, choose the word or phrase that is most closely associated with the given item. You may use a choice more than once, or not at all. Eliminate those choices that you think to be incorrect and mark the letter of your choice on the answer sheet.

Questions 1-4:

(A) Possesses hydrolytic enzymes
(B) Functions in protein synthesis
(C) Condenses (packages) secretory products
(D) Functions in energy production

1. Mitochondria
2. Lysosome
3. Golgi apparatus
4. Rough endoplasmic reticulum

Questions 5-10:

(A) Thyroid
(B) Parathyroid
(C) Thymus
(D) Adrenal

5. Regulates the resorption of calcium from bone
6. Produces mineralocorticoids and glucocorticoids
7. Removal results in muscle spasms, tetany, and death
8. Oversecretion can cause an individual to have bulging eyeballs
9. Insufficiency can lead to mental and physical sluggishness
10. Plays a dominant role in the development of a competent immune system

---

*Explanations for science answers can be found on p. 253.

Questions 11-14:

(A) Pepsin
(B) Trypsin
(C) Pancreatic amylase
(D) Chymotrypsinogen

11. A zymogen or enzyme precursor

12. A proteinase with a pH optimum around 2

13. Chloride ion is an activator ion for the enzyme

14. Can be activated by trypsin because of splitting of a single peptide bond

DIRECTIONS: Each of the statements or questions is followed by four or five suggested completions or answers. Choose the one that best completes the statement or answers the question, and mark the letter of your choice on the answer sheet.

15. Hydra usually reproduce by the process known as budding. This form of reproduction is called as
(A) cleavage reproduction.
(B) vegetative reproduction.
(C) binary fision (mitosis).
(D) parthenogenesis.
(E) sexual reproduction.

16. The term "limey," as applied to British individuals, refers to the
(A) early dietary approach to the prevention of scurvy in the British navy.
(B) large numbers of lime trees transplanted from Spain to southern Wales in the eighteenth century.
(C) practice of adding lime slices to the gin drinks ordinarily consumed by British soldiers in India.
(D) pale green skin seen in many individuals in the British Isles as a result of a combination of diet and insufficient exposure of the skin to sunlight.
(E) early dietary approach to the prevention of rickets in the British navy.

17. Blood in the pulmonary veins is rich in
(A) oxyhemoglobin.
(B) carbaminohemoglobin.
(C) hemoglobin.
(D) uric acid.
(E) carbon dioxide.

18. Fertilization in the human female usually takes place in the upper one-third of the oviduct while implantation occurs in the
(A) lower one-third of oviduct.
(B) Mullerian duct.
(C) vagina.
(D) peritoneum.
(E) uterus.

19. A common experiment carried out in the physiology laboratory on the turtle heart involves first destroying the S-A node, observing the heart and then destroying the A-V node and observing and recording the results. After these procedures it is found that the heart now
(A) beats faster.
(B) exhibits no change in heart rate.
(C) beats slower.
(D) will stop beating.

20. Messenger RNA receives its instructions from
(A) ribosomes.
(B) endoplasmic reticulum.
(C) DNA in the nucleus.
(D) cytoplasm.
(E) Golgi zone.

21. Undigested food is eliminated from the body by the process of
(A) exocytosis.
(B) excretion.
(C) egestion.
(D) catabolism.
(E) assimilation.

22. The most sensitive tests developed for the accurate detection of very small amounts of hormones to date are
(A) bio-assays.
(B) immuno-assays.
(C) ascorbic acid depletion tests.
(D) fluorometric assays.
(E) chromatographic assays.

23. The diagnostic tests for pregnancy utilize the presence of
(A) progesterone.
(B) estrogen.
(C) chorionic gonadotropin.
(D) oxytocin.
(E) luteinizing hormone.

24. Photoperiodism is
(A) the ability to perceive color by the cones of the retina.
(B) the physiological response of an organism to light and dark periods (cycles).
(C) the ability to utilize CO_2 to produce O_2.
(D) not a factor of biological significance.
(E) the ability to perceive black and white shades by the rods of the retina.

25. The part of the neuron that conducts impulses away from its cell body is called the
(A) axon.
(B) dendrite.
(C) node of Ranvier.
(D) Schwann sheath.
(E) nucleus.

26. After fertilization the zygote will develop into a male organism if the
(A) egg possesses a Y-chromosome.
(B) sperm possesses an X-chromosome.
(C) zygote possesses two X-chromosomes.
(D) zygote possesses two Y-chromosomes.
(E) sperm possesses a Y-chromosome.

27. Fetal blood is carried to the placenta for oxygenation by the
(A) umbilical arteries.
(B) ductus venosus.
(C) ductus arteriosus.
(D) foramen ovale.
(E) umbilical veins.

28. A characteristic of intestinal parasites such as *Ascaris* is a tough protective cuticle which
(A) protects the parasite from the host's enzymes.
(B) protects the parasite from other parasites the host carries.
(C) protects the host from the parasite's enzymes.
(D) keeps the parasite in a dormant state.

29. Of the following which is the incorrectly paired one?
(A) Robert Hooke—cell wall
(B) Schleiden and Schwann—cell theory
(C) Robert Brown—nucleus
(D) Watson and Crick—DNA model
(E) Virchow—spontaneous generation of living cells

30. Running to catch the bus to go to work has produced a rapid heart rate, an increase in the respiratory rate, and an increase in blood pressure in an individual. We can attribute these changes to
(A) the peripheral nervous system.
(B) the central nervous system.
(C) the parasympathetic component of the autonomic nervous system.
(D) increased metabolic rate.
(E) the sympathetic component of the autonomic nervous system.

31. Homologous structures have
(A) common embryonic origins.
(B) similar structures and shapes only in ontogeny.
(C) different embryonic origins.
(D) common functions but different shapes.
(E) different functions but the same shapes.

32. In rabbits, rough coat is dominant over smooth coat. Brown is dominant over gray fur color. A rough, brown male is mated to a couple of smooth, gray females. The offspring present the following ratios: 18 rough, brown; 21 rough, gray; 16 smooth, brown; 24 smooth, gray. If this male had been mated to a female of his own genotype, what proportion of the offspring would have exhibited rough, gray coats?
(A) 4 out of 16
(B) 3 out of 32
(C) 3 out of 16
(D) 12 out of 16
(E) 1 out of 16

33. Which of the following is mismatched?
(A) nervous system—reception, conduction, integration, effect
(B) skeletal system—posture, protection, locomotion, blood cell production
(C) epidermis—support, integration, exchange, filtration
(D) gastrointestinal system—absorption, secretion, digestion, egestion

34. Which of the following muscle types is not under the control of the autonomic (involuntary) nervous system?
(A) heart (cardiac)
(B) smooth
(C) skeletal (striated)
(D) arrector pili

35. In animals, cell division takes place throughout the body. In higher plants cell division occurs in localized ________ regions. These regions are found at the apices and as cambiums of roots and stems.
(A) young
(B) immature
(C) differentiated
(D) meristematic
(E) growth cone

Questions 36-38:

Mesoderm gives rise to ____(36)____, while ectoderm gives rise to ____(37)____ and endodermal derivation can be ascribed to ____(38)____.

36. (A) gall bladder
(B) appendix
(C) lungs
(D) muscle

37. (A) skin
(B) lens of the eye
(C) central nervous system
(D) all of the above

38. (A) lining of gut
(B) pituitary
(C) lining of respiratory system
(D) A and C above

STOP. If you finish before the time limit is up, go over your work for this section. DO NOT look at any other sections of the model examination. When your time limit is up, go on to the next section.

Chemistry

DIRECTIONS: In the following questions, four choices are presented that have been labeled A-D. For each question, choose the alternative that is most closely associated with the given item. You may use a choice more than once, or not at all. Eliminate those choices that you think to be incorrect, and mark the letter of your choice on the answer sheet.

Questions 1-3:

Consider the reaction below:

$$\underset{(A)}{A + B + C} \xrightarrow[(B)]{E\ (enzyme)} \underset{(C)}{ABCE} \longrightarrow \underset{(D)}{D + F} + \underset{(B)}{E}$$

1. The enzyme substrate complex
2. The reactants
3. The end product

Questions 4-7:

(A) Ionic bond
(B) Covalent bond
(C) Peptide bond
(D) Hydrogen bond

4. Formed by transfer of an electron from one atom to another
5. Formed by sharing electrons between two carbon atoms
6. Type of bond in molecules of KF
7. Type of bond in hydrogen molecule

DIRECTIONS: Each of the statements or questions is followed by four or five suggested completions or answers. Choose the one that best completes the statement or answers the question, and mark the letter of your choice on the answer sheet.

8. The development of our solar system is thought to have proceeded from the condensation of gases composed primarily of
(A) hydrogen.
(B) oxygen.
(C) carbon.
(D) argon.
(E) nitrogen.

9. Most enzymes are named to indicate the reaction they catalyze and have the suffix
(A) -ide.
(B) -ogen.
(C) -ase.
(D) -ose.
(E) -ade.

Questions 10, 11, 12:

Phenylamine is cooled to 0°C and treated with HCl and $NaNO_2$. After a few minutes of reaction time cuprous bromide is added, and the solution is heated.

10. The solution was cooled because
(A) the desired reaction proceeds too quickly above 0°, and thus an overreaction may result.
(B) the intermediate produced at the 0° temperature is unstable at higher temperature.
(C) HCl and $NaNO_2$ react only at low temperature.
(D) phenylamine is quite volatile and would evaporate at temperatures above 10°C.

11. The final aromatic product would contain about ______________ percent nitrogen.
(A) 20
(B) 15
(C) 8
(D) 90
(E) 0

12. The final product would primarily be a (an)
(A) azo dye.
(B) organometallic compound.
(C) monosubstituted benzene containing no metal.
(D) disubstituted benzene.
(E) enzyme.

13. Enzymes are
(A) proteins that catalyze chemical reactions, but they do not have the usual chemical and physical properties of proteins.
(B) proteins containing a high concentration of D-amino acids.
(C) compounds of amino acids, but they cannot be hydrolyzed to form free amino acids.
(D) proteins and may be considered as such chemically and physically.
(E) metallic compounds.

14. A covalent bond
(A) is one in which an orbital electron has been completely transferred from one atom to another.
(B) is one in which a pair of orbital electrons are shared between two atoms.
(C) occurs only in inorganic or organometallic compounds.
(D) occurs only in organic compounds.
(E) is a very unstable bond.

15. A metabolic process that produces energy to convert ADP^+ phosphate into ATP is the
(A) production of fructose and glucose from sucrose.
(B) production of fatty acids and glycerol from triglycerides.
(C) production of CO_2 and water from fatty acids.
(D) production of steroids from acetate.
(E) production of N_2 from fatty acids.

16. A solution is said to be of ____________ pH if it contains equal concentrations of hydroxyl and hydrogen.
(A) around 14
(B) around 0
(C) neutral
(D) just very slightly acidic
(E) just very slight basic

17. A molecule possessing NH_2 and COOH groups is classified as a (an)
(A) glycerol.
(B) protein.
(C) amino acid.
(D) carbohydrate.
(E) fat.

18. When CO_2 is dissolved in water, the end product will be
(A) carbon hydrate.
(B) carbon trioxide.
(C) carbon hydroxide.
(D) carbonic acid.
(E) carbon tetrachloride.

19. About twenty of all the elements known are regularly found in protoplasm; this may vary. Choose the item below that is present in the smallest quantity (percentage by weight).
(A) oxygen
(B) carbon
(C) hydrogen
(D) iron
(E) nitrogen

20. Where is messenger RNA synthesized in a cell?
(A) nucleus
(B) mitochondria
(C) ribosomes
(D) endoplasmic reticulum
(E) Golgi apparatus

21. A colloidal solution is influenced greatly by all of the following except
(A) electric charges.
(B) particle size.
(C) Brownian movement.
(D) gravitational forces.

22. Heating of benzaldehyde with NaOH produces
(A) no reaction.
(B) a long chain polymer by aldol condensation.
(C) benzoic acid and benzyl alcohol.
(D) benzoic acid and methyl alcohol.
(E) benzene and sodium carbonate.

23. The Lambert-Beer law
(A) was developed to explain the nonlinear production of alcohol by yeast in the brewing industry.
(B) describes the reproduction characteristics of yeast.
(C) relates the wave length of light to the light absorption of a solution at different wavelengths.
(D) relates changes in the light absorption at a particular wavelength to changes in thickness and/or concentration of a solution in the light path.
(E) may be explained in part by all of the statements.

24. Phenol is most soluble in
(A) aqueous NaOH.
(B) aqueous $NaHCO_3$.
(C) aqueous HCl.
(D) pure water.
(E) distilled water.

25. The metabolism of which of the following food components produces the greatest energy yield per gram?
(A) triglyceride
(B) glucose
(C) fructose
(D) protein
(E) carbohydrate

26. 1,3-Butadiene is a
(A) cumulative diene.
(B) conjugated diene.
(C) isolated diene.
(D) product of the reaction of calcium carbide with water.

27. An important chemical method for resolution of a racemic mixture utilizes the formation of
(A) a meso compound.
(B) geometric isomers.
(C) diastereomers.
(D) enantiomers.
(E) racemers.

28. The four deoxyribonucleotides which make up DNA are
(A) adenine, guanine, thymine, cytosine.
(B) adenine, guanine, cytosine, uracil.
(C) adenine, polyamine, thymine, cytoplasm.
(D) guanine, adenine, transfer RNA, cytosine.
(E) adenine, guanine, cytosine, nuclear RNA.

29. The base-catalyzed reaction below produces

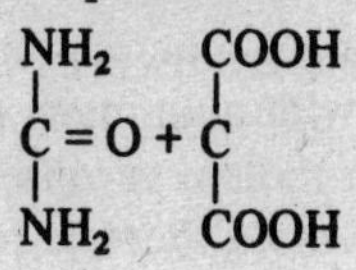

(A) cyclamate.
(B) nylon.
(C) barbital.
(D) saccharin.
(E) amphetamine.

30. The mechanism of enzymatic action involves
(A) slow degradation of the enzyme to form an enzyme-substrate complex.
(B) temporary union of enzyme with substrate.
(C) no specificity for a given substrate.
(D) resistance to deactivation by high temperatures.
(E) rapid degradation of the enzyme to form an enzyme-substrate complex.

31. DNA and RNA are both nucleic acids found in the nucleus; however, DNA differs from RNA in that DNA has
(A) fewer phosphate components.
(B) uracil instead of adenine as a nitrogenous base.
(C) a ribose instead of deoxyribose as a sugar.
(D) a deoxyribose instead of a ribose as a sugar.
(E) a shorter chain sugar.

32. The rate with which small molecules enter or leave cells is dependent on several factors, among them is (are)
(A) the charge they possess.
(B) their solubility (in lipid, etc.).
(C) their molecular size.
(D) all of the above.

33. A compound with the structure $H_2C=\underset{\displaystyle H}{\underset{|}{C}}-CH_2-\underset{\displaystyle H}{\underset{|}{C}}=O$ is
(A) an acid.
(B) an anhydride.
(C) a ketone.
(D) none of the above.

34. An element ordinarily found in monoatomic form is
(A) helium.
(B) argon.
(C) neon.
(D) all of the above.

35. Hydrolysis of sucrose produces an equimolar mixture of
(A) fructose and glucose.
(B) glucose and either ribose or deoxyribose.
(C) galactose and glucose.
(D) glucose and maltose.
(E) none of the above.

36. A compound with the formula C_3H_6 could be
(A) propane.
(B) propyne.
(C) cyclopropane.
(D) none of the above.

37. An example of a polyester is
(A) nylon.
(B) dacron.
(C) polyethylene.
(D) polymixin B.
(E) achromycin.

38. Most home units for softening water
(A) remove ions such as calcium and replace them with sodium ions.
(B) remove virtually all ions, producing water of the same chemical purity as distilled water.
(C) remove primarily anions such as sulfur.
(D) add small quantities of soap to produce water that feels soft.
(E) function by osmosis.

39. The Hall Process for the production of metallic aluminum utilizes
(A) the reaction of metallic sodium with aluminum salts.
(B) electrolysis of aluminum salts in molten cryolite.
(C) heating of aluminum salts in an atmosphere of hydrogen.
(D) heating aluminum salts with suspended carbon particles.
(E) heating of aluminum salts in an atmosphere of nitrogen.

40. In the usual industrial process, electrolysis of brine produces ______________ respectively at the two electrodes.
(A) chlorine and steam
(B) chlorine and sodium
(C) chlorine and sodium hydroxide
(D) sodium hydroxide and hydrochloric acid
(E) bromine and steam

41. The gas responsible for the rising of bread is
(A) hydrogen.
(B) carbon dioxide.
(C) nitrogen.
(D) oxygen.
(E) ozone.

42. The major component of permanent type antifreeze for automobile cooling systems is
(A) glycerol.
(B) methanol.
(C) ethylene glycol.
(D) isopropyl alcohol.
(E) ethyl alcohol.

43. Upon the addition of ammonium chloride to water, the temperature of the liquid is observed to decrease. This is best explained by
(A) a broken thermometer.
(B) the heat of solution.
(C) salting out of organic contaminants.
(D) none of the above.

44. All macromolecules (proteins, polysaccharides, etc.) must be ______________ before they can be absorbed by the intestines.
(A) emulsified
(B) detoxified
(C) pasteurized
(D) hydrolyzed
(E) oxydized

45. To accomplish the conversion of carbohydrates into CO_2, H_2O, and ATP the Krebs cycle must operate properly. In addition
(A) the carbon cycle and CO_2 must be present.
(B) glycogen synthesis must supply the energy.
(C) cholesterol synthesis must be carried on.
(D) oxygen and electron transport reactions must be present.
(E) fluoroacetate must be available.

46. When glucose enters a cell, it is converted into ______________ before it undergoes any other chemical transformations.
(A) galactose-6-phosphate
(B) glycogen
(C) maltose-6-phosphate
(D) glucose-6-phosphate
(E) all of the above

47. The least basic amine listed below is
(A) aniline.
(B) p-nitroaniline.
(C) p-methylaniline.
(D) p-methoxyaniline.

48. Biological compounds containing carbon, hydrogen, and oxygen but little or no nitrogen include
(A) fats (triglycerides).
(B) carbohydrates.
(C) proteins.
(D) fats (triglycerides) and carbohydrates.
(E) all of the above.

49. An alkyl chloride, e.g., $CH_3—CH_2—CH_2Cl$, is best prepared by reacting the corresponding alcohol with
(A) Cl_2.
(B) PCl_3.
(C) HOCl.
(D) HCl.

STOP. If you finish before the time limit is up, go over your work for this section. DO NOT look at any other sections of the model examination. When your time limit is up, go on to the next section.

Physics

DIRECTIONS: Each of the statements or questions is followed by five suggested completions or answers. Choose the one that best completes the statement or answers the question, and mark the letter of your choice on the answer sheet.

1. A car travels at 30 kilometers/hour for 15 kilometers. It then increases its average speed to 60 km/hr. for the next 30 kilometers. The overall average speed for the 30 km is:
(A) 30 km/hr.
(B) 35 km/hr.
(C) 40 km/hr.
(D) 45 km/hr.
(E) 50 km/hr.

2. If we neglect friction, the acceleration of a free-falling body near the surface of the earth is about 9.8 m/sec^2. This means that the
(A) velocity at the end of one second will be 19.6 m/sec. if the body started at rest.
(B) velocity of a freely falling object increases 9.8 m/sec. for each second that the object is falling.
(C) body would drop 9.8 m in the first second.
(D) velocity does not change as the body falls.
(E) motion is nonuniform.

3. A gas under 1 atmosphere absolute pressure occupies a 2 cubic meter volume at 293°K. What will the temperature be if the volume is increased to 3 cubic meters and the pressure is 4 atmospheres absolute?
(A) 0°K
(B) 273°K
(C) 373°K
(D) 1119°K
(E) 1758°K

4. Which one of the statements below is false?
(A) An endothermal reaction requires the addition of energy before it can occur.
(B) An exothermal reaction converts chemical energy to another form.
(C) The concepts of exothermal and endothermal reactions are relevant in discussing nuclear reactions.
(D) After an exothermal reaction the final temperature of the components is unchanged.
(E) During an exothermal reaction heat is released.

5. Isotopes of a given element have the same atomic number but have a different mass number. Which of the statements below is true?
(A) Isotopes of a given element have a larger number of electrons and protons.
(B) Isotopes of a given element have a smaller number of electrons and protons.
(C) Isotopes of a given element have a different number of nucleons in the nucleus.
(D) All elements have isotopes.
(E) Isotopes are indistinguishable from one another.

6. The density of a given steel block is 7.8 gm/cm^3. What is the mass of a steel block whose dimensions are 2 meters by 3 meters by 5 meters?
(A) 234×10^6 gm
(B) 1234 gm
(C) 7.8×10^6 gm
(D) 178 gm
(E) 30 gm

7. What is the kinetic energy possessed by a 100-gram projectile moving with a velocity of 60 m/sec.?
(A) 60 joules
(B) 180 joules
(C) 360 joules
(D) 3600 joules
(E) 6000 joules

8. The basic unit of force in the metric system is a newton which implies that mass and acceleration are
(A) gm and m/sec.
(B) kg and m/sec.^{2}.
(C) lb. and ft./sec.^{2}.
(D) kg and m/sec.
(E) lb. and m/sec.^{2}.

9. In uniform circular motion, the radially inward-directed force to maintain the body in a circular motion is known as
(A) centrifugal force.
(B) kinetic friction.
(C) moment of inertia.
(D) universal gravitation.
(E) centripetal force.

10. A 5 kg object is raised 10 meters from the floor. Compute the work done in joules.
(A) 5 joules
(B) 50 joules
(C) 98 joules
(D) 490 joules
(E) 980 joules

11. A man 2 m tall stands 3 m from an intense source of light at the level of his feet. The man's shadow appears on a wall 15 m from the source of light. How tall is the shadow?
(A) 6 m
(B) 10 m
(C) 12.5 m
(D) 17.5 m
(E) 22.5 m

12. When water waves approach the shore at an angle, they will be slowed down in the shallower positions rather than the deeper positions. The portion of the wave in deeper water will consequently swing around until the entire wave train is almost parallel to shore. This phenomenon of wave action is called
(A) reflections.
(B) diffraction.
(C) dispersion.
(D) retardation.
(E) refraction.

13. A car's electric light system is a constant voltage system and not a constant current system. If the resistance in this system is tripled, the resulting power (P) is
(A) $1/3P$.
(B) $1/2P$.
(C) P (same).
(D) $2P$.
(E) $3P$.

DIRECTIONS: Listed below are five laws of physics and five phrases of definition. Match the correct definition with the appropriate law.

Questions 14-18:

(A) The induced emf in a circuit is equal to the rate of decrease of flux through the circuit.
(B) The relationship between volume and temperature of a nearly ideal gas where the pressure is kept constant is such that the volume is proportional to the absolute temperature.
(C) When a body exerts a force on another body, the second body exerts an equal and opposite force on the first body.
(D) At the same temperature and pressure, equal volumes of different gases contain equal numbers of molecules.
(E) Every body in the universe attracts every other body with a force that is directed along a line connecting them and varies directly with their masses and inversely with the square of distance between them.

14. Charles' law
15. the Faraday law
16. the law of universal gravitation
17. Newton's third law of motion
18. Avagadro's law

19. A ball is at the crest of a hill. The ball moves to a new position after a small amount of displacement. Initially, the ball was in
(A) stable equilibrium.
(B) neutral equilibrium.
(C) positive equilibrium.
(D) unstable equilibrium.
(E) productive equilibrium.

20. A body is submerged in water. The upward force acting upon this body is
(A) equal to its weight.
(B) equal to the weight of the displaced fluid.
(C) the absolute pressure at the surface of the fluid.
(D) dependent upon its center of gravity.
(E) directly proportional to its length.

21. The energy of a water wave is directly proportional to the square of its amplitude. If the amplitude is doubled, what occurs to the wave energy?
(A) It is doubled.
(B) It is tripled.
(C) It is quadrupled.
(D) It is halved.
(E) It remains the same.

22. Using the vector diagram below, determine the resultant vector.

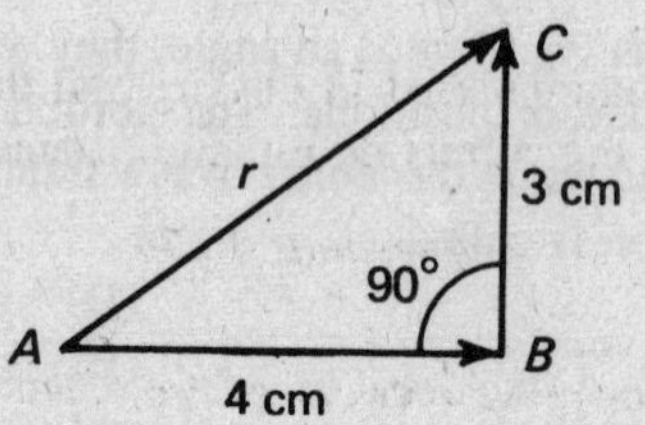

(A) 5 cm at 37°
(B) 5 cm
(C) 5 cm at 45°
(D) 8 cm at 45°
(E) 8 cm at 90°

23. In uniformly accelerated motion, the following relationship holds:

$$v = v_0 + at$$
$$x = v_0 t + \frac{1}{2}at^2$$

where x = distance moved, t = time, a = acceleration, v_0 = velocity at start, and v = velocity at end. What is the acceleration of a body whose initial velocity of 1340 cm/sec. increases to 2690 cm/sec. in 348 m within 15 seconds?
(A) 15 cm/sec.^{2}
(B) 30 cm/sec.^{2}
(C) 45 cm/sec.^{2}
(D) 60 cm/sec.^{2}
(E) 90 cm/sec.^{2}

24. What is the radius of a curve if the curve is properly banked for a car traveling at 2500 cm/sec. and $\tan \theta = v^2/ra$, where r = radius, v = velocity, a = acceleration, and $\tan \theta = 1$?
(A) 16 m
(B) 32 m
(C) 48 m
(D) 64 m
(E) 80 m

25. There are two absolute temperature scales, the Kelvin scale and the Rankin scale. Which statement below is correct?
(A) The Kelvin scale is measured in centigrade degrees.
(B) Absolute zero is the zero point for each scale and not the freezing point.
(C) The Rankin scale uses Fahrenheit degrees.
(D) The boiling point of water on the Kelvin scale is 373 K° and 672°R.
(E) All of the above.

26. Under certain conditions, solids will go directly from the solid state to the gaseous state without going through the liquid state. This process is called
(A) melting.
(B) freezing.
(C) vaporization.
(D) condensing.
(E) sublimation.

27. The velocity of sound in air is 332 m/sec. at 0°C. What is the velocity of sound in air at 20°C?
(A) 344 m/sec.
(B) 1268 m/sec.
(C) 1420 m/sec.
(D) 1484 m/sec.
(E) 4975 m/sec.

28. The velocity of sound in water is 1435 m/sec. and the velocity of sound in air is 332 m/sec. at 0°C. If a tuning fork vibrating at 410 cycles per second is placed in water at 0°C, what is the wavelength of the sound waves that are produced?
(A) 1.0 m
(B) 2.5 m
(C) 3.5 m
(D) 4.5 m
(E) 6.0 m

29. A man 2 m tall stands 5 m in front of a plane mirror. How tall is his image?
(A) 0.5 m
(B) 1.0 m
(C) 1.5 m
(D) 2.0 m
(E) 2.5 m

DIRECTIONS: Five basic equations used in physics and their definitions or names are given below. Match the equation with the correct definition or name.

Questions 30-34:

(A) Bernoulli's equation
(B) Lens-maker's equation—the focal length of a lens is directly related to the index of refraction of the glass and the radius of curvature of each face.
(C) Law of universal gravitation states that every body in the universe attracts every other body with a force that is directed along a line connecting them and that varies directly with their masses and inversely with the square of the distance between them.
(D) Snell's law
(E) The general gas law—a relationship which relates the pressure, volume, and temperature of a gas.

30. $1/f = (n - 1)(1/R_1 + 1/R_2)$

31. $PV/T = P_0V_0/T_0$

32. $h_1 + P_1/w + V_1^2/2a = h_2 + P_2/w + V_2^2/2a$

33. $F = G(m_1m_2/d^2)$

34. $\sin\theta_i/\sin\theta_r = n_r/n_i$

35. The half-life of a radioactive element is 10 years. How much of the original element remains at the end of 80 years?
(A) $\frac{1}{32}$
(B) $\frac{1}{64}$
(C) $\frac{1}{128}$
(D) $\frac{1}{256}$
(E) $\frac{1}{512}$

36. All but one of the terms listed below are elementary particles of an atom. Which one is not?
(A) boron
(B) electron
(C) neutron
(D) positron
(E) proton

37. The energy emitted per unit of time by a radiating object is called radiant power. That part of the radiant power in the visible range is known as
(A) illuminance.
(B) reflection.
(C) luminous flux.
(D) conductance.
(E) induction.

38. Charging a body without making contact with the body is called charging by
(A) capacitance.
(B) lightning
(C) conductance.
(D) induction.
(E) resistance.

STOP. If you finish before the time limit is up, go over your work for this section. DO NOT look at any other sections of the model examination. When your time limit is up, go on to the next section.

SCIENCE PROBLEMS

85 MINUTES
66 QUESTIONS

The following questions require you to use your knowledge of science to solve problems.

DIRECTIONS: The following questions are in groups. Preceding each series of questions is a paragraph or a short explanatory statement, a formula or set of formulas, or a definition. Read the written material and then answer the questions. Eliminate those choices that you think to be incorrect and mark the letter of your choice on the answer sheet.

For uniformly accelerated angular motion, the following equations hold:

$$w = w_0 + \alpha t$$
$$\theta = w_0 t + \tfrac{1}{2}\alpha t$$

where w = angular velocity, α = angular acceleration, t = time, θ = angular distance, and subscript $_0$ indicates initial condition. A wheel at rest starts rotating with an angular acceleration of 10 radians/sec./sec.

1. What is its angular velocity at the end of 4 seconds?
   (A) 8 radians/sec.
   (B) 16 radians/sec.
   (C) 24 radians/sec.
   (D) 32 radians/sec.
   (E) 40 radians/sec.

2. How many revolutions has the wheel made at the end of 4 seconds?
   (A) 3.2 revolutions
   (B) 6.4 revolutions
   (C) 9.6 revolutions
   (D) 12.7 revolutions
   (E) 15.9 revolutions

3. If the angular velocity of the wheel at the end of the 4 seconds increases to 60 radians/sec. in the next 4 seconds, the magnitude of the angular acceleration changes to
   (A) 5 radians/sec./sec.
   (B) 10 radians/sec./sec.
   (C) 15 radians/sec./sec.
   (D) 20 radians/sec./sec.
   (E) 25 radians/sec./sec.

A protein is least soluble at its isoelectric point since it has an equal number of positive and negative charges. The amino acid residues with their functional groups such as $-NH^+$ or $\overset{O}{\overset{\|}{C}}-OH$ or $\overset{O}{\overset{\|}{C}}-O^-$ would, therefore, not have repulsion effects to separate the protein molecules. Increasing turbidity is an indication of insolubility. At a pH below the isoelectric point, more $\overset{O}{\overset{\|}{C}}-O^-$ would be protonated.

4. Given the table below with increasing + indicating increasing turbidity, which is the isoelectric point of the protein?

pH AND SOLUBILITY OF A PROTEIN

pH	5.9	5.6	5.5	5.2	5.0	4.8
Turbidity	0	+	+	++	+	0

   (A) 5.9 or 4.8
   (B) 7
   (C) 5.6
   (D) 5.0
   (E) 5.2

5. What is the net charge on the protein from the previous question?
(A) 0
(B) +2
(C) −2
(D) +5
(E) 5.2

6. At pH 4.8 net charge on the protein from above is
(A) zero.
(B) positive.
(C) negative.
(D) not enough information given.
(E) equal number of positive and negative charges.

An unknown compound is composed solely of nitrogen, carbon, and hydrogen. An analysis for nitrogen reveals 45.2%. Complete combustion of 0.100 g of the compound produced 0.145 g of water and 0.142 g of carbon dioxide.

7. The empirical formula of the compound is
(A) CHN.
(B) CHNO.
(C) CH_5N.
(D) C_2H_4N.
(E) $C_2H_2N_3$.

8. The compound could be a (an)
(A) olefin.
(B) organic nitrate.
(C) substituted pyridine.
(D) amine.
(E) nitrile.

9. If it is found that the molecular weight is twice that of the empirical formula, it is possible to write the
(A) structural formula.
(B) formula with functional groups indicated.
(C) molecular formula as $C_2H_{10}N_2$.
(D) molecular formula as $C_4H_4N_6$.
(E) none of the above.

The following experiments are designed to illustrate several phenomena. The instructor in a general biology class demonstrates these in the following manner.

Experiment 1: A piece of spaghetti measuring 3 inches in length is placed in a bowl of warm water and measured after 15 minutes. Its length has increased to 3.7 inches.

10. The increase in length is due to the absorption of water by a (an)
(A) inert substance.
(B) semipermeable substance.
(C) colloidal substance.
(D) isotonic substance.
(E) hypertonic substance.

11. The forces observed are substantial and might explain
(A) the splitting of a concrete driveway by mushrooms.
(B) the splitting of a sidewalk by the roots of trees.
(C) the damage (crumbling of rock) observed on a mountainside due to the growth of vegetation.
(D) all of the above.
(E) none of the above.

12. The phenomenon demonstrated may best be defined as
(A) imbibition.
(B) osmosis.
(C) concentration.
(D) turgor.
(E) plasmolysis.

Experiment 2: Study the illustration below to answer the following three questions.

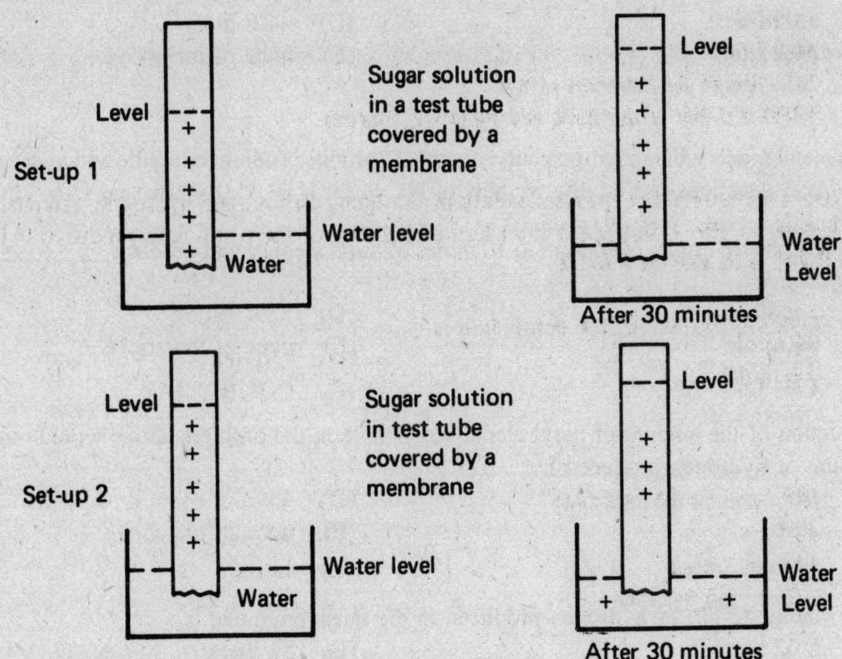

13. From your observation you deduce that the test tubes were placed in a (an) ______ medium.
(A) hypertonic
(B) hypotonic
(C) isotonic
(D) inert
(E) saturated

14. Set-up 1 demonstrates the phenomenon of
(A) imbibition.
(B) osmosis.
(C) turgor.
(D) plasmolysis.
(E) cyclosis.

15. Set-up 2 demonstrates the phenomenon of
(A) imbibition.
(B) osmosis.
(C) diffusion.
(D) turgor.
(E) plasmolysis.

Avogadro's number may be given as 6.02×10^{23}. Standard temperature and pressure (STP) are 273°K and 760 mm mercury (760 torr).

16. At STP the number of molecules in 1 mole of glucose is
(A) 22.4×10^{12}.
(B) 22.4×10^{15}.
(C) 3.01×10^{20}.
(D) 6.02×10^{23}.
(E) 9×10^{23}.

17. Reducing the pressure from 760 to 380 torr would change the number of molecules in one mole of glucose to
(A) 10% of its former value.
(B) 30% of its former value.
(C) 50% of its former value.
(D) 75% of its former value.
(E) none of the above.

18. If a sample contains 3.01×10^{23} molecules of hydrogen in a container at 273°K and a pressure of 760 torr, the volume will be
(A) 6.02 liters.
(B) 11.2 liters.
(C) 22.4 liters.
(D) 44.8 liters.
(E) none of the above.

Sodium metal reacts with anhydrous butyl alcohol to produce sodium butoxide and hydrogen. For the following 3 questions use atomic weights of Na = 23; H = 1; 0 = 16; and C = 12.

19. The addition of 1 mole of sodium to 10 moles of butyl alcohol will produce ____________ of hydrogen.
(A) 1 mole
(B) 0.1 mole
(C) 0.5 moles
(D) 22.4 moles
(E) none of the above

20. Reduction of the amount of butyl alcohol to 1 mole in the problem above would reduce the amount of hydrogen produced by
(A) 10%.
(B) 20%.
(C) 40%.
(D) 45%.
(E) none of the above.

21. The volume (STP) of hydrogen produced in the question above is
(A) 6.02 liters.
(B) 11.2 liters.
(C) 22.4 liters.
(D) 52 liters.
(E) none of the above.

Boyle's law states that the volume of a confined gas varies inversely with the absolute pressure provided that the temperature remains constant. Using this information, apply it to the questions below.

1 liter of oxygen at a pressure of 4 atmospheres is mixed with 5 liters of nitrogen at 2 atmospheres. The mixture is then subjected to 5 atmospheres absolute pressure.

22. What is the pressure of the oxygen in the mixture?
(A) 5.0 atm
(B) 4.0 atm
(C) 3.33 atm
(D) 1.67 atm
(E) 0.67 atm

23. Compute the total pressure of the new mixture.
(A) 0.67 atm
(B) 1.67 atm
(C) 2.34 atm
(D) 3.00 atm
(E) 3.67 atm

24. Calculate the volume of the mixture after it is subjected to 5 atmospheres pressure.
(A) 0.5 liters
(B) 1.0 liters
(C) 1.8 liters
(D) 2.8 liters
(E) none of the above

It has been known for some time that chronic (or in some cases acute) exposure of animals to certain agents results in a fatty degeneration of the liver. Fatty degeneration or fatty liver means an abnormal accumulation of lipid (organic solvent soluble) has occurred. This is a common response of the liver to injury and most often involves an abnormal accumulation of triglyceride (ester of 3 moles of a carboxylic acid and glycerol). Agents capable of producing this effect include such diverse compounds as salts of cerium and other rare earths, carbon tetrachloride, ethyl alcohol, and certain antibiotics. Fatty livers may result from (1) increased liver synthesis of lipid, (2) decreased liver metabolism of lipid, (3) decreased liver secretion of lipid into the blood (as lipoproteins) or combinations of these factors.

25. Long term ingestion of ethyl alcohol can result in liver damage possibly due to
(A) accumulation of triglycerides.
(B) increased breakdown of lipids.
(C) increased secretion of lipid into the blood.
(D) increased metabolism of lipid.
(E) all of the above.

26. A person who by profession was a rug cleaner and who still used older methods, such as carbon tetrachloride as a cleaning agent, died under unusual circumstances. On autopsy, organic chemical extract of normal liver showed 1.5% lipid. What might be a reasonable value for an organic chemical extract from the rug cleaner's liver?
(A) no reason to expect any different from normal
(B) 1.5% lipids
(C) 0.5% lipids
(D) 6% lipids
(E) zero % lipids

27. For a rat treated with hydrazine and injected with ^{14}C-labeled carboxylic acid after 6 hr., 50 μg/100 μg lipoprotein (normal animals injected similarly showed 25μg/100 μg) was found. This experiment would rule out ______________ as being a cause for fatty liver.
(A) increased liver synthesis of lipid
(B) decreased liver metabolism
(C) decreased secretion of lipid
(D) all of the above
(E) hydrazine

A balloon has been filled with an unknown gas. Having no sophisticated equipment at hand, it is decided to bubble the gas through calcium hydroxide.

28. If a precipitate forms, the gas is identified as
(A) sulfur dioxide.
(B) sulfur trioxide.
(C) carbon monoxide.
(D) butane.
(E) none of the above.

29. Another portion of the unknown gas is passed over a flame. If the gas ignites, this information coupled with the information from the previous question tells us that the gas is
(A) carbon monoxide.
(B) butane.
(C) butadiene.
(D) an ideal gas.
(E) a mixture.

30. A portion of the gas is cooled and then used to fill a beaker. When a lighted splint is inserted into the beaker, the splint is extinguished. This tells us that the gas does not contain a high concentration of
(A) CO_2.
(B) N_2.
(C) N_2O.
(D) C_2F_6.
(E) O_2.

Electrolysis is an important industrial method for the preparation of various chemicals. Electrolysis may be accomplished in aqueous solution or in fused salt depending on the products desired.

31. Electrolysis of aqueous sodium chloride will allow the collection of ____________ at the anode.
(A) chlorine
(B) sodium
(C) hydrogen
(D) sodium hydroxide
(E) none of the above

32. Electrolysis of fused sodium chloride will allow the collection of ____________ at the cathode.
(A) chlorine
(B) sodium
(C) hydrogen
(D) sodium hydroxide
(E) none of the above

33. Electrolysis of aqueous sodium chloride allows the collection of ____________ at the cathode.
(A) sodium
(B) sodium hydroxide
(C) hydrogen
(D) B and C
(E) none of the above

Given the circuit diagram below where Ra, Rb, and Rc are respectively the resistances in series.

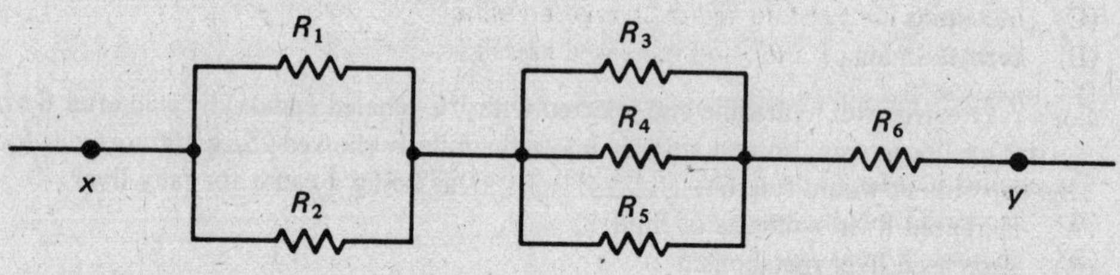

34. The resistance across the parallel resistors R_1 and R_2 can be correctly expressed as
(A) $Ra = R_1 + R_2$.
(B) $1/Ra = 1/R_1 + 1/R_2$.
(C) $Ra = (R_1)(R_2)$.
(D) $Ra = R_1/R_2$.
(E) none of the above.

35. If one resistor (Rs) were to replace the entire group of resistors above, its value would be equal to
(A) $Rs = 1/Ra + 1/Rb + 1/Rc$.
(B) $Rs = (Ra)(Rb)(Rc)$.
(C) $Rs = RaRb/Rc$.
(D) $Rs = Ra - Rb/Rc$.
(E) $Rs = Ra + Rb + Rc$.

36. If total resistance from x to y is 60 ohms and the circuit current of 2 amps is flowing, what is the potential difference across this resistance?
(A) 30 volts
(B) 60 volts
(C) 120 volts
(D) 180 volts
(E) none of the above

Blood, in arteries, exists as a heterogeneous mass which has resistance properties. With this in mind, it is understandable that the greatest rate of flow is experienced in the center of the artery with a concomitant decrease in flow as one approaches the periphery.

37. One can attribute a drop in blood pressure within an artery to
(A) friction resulting from blood flowing against the wall of an artery.
(B) the summation of individual shear forces within layers of blood throughout the artery.
(C) gradual change in the histological construction of the innermost surface of the artery.
(D) none of the above.
(E) all of the above.

38. Blood flow is a function of
(A) the amount of elasticity of the arterial wall at a particular point.
(B) the physiological status of the blood.
(C) its compactness as visualized by its radius.
(D) none of the above.

39. Given that the cross-sectional area influences flow by the fourth power of the radius, the flow of a large blood vessel whose diameter is reduced by 50% is in turn reduced to
(A) 1/2.
(B) 1/16.
(C) 1/4.
(D) 1/32.
(E) 1/50.

Reaction equilibria may be affected by temperature or pressure. Consider the reaction

$$X_2 \text{ (gas)} + Y_2 \text{ (gas)} \rightarrow X_2Y_2 \text{ (gas)}$$

which is exothermic in the direction in which it is written.

40. The equilibrium could be shifted in the direction of X_2Y_2 by
(A) increased temperature.
(B) increased pressure.
(C) increased temperature and decreased pressure.
(D) decreased temperature and increased pressure.
(E) none of the above.

41. The equilibrium could be shifted in the direction of X_2 and Y_2 by
(A) decreased temperature.
(B) decreased pressure.
(C) increased temperature and increased pressure.
(D) decreased temperature and decreased pressure.
(E) none of the above.

42. A combination of increased temperature and increased pressure would cause the equilibrium to shift
(A) markedly to the left.
(B) slightly to the left.
(C) markedly to the right.
(D) slightly to the right.
(E) with direction and magnitude unknown or not shift at all.

The half-life of a radioactive element is the time required for one-half of a given amount of an element to disintegrate. The fraction remaining F in equation form is $F = (\frac{1}{2})^{\frac{t}{T}}$ where t = time interval and T = half-life.

43. The half-life of a particular element is 10 seconds. What amount of 10^9 atoms remains after 90 seconds?
(A) 10^9 atoms
(B) 2×10^9 atoms
(C) 2×10^6 atoms
(D) 2×10^3 atoms
(E) 2 atoms

44. What percentage of the original atoms have disintegrated in the 90 seconds?
(A) 99.8%
(B) 50.4%
(C) 41.7%
(D) 49.6%
(E) 0.2%

45. Select the best statement below about elements with a half-life on the order of microseconds.
(A) Those elements will never totally disintegrate.
(B) The half-life concept does not apply to them as it does to longer half-life elements.
(C) Their half-life is adversely influenced by pressure, temperature, and volume.
(D) They need to be continuously generated through radioactive decay of heavier elements to continue to exist.
(E) None of the above.

Newton's law of universal gravitation expressed mathematically is $F = G\frac{M_1M_2}{d^2}$ where G = universal physical constant = to $6.67 \times 10^{-11} \frac{\text{Newton} - M^2}{kg^2}$, M_1 and M_2 are masses of particles attracted, and d is the distance between them.

46. Knowing this law enables us to
(A) calculate the mass of the earth.
(B) determine what a person would weigh on the surface of another planet.
(C) state that the force of attraction of a person of mass m varies directly with radius of another planet of equal density.
(D) state that all of the above are true.

47. What is the force of attraction, in newtons, between two bodies separated by 20 m and having masses of 1 kg and 5 kg respectively?
(A) 7×10^{-11}
(B) 8×10^{-13}
(C) 9×10^{-12}
(D) 2×10^{-9}
(E) none of the above

48. A variation of the law can be written as $F = \frac{4}{3}\pi\ G\ M_1\ rD$ where $G = 6.67 \times 10^{-11} \frac{\text{Newton}\ M^2}{kg^2}$, r = radius of planet, D = density of sphere, and M_1 = mass on the planet of a given object. Using this calculate the mass of an object weighing 70 kg on earth after it has been transported to a planet that has the same density as the earth but whose radius is ¼ that of the earth (radius of earth = 6380 km).
(A) 70 kg
(B) 140 kg
(C) 210 kg
(D) 280 kg
(E) 350 kg

The rate of a reaction is related to the rate constant as well as the concentrations of the reactants. An example is the reaction $A + 2B \rightarrow C + 2D$.

49. The rate of the reaction could be calculated as
(A) $2k\ [A]\ [B]$.
(B) $k^2\ [A]\ [B]$.
(C) $2k[C]\ [D]$.
(D) $k^2\ [C]\ [D]$.
(E) none of the above.

50. The greatest increase in the reaction rate as shown would be caused by doubling the concentration of
(A) A.
(B) B.
(C) C.
(D) D.
(E) A and C.

51. Doubling the concentration of A and halving the concentration of C would change the reaction rate to ____________ of its former rate.
(A) 100%
(B) 75%
(C) 50%
(D) 200%
(E) none of the above

The strong acid H_2X is allowed to react with the base ZOH.

52. Twenty milliliters of a 0.5 *N* solution of H_2X will be neutralized by ____________ of a 1 *N* solution of ZOH.
(A) 20 ml
(B) 10 ml
(C) 5 ml
(D) 40 ml
(E) >50 ml

53. The number of milliequivalents in 120 ml of the 0.5 *N* solution of H_2X is ____________ that in 120 ml of the 1 *N* ZOH solution.
(A) half
(B) twice
(C) equal to
(D) one-fourth
(E) four times

54. The greatest number of milliequivalents below (acid or base) is in 500 ml of
(A) 1 *N* solution of H_2X.
(B) 1 *N* solution of ZOH.
(C) 1 *M* solution of H_2X.
(D) 1 *M* solution of ZOH.
(E) choices A and C.

The specific gravity of lead is 11.3.

55. What is the density of lead in gm/cm^3?
(A) 1.0
(B) 2.7
(C) 7.8
(D) 11.3
(E) 13.6

56. What is the volume of a block of lead whose mass is 600 kg?
(A) 11.3×10^3 cm^3
(B) 53.1×10^3 cm^3
(C) 60×10^3 cm^3
(D) 67.8×10^3 cm^3
(E) none of the above

57. What is the density of lead in $lb./ft.^3$?
(A) 113.25
(B) 600.75
(C) 786.25
(D) 1678.25
(E) none of the above

$$2H_2O \rightleftharpoons \underset{\text{a hydrated proton (hydronium ion)}}{H_3O^+} + \underset{\text{hydroxyl ion}}{OH^-}$$

The reaction above is directed so that the predominant form at equilibrium is undissociated water. Expressed as a special chemical equilibrium with an equilibrium constant, K_w:

$$K_w = [H_3O^+][OH^-] = 1 \times 10^{-14}$$

58. At equilibrium for H_2O
(A) there are equal concentrations of H_2O, H_3O^+ and ^-OH.
(B) the concentration of $H_3O^+ \times {}^-OH$ is equal to that of H_2O.
(C) the concentrations of H_3O^+ and ^-OH are equal.
(D) the K_w is neutral.
(E) there is twice as much H_2O at equilibrium as OH^- or H_3O^+.

59. When the H_3O^+ concentration equals 10^{-7}, then
(A) the ^-OH concentration is 10^{-14}.
(B) the ^-OH concentration is 10^{-7}.
(C) the ^-OH concentration plus the H^+ is 10^{-14}.
(D) the K_w is neutral.
(E) the K_w equals the H_3O^+ minus the OH^-.

60. When OH^- was added to increase the OH^- to OH^{-4},
(A) the K_w would change to 10^{-1}.
(B) the H^+ would change to 10^{-4}.
(C) the H^+ would change to 10^{-10}.
(D) the K_w would be neutral.
(E) this is an impossible condition since H^+ must equal ^-OH.

Steam distillation is a technique by which an immiscible higher boiling liquid may be distilled at a lower temperature as one component of a binary azeotrope with water.

61. Compound Z is steam distilled at a pressure of 760 torr and a temperature of 90°C. If the vapor pressure of water at 90°C is 526 torr, then the vapor pressure of compound Z is
(A) 760 torr.
(B) 526 torr.
(C) 234 torr.
(D) 144 torr.
(E) none of the above.

62. This technique is particularly helpful if compound Z is
(A) hygroscopic.
(B) highly volatile.
(C) highly sensitive to elevated temperatures.
(D) water soluble.
(E) none of the above.

63. After steam distillation the 2 components of the product may be separated by
(A) distillation.
(B) removing one liquid layer.
(C) filtration.
(D) choices A and C.
(E) none of the above.

Enzymatic actions are necessary for certain processes to take place. Study the results of the following experiments to answer the questions below.

Experiment 1:
Test tube 1. Compound A + water — after 1 hour no reaction
Test tube 2. Compound B + Compound A — after 1 hour there is a noticeable color change
Test tube 3. Compound B + Water — after 1 hour no reaction

Experiment 2:
Test tube 1. Compound X + Compound Y + Water — no reaction
Test tube 2. Compound X + Acid + Water — no reaction
Test tube 3. Compound X + Compound Y + Acid — reaction product
Test tube 4. Compound X + Compound Y + Solution of bicarbonate — no reaction

Experiment 3:
Test tube 1. Compound Z + Compound W; examined after being left at room temperature for 30 minutes — some reaction product
Test tube 2. Compound Z + Boiled Compound W; examined after being left at room temperature for 30 minutes — no reaction product
Test tube 3. Compound Z + Compound W; examined after being left in an ice bath for 30 minutes — some reaction product

64. In experiment 1, test tube 2 contained the enzyme.
(A) True
(B) False

65. The object of experiment 2 was to establish that enzymes are influenced by
(A) pressure.
(B) temperature.
(C) pH.
(D) all of the above.
(E) none of the above.

66. Experiment 3 demonstrated that ______________ affected the enzymatic reaction.

(A) pressure
(B) temperature
(C) boiling
(D) pH
(E) all of the above

STOP. If you finish before the time limit is up, go over your work for this section. DO NOT look at any other sections of the model examination. When your time limit is up, go on to the next section.

SKILLS ANALYSIS: READING

85 MINUTES
68 QUESTIONS

The following questions are to be answered based on your careful reading of selections from scientific writings.

DIRECTIONS: Read each passage carefully, then answer the questions following it. Consider only the material within the passage in answering the questions. Eliminate those choices that you think to be incorrect and mark the letter of your choice on the answer sheet.

It has become obvious in recent years that the decision making power in many school districts is shifting, and is becoming more liberalized as both teachers and parents realize that they are an important facet in the total school operation. They know that without their support and cooperation the system cannot continue to function smoothly.

Consequently, today's educator is no longer content to sit in the background and let decisions be made and programs formulated. New teachers want a voice, they demand a piece of the action, and they are daring enough to question the judgments of the system in their desire to achieve a better educational experience for their students as well as a more economically realistic position for themselves.

Not too many years ago, perhaps as little as a decade in some areas, the decision making power in a school system could have been observed by quickly glancing at an organizational chart which would most probably have looked like this;

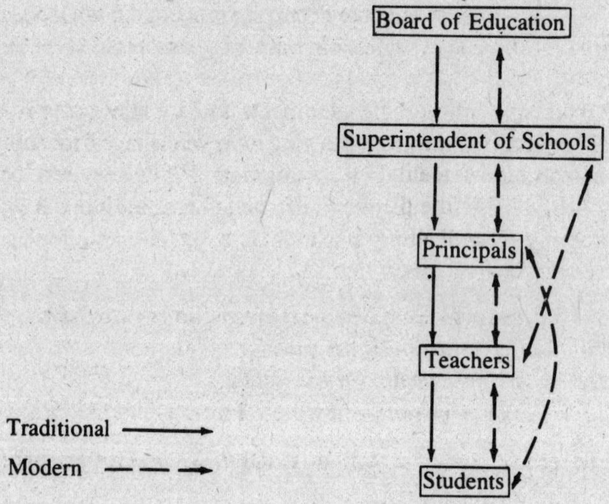

Although much simplified, the chart indicates a flow of power from the school board to the superintendent of schools down to the individual school principals and from there to the teachers and, finally, a minimal involvement of the students themselves.

The board of education was naturally found at the top, for it was assumed that this body represented the taxpaying community. Next in importance was the superintendent, whose word was considered to be law and who would, if so disposed, allow the principal some freedom to make decisions.

By the same token, those principals that prided themselves in being of a democratic nature, would then allow teachers to have a voice in selected matters and would even possibly afford students the opportunity of making minute decisions in appropriate areas.

Within the confines of the individual school, the principal was looked upon as the one person who knew more about educational matters than any other member of the staff. Therefore, he or she was spotlighted not only as the chief administrator, but as the supreme educational leader of the complex. Teachers occupied the place of facilitators, whose main job it was to take the programs that were handed down to them and see that they were carried out satisfactorily. The students were viewed as receptacles for receiving and digesting information. Their major contribution rested in being accepted to an institution of higher learning, thus making the system look good and giving the taxpayers the feeling that the money they spent was, after all, worthwhile.

The entire pattern of decision making, as presented, was based on the very real fact that the board of education controlled the purse strings of a school system. Since money has always been of supreme importance, it was considered the most logical path to follow. Few people thought to question its wisdom or bothered to seek alternatives.

The modern public has slowly come to realize that even though money is still the most crucial factor in operating an efficient school system, there are also other vital and important elements that contribute to its success.

For example, parents are demanding a voice in the operation of local schools. They favor an open door policy which affords them the opportunity to see what is going on in the classrooms and allows many of them to get involved on a parent-volunteer basis. Parents speak out in many cases by manipulating a very vital school input, over which they have strict control, namely their children. Thus we read of such things as parents keeping their offspring out of school to protest situations that they find unsuitable and intolerable. Even though these actions may not in themselves solve the problems, they do cause those in authority to sit up, take notice, and search for possible solutions at a speedy rate.

Every bit as important as the public's realization of its powers, is the teachers' realization that they too have a commodity that is of supreme importance to the system, and that is themselves. When teachers join forces and remove this vital input, school systems are forced to close and the educational machine comes to a halt. Teachers' strikes are now occurring more and more frequently in all areas of the country, and the threat of the entire profession becoming unionized is no longer a laughing matter.

Today's wise school systems have made note of these developments and are attempting to deal with them reasonably. Sharing the decision making power by allowing more realistic and meaningful input from both parents and teachers has become a reality in many districts. While a revised look at the power flow chart today would probably show the players in the same basic positions it would certainly have the arrows of decision coming not only down in a direct line, but also pointing up and out, allowing for a much more liberalized flow of communication and ideas.

The following statements are related to the passage. Based on the information given, select:

(A) if the statement is *supported by* the information in the passage.
(B) if the statement is *contradicted by* the information in the passage.
(C) if the statement is *neither supported nor contradicted by* the information in the passage.

1. Economics constitutes the prime reason today's teacher clamors for a greater voice in educational decision making.
2. Parents are becoming increasingly more involved in school situations because they are anxious to determine whether teachers are worth the tax dollars invested in them.
3. Teachers are more willing than ever to speak out concerning the development of new programs and policies.
4. Since money is the key factor in operating an efficient school system, and since the board of education holds the purse strings, it stands to reason that the latter should have absolute power over all facets of the educational machine within a district.
5. The realization that they are of vital importance to the school system has caused teachers to adopt a militant, unionistic attitude.
6. The National Education Association represents modern educators throughout the United States.
7. Today's students are radical and demand a share in the decision making process of local school systems.

8. Although a modern organizational chart might resemble one of the past as far as the position of its components is concerned, the flow of power has become more liberalized.

9. Parent-volunteer programs are one avenue of public involvement in local schools.

10. School-systems of the future will probably see an equal division of powers among the board of education, the teachers, and the public.

Performance appraisals— "Who needs them? I'm doing a good job, so why does someone need to sit and put it in writing, then waste my time and theirs talking about it? If I'm doing something that they don't like, let them tell me about it when it happens." This is a typical comment heard from many employees.

The performance appraisal, if completed properly, can be one of the most useful tools a manager can use in developing and training subordinates regardless of what some employees may express. It is a compilation of the employee's strengths and weakness in one concise form. It serves to show the employee the areas in which a good job is being done and also indicates which areas need improvement. The appraisal serves as a permanent record which documents the employee's growth and progress or shows why a promotion is not offered. A performance appraisal forces a manager to discuss an employee's performance on a one-to-one basis and find out more about what the employee's opinions and aspirations might be. This area is often overlooked in the busy day-in and day-out routine of business. It also gives the employee a chance to see what the boss really thinks about his or her work.

An interesting and often very beneficial way of handling a performance appraisal is to give employees a blank evaluation form a few days before the appraisal interview and ask that they rate themselves. When the appraisal takes place, the manager and employee compare their evaluations and work out the areas of disagreement so that each understands the other's position. An unusual result often takes place. Not only do the manager and employee end up with a better knowledge of each other, but they often find that their evaluations are very close to being in agreement. If anything, the employees usually find that they have under-rated themselves. An exception to this result, which the manager must be alert to recognize, is that an unsatisfactory performer may evaluate his or her performance higher than does the manager. The appraisal interview in this situation can often be more valuable than that of the satisfactory performer. It gives the manager an opportunity to counsel an already trained employee and turn around the performance rather than having to seek out and train a replacement. The manager must evaluate the time, expense, and attitude of the present employee against the time and expense of hiring and training a new employee.

Performance appraisals, properly administered, can cut down on turnover and greatly increase the morale of a department. The end result is increased productivity which is really what we are all striving to accomplish.

The following statements are related to the passage above. Based on the information given, select:

(A) if the statement is *supported by* the information in the passage.

(B) if the statement is *contradicted by* the information in the passage.

(C) if the statement is *neither supported nor contradicted by* information in the passage.

11. Managers feel that performance appraisals are a waste of time.

12. A satisfactorily performing employee will rate himself or herself higher than the manager.

13. A performance appraisal only points out the weak areas of performance.

14. The performance appraisal gives the employee and the manager a time to discuss the employee's future in private.

15. Employees and managers can usually work out their differences during the appraisal interview.

16. All performance appraisals are preceded by giving employees blank forms to rate themselves.

17. Performance appraisals often lead to a better understanding between managers and employees and can eventually lead to increased productivity.

18. Most large companies are now using the performance appraisal method because it has been proven a highly effective tool for dismissing unsatisfactory employees.

Time waits for no one. How often we have heard this statement; yet very few of us really pay attention to what it means. We are so busy with all of the things we have to do that we never stop to realize how much we have left undone, or how our priorities have become confused.

It is never too late to learn how to effectively manage our time. The most common response from most people to this suggestion is that they do not have time to learn how to manage their time. These are the people that need time management the most.

Measuring one's time is not as difficult as one might imagine. It merely requires the listing of every activity, regardless of how small, on a piece of paper each day for a week. If there are recurring items, a column can be so headed which will only require a check mark rather than writing out the activity. At the end of the work week, each of the five (5) papers are reviewed to see where time was wasted. These are the main items to be concentrated on during the next week. A side benefit of this analysis may reveal some items which may be delegated to subordinates or eliminated completely.

Another way of managing one's time, is to list all of the essential activities which must be completed within the next week. Once this list is compiled, go back and organize the activities. Begin with the most important priority and continue it until it is completed, then proceed to the next one and so on. At the end of the week, there may be some items left over which were not completed. Incorporate these in the next week's schedule. They may have moved up in the priority ranking by this time or they may have taken care of themselves and can be eliminated. It is amazing how much can be accomplished with this system. Eventually, the priority items will decrease and there will be available time to be used for other purposes.

You have the essential tools to help you get everything done that you hope to accomplish. Every minute that passes is gone forever.

The following statements are related to the passage above. Based on the information given, select:

(A) if the statement is *supported by* the information in the passage.

(B) if the statement is *contradicted by* the information in the passage.

(C) if the statement is *neither supported nor contradicted by* information in the passage.

19. Time management is only necessary for experienced managers.

20. Time management is time consuming if it is done properly.

21. Time management can be an aid to identify items to be delegated.

22. With the amount of paper work most people must process, time management is the only way to get things done on time.

23. Time management helps to identify priorities.

24. Managing one's time is best learned *before* embarking upon a career.

With the coming of age of the diet generation, amphetamine has taken a place among the most frequently prescribed drugs. It is the chemical structure of amphetamine which gives it resistance to enzymatic destruction and makes it effective after oral ingestion. The compound also exhibits a prolonged ability to activate and stimulate the nervous system. Three forms of the compound exist, with the levorotatory form being the most potent. This is a deviation from usual pharmacodynamic principles since, in most instances, the dextrorotatory form is the most active. Amphetamine is a potent stimulator which mimics many of the actions of the sympathetic nervous system. Adrenalin, the compound released by the sympathetic nervous system, elicits its effect as a result of direct action upon receptors in muscle and glands; amphetamine probably utilizes the same receptor sites as adrenalin. Amphetamine, however, differs from adrenalin in the fact that repeated administration results in a decreasing response of the organism to the drug. If both drugs are administered simultaneously, their action is of an additive nature. The stimulatory response of amphetamine results in an elevated blood pressure, cardiac output, respiratory activity, and basal metabolic rate and hyperirritability. Animals that receive very high doses of the drug become restless, agitated, and sleepless and exhibit tremors but no seizures have been reported. Students during examination week might ingest amphetamine to increase their psychomotor activities. Administration of the drug will result in alertness, and enhancement of initiative, mood, confidence, concentration and expression; however, it has been shown that while the drug allows us to function for longer time periods, it does not enhance the overall performance. Mental ability is not affected by amphetamine.

The following statements are related to the information presented previously. Based on the information given, select:

(A) if the statement is *supported by* the information in the passage.
(B) if the statement is *contradicted by* the information in the passage.
(C) if the statement is *neither supported nor contradicted by* information in the passage.

25. Repeated administration of adrenalin results in a decreasing response of the organism to the drug.

26. Amphetamine can be used to treat mental depression.

27. Chemically most compounds exhibit increased action if they are present in the levorotatory form.

28. Amphetamine is a short acting drug.

29. Adrenalin and amphetamines probably have a similar mechanism of action.

30. Amphetamine has no effect upon the circulatory system.

31. Amphetamine may be used in the treatment of certain types of epilepsy.

32. The overall initiative rather than the ability to do mental tasks is increased by amphetamine.

33. Considerable danger lies in the promiscuous use of amphetamine.

34. Psychological and social factors must be considered as components of therapeutic processes.

Tooth development, or odontogenesis, begins at 6½ weeks postconception in the human embryo, and continues for the next 20 years of life. It is initiated as a horseshoe-shaped epithelial thickening in the maxillary and mandibular arches, which sinks into the underlying mesenchyme, and is known as the dental laminae. At 10 discrete regions on this epithelial band of both arches, inductive activity produces lingually oriented outgrowths, known as buds. These buds will then give rise to the enamel organ—the epithelially derived structure that will be responsible for the formation of enamel, as well as for the shape, size, and number of roots the tooth will possess. The mesenchymal tissue of the region surrounding the bud will begin to interact with the epithelially derived bud in several ways. First, a mesenchymal condensation, at the inferior aspect of the bud will direct the future downgrowth of the bud so that a condensation of mesenchymal cells will be surrounded and almost completely enveloped by this epithelial structure. This mesenchymal condensation, the dental papillae, is responsible for the formation of dentin, and will eventually give rise to the pulp of the tooth. The mesenchyme surrounding the rest of the bud will envelop the growing bud and will give rise to the future periodontal ligament and the cementum of the root.

The following statements relate to the passage above. Based on the information given, select:

(A) if the statement is *supported by* the information in the passage.
(B) if the statement is *contradicted by* the information in the passage.
(C) if the statement is *neither supported nor contradicted by* information in the passage.

35. Tooth development is initiated earlier in females than in males.

36. The bud is the first sign of odontogenesis.

37. Enamel is mesenchymally derived.

38. The enamel organ's only function is to determine the shape, size, and number of roots.

39. The dental papilla is responsible for the formation of dentin and will also give rise to the future pulp of the tooth.

40. Since enamel is epithelially derived, it is the hardest tissue in the body.

41. Dentin, pulp, enamel, and periodontal ligament are all derived from the mesenchyme.

42. Each dental lamina will have 10 buds.

The formation of the palate occurs in several steps. The primary palate, that which contains the five incisors, is formed by the fusion of the globular process of the median nasal process with the right and left lateral palatine shelves of the maxillary process. The secondary palate, or the rest of the hard palate and soft palate, is formed by the fusion of the lateral palatine shelves with each other. Prior to the formation of the palate, the lateral palatine shelves are in the vertical position and the tongue is intervened between them in such a fashion that the tongue occupies both the nasal and oral cavities. At a particular time in development the tongue descends into the prospective oral cavity; and the lateral palatine shelves elevate so that now they are horizontally positioned and in fact act as a dividing plate, separating, almost completely, the oral cavity from the nasal cavity. The two shelves grow medially, contact each other, and fuse. This process is initiated at the middle of the hard palate and spreads both anteriorly and posteriorly, until the secondary palate is completed. If fusion does not occur, cleft palate results. Such clefts may involve the primary palate only, the secondary palate only, a portion of the secondary palate only, or both primary and secondary palates. Additionally, clefts of the primary palate may involve the right side only, the left side only, or both right and left sides, in which case it is referred to as bilateral cleft of the primary palate.

The following statements are related to the passage. Based on the information given, select:
(A) if the statement is *supported by* the information in the passage.
(B) if the statement is *contradicted by* the information in the passage.
(C) if the statement is *neither supported nor contradicted by* information in the passage.

43. Fusion of the secondary palate occurs first in the middle of the soft palate.

44. The primary palate is derived from the lateral palatine shelves and the globular process.

45. Clefts of the secondary palates may be bilateral.

46. The palate separates the nasal and oral cavities from each other.

47. Clefts of the palate are much more common than harelip.

48. The tongue descends into the oral cavity before the palatine shelves elevate.

49. Clefts of the secondary palate are more common than clefts of the primary palate.

50. The lateral palatine processes fuse with each other prior to elevation to the horizontal position.

In long-term care facilities, the medical records department assists the attending physician and the administration of the facility in documenting the course of the patient's illness and medical treatment while an inpatient. It also aids the professional staff in providing good patient care planning. Responsibilities for accurate record keeping and documentation rest with the administration and medical staff, both professional and nonprofessional.

A separate medical record must be maintained for each patient admitted to the facility and kept inviolate and preserved for a statutorily specified period of time after patient's discharge. The medical staff maintains an active clinical record of the resident as documentation of the diagnostic history, medications and treatments provided and their corresponding results, and inpatient care planning. The chart is a tool by which the staff communicates patient care and will serve as documentation to be used in legal proceedings.

For those long-term care facilities participating in federal and state health programs, there are specific requirements relative to the documentation of a resident's plan of care and the skills and training of the personnel executing the documentation and participating in the development of the overall plan of care.

51. From the above passage it can be inferred that
(A) medical records are a communication tool.
(B) medical records are legal documents recognized in legal proceedings.
(C) long term care facilities serve as protectors of patient's rights.
(D) A and B.
(E) B and C.

52. The phrase that best conveys the central idea of the above passage is
(A) clinical records are inviolate.
(B) medical records serve as a integral and important function in patient care planning.
(C) documentation of total patient care is vital in long-term care facilities.
(D) accurate charting makes patient care planning more effective.
(E) discharge plans are limited to professional judgments.

53. The writer does not state that
   (A) documentation in the clinical records is a responsibility shared by professional and nonprofessional staff.
   (B) discharged medical records are retained for a statutorily specified period of time.
   (C) clinical records are a communication tool.
   (D) release of information from a patient's clinical record is restricted.
   (E) previous diagnoses are to be included in the current clinical record.

54. The clinical record serves all of the following purposes except as
   (A) a tool in patient care planning.
   (B) a legal document.
   (C) proof that the best treatment was provided.
   (D) documentation of diagnostic history while an inpatient.
   (E) a means by which a physician orders a treatment plan for a patient.

The limitations of a state's territorial domain are determined by definite boundary lines which mark the extent of the property rights of the state and of its jurisdiction over persons. The existing boundary lines of states have been determined for the most part by definite international conventions. Many of these conventions have materialized as peace treaties following territorial disputes or wars of conquest while still others have been in the form of voluntary agreements between nation states which have brought about an amicable settlement of boundaries.

With respect to constitutional law in the United States, the individual maintains sovereignty not only over the plot of earth that one owns, but, in addition, retains jurisdiction over the acreage in a three-dimensional interpretation. That is, subject to governmental control for aeronautical usage either by the government or by commercial traffic, the sky is the limit. Likewise, retention of mineral rights and subterranean activity is the jurisdiction of the property owner.

It does not necessarily follow, however, that nation states are to follow the same dictum. Unless nation states are participants to binding agreements—made either through international conventions, wars of conquest, or peace treaties—the adjudicatory process lies through international courts of justice or negotiators recognized by and acting on behalf of the parties involved.

55. The subject of this passage is
   (A) determination of boundary lines between nation states.
   (B) individual property rights guaranteed under the Constitution.
   (C) limitations of territorial domain.
   (D) national sovereignty in international boundary disputes.
   (E) origin of property rights.

56. The writer states that
   (A) territorial rights as interpreted from the Constitution are three dimensional.
   (B) international law is derived from participatory judgments of the consenting states.
   (C) periodic international conventions are held to solve boundary disputes between nation states.
   (D) boundary disputes between nation states must be submitted to international courts of justice.
   (E) the best means of determining boundary lines is to fight it out.

57. A method of determining boundary lines not mentioned in the above passage is by
   (A) international convention.
   (B) the Constitution.
   (C) peace treaties.
   (D) voluntary agreements between nation states.
   (E) wars of conquest.

58. Based on the information given in the passage, which of the following is NOT a true statement?
(A) Boundary lines determine the limitations of a state's territorial domain.
(B) International boundary lines are generally determined by international conventions.
(C) Control over the skies is retained by individual nation states.
(D) Parties to a boundary dispute can take action through international courts of justice to have the dispute resolved.
(E) All of the above.

With the current emphasis on development of reading skills across the United States (in particular, the standards of quality enacted by the general assembly of the Commonwealth of Virginia and the initiation of the Supplemental Skills Development Program by the Virginia State Department of Education), each school needs to be aware of those areas of reading in which students demonstrated consistent skill weaknesses and, if possible, identify the basic reasons for disparities between ability and achievement in order to develop a supplemental skills program that will improve reading skills.

There are several standardized reading achievement tests and tests measuring educational ability which can be administered that will assist in identifying students who exhibit disparities between levels of ability and of achievement and in what areas of reading weaknesses can be categorized for remediation.

Analysis of information—gleaned from individual student cumulative folders; from interviews with the administrative staff and teachers, former and present, of students identified for remediation and intensification; and by examination of testing materials and testing conditions—may be used as a basis for a quantitative and qualitative study leading to a meaningful intensification program.

59. The central idea conveyed in the above passage is that
(A) reading skill weaknesses in elementary school children can be attributed to environmental circumstances.
(B) disparities between achievement and ability levels should be identified before instituting remediation or intensification programs in reading skill development.
(C) subjective judgments made by educators are prejudicial to identification of a learner's reading weaknesses.
(D) selection of testing materials will vary disparities in achievement and ability levels.
(E) enactment of standards of quality will provide the avenue by which reading success may be achieved.

60. The passage specifically states that
(A) local schools need to identify reading disparities.
(B) cumulative folders provide valuable information which can be used in a qualitative and quantitative study.
(C) examination of testing materials and conditions must be used as a basis for quantitative and qualitative study.
(D) the Supplemental Skills Development Program was enacted by the general assembly.
(E) student demographic data must be collected to provide a basis for possible study.

61. The writer implies that
(A) most elementary school age children in Virginia are below the national reading norms.
(B) Virginia schools are inferior to all other southern school systems.
(C) standards of quality serve as models for optimum performance by the local school districts in Virginia.
(D) subjective assessments of a child's home life are valid in determining causative disparities in reading levels.
(E) remediation programs in reading can be successful if properly developed.

62. The writer mentions each of the following sources of information for qualitative study EXCEPT
(A) cumulative folders.
(B) testing materials.
(C) parental interviews.
(D) testing conditions.
(E) teachers and administrative staff.

Just about anyone you talk to nowadays complains about the cost of his automobile insurance. It's about time that someone came to the defense of the insurance companies.

We are all familiar with the effects of inflation, but most people forget that the insurance companies are affected, too. An interesting point should be noted. Even though the total costs of producing a policy have been increasing because of increased salaries, paper cost, equipment replacement, etc., the insurance companies' expense ratios have been going down.

If expenses are reduced, then why are premiums going up? Let's look at what makes up the rates that the insurance companies must charge. Automobile repair rates for labor have risen about 20% in the last year and a half. In addition, it has been shown that a new automobile costing $5,000 would cost $20,000 if it were to be repaired with replacement parts (not including the engine). During this same period, a semiprivate hospital room has increased in cost over 22% and physicians' and surgeons' fees have increased 20%. Lawyers continue to ask for larger awards, and the courts are granting them. How can insurance companies continue to pay amounts inflated in this manner without reflecting the increase in their rates?

It is a real shame that the insurance companies don't make these facts known more widely to their customers. A widespread advertising campaign would help to explain their position and make it more tolerable when that next bill comes and has once again increased.

The following statements are related to the passage above. Based on the information given, select:
(A) if the statement is *supported by* the information in the passage.
(B) if the statement is *contradicted by* the information in the passage.
(C) if the statement is *neither supported nor contradicted by* information in the passage.

63. Insurance company expense ratios are continuing to rise with inflation.

64. A car repaired with replacement parts would cost four (4) times as much as a new car.

65. The public is fully aware of why their insurance premiums are increasing.

66. Automobile insurance premiums have risen mainly because of larger awards in law suits.

67. Inflation is affecting the insurance industry and the rates that are charged.

68. Insurance companies are involved in a widespread advertising campaign to make their customers aware of the inflationary problems that have caused rates to rise.

> STOP. If you finish before the time limit is up, go over your work for this section. DO NOT look at any other sections of the model examination. When your time limit is up, go on to the next section.

SKILLS ANALYSIS: QUANTITATIVE

85 MINUTES
68 QUESTIONS

The following questions are to be answered based on your knowledge of basic mathematical principles and relationships.

DIRECTIONS: Read each passage carefully, study each table or chart, then answer the questions following it. Consider only the material presented in answering the questions. Eliminate those choices that you think to be incorrect and mark the letter of your choice on the answer sheet.

Using a syringe containing heparin, fifty milliliters of blood were drawn from a healthy male volunteer. Following centrifugation, the "buffy coat" was removed and a lymphocyte rich cell population was obtained by sedimentation through 2% Dextran. After washing in 0.9% saline the lymphocytes were placed in cell culture tubes at a concentration of 5×10^6 cells/ml cell culture medium/tube. To one-half of the tubes was added 5 μg of phytohaemogglutinin, a substance which causes lymphocytes to undergo mitosis. The other half of the tubes received no phytohaemogglutinin. Radioactive tracers for RNA, DNA, and protein synthesis were then added to all tubes and aliquots removed at selected intervals. The following data were obtained:

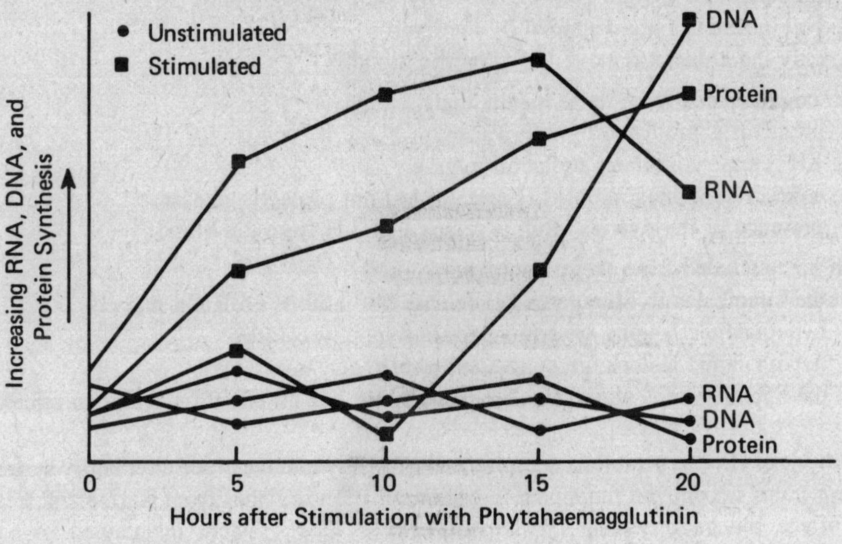

1. The purpose of this experiment was to
   (A) determine the role of heparin in blood cotting.
   (B) determine the sequence of events in cells stimulated to undergo mitosis, and to compare these data to those gathered from unstimulated cells.
   (C) isolate a pure population of lymphocytes.
   (D) determine the life-span of lymphocytes.

2. From these data it can be seen that increased
   (A) RNA synthesis precedes increased protein synthesis.
   (B) DNA synthesis precedes increased protein synthesis.
   (C) protein synthesis precedes increased RNA synthesis.
   (D) DNA synthesis precedes increased RNA synthesis.

3. It may also be assumed that
   (A) DNA synthesis is dependent on previous RNA synthesis.
   (B) protein synthesis is dependent on previous RNA synthesis.
   (C) RNA synthesis is dependent on previous protein synthesis.
   (D) unstimulated lymphocytes synthesize RNA, DNA and protein at a low rate.

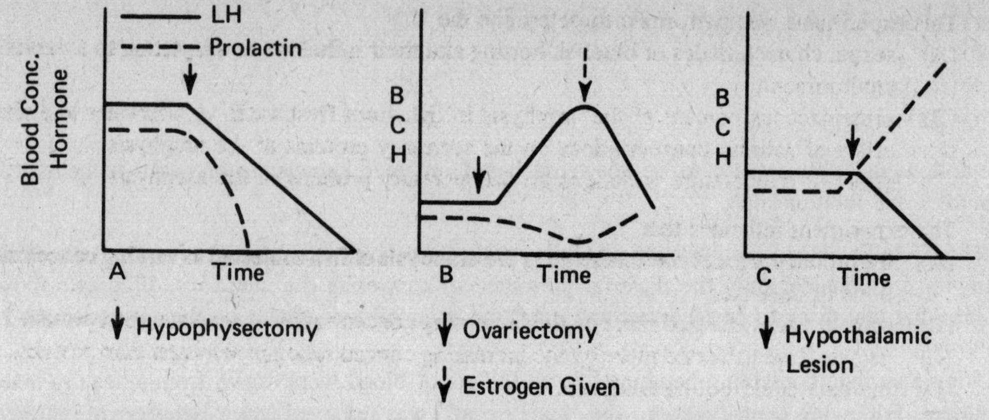

The graphs represent experimental results obtained when the pituitary gland was removed (A), the ovaries were removed (B) and lesions were placed in the hypothalamus (C), that part of the brain most closely related to the pituitary gland. The hormones LH and prolactin were measured in blood by radioimmunoassay.

4. It can be concluded from these results that
(A) prolactin and LH are removed from the blood at the same rate.
(B) prolactin and LH are both produced by the pituitary gland.
(C) both hormones are degraded by the liver.
(D) only the kidneys remove LH from the blood.

5. It can be concluded from these results that
(A) prolactin is produced by the ovaries.
(B) LH release stimulates prolactin release.
(C) ovarian hormones inhibit LH release, but not prolactin release.
(D) presence of the ovaries inhibits removal of LH from the blood.

6. It can be concluded from these results that
(A) the hypothalamus stimulates LH release but inhibits prolactin release.
(B) hypothalamic lesions are equivalent to hypophysectomy.
(C) hypothalamic lesions are equivalent to estrogen injections.
(D) the hypothalamus stimulates LH release, but has no effect on prolactin release.

The urophysis of teleosts secretes a neurohormone directly into the blood circulatory system. This secretory apparatus is believed functional in osmoregulation in fishes from marine and freshwater habitats. Fifteen blueback herring (*Pseudoharengus aestivalis*) were maintained in a marine aquarium at temperatures of 40°-45°. The fish were subjected to increasing salt concentration to a final concentration equal to twice that of seawater. At each concentration four to twelve urophyses were dissected and extracted, and electrophoresis on polyacrylamide gels was performed. Two specific bands of protein were identified as being specific to the urophysis. The amount of protein was determined by microdensitometry. The results are shown in the graph.

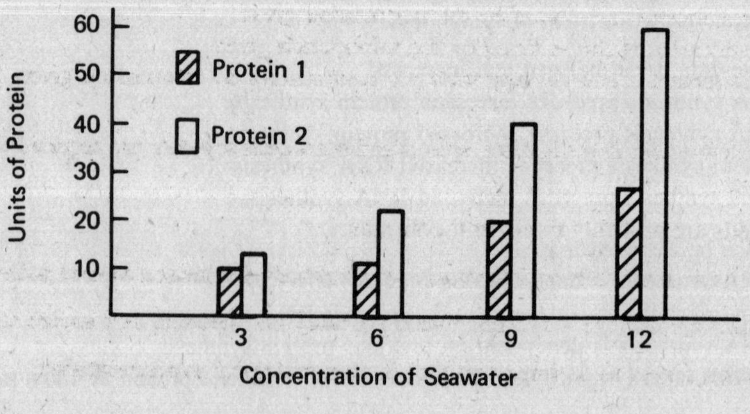

7. This experiment was performed to determine the
   (A) sexual characteristics of bluefish herring and their influence on adaptation to a varying environment.
   (B) proteinaceous content of the urophysis in fish from freshwater vs. saltwater habitats.
   (C) effect of salinity concentrations on the secretory proteins of the urophysis,
   (D) effect of temperature variations on the secretory proteins of the urophysis.

8. The experiment indicates that
   (A) the protein material was unaltered in the urophysis of fish subjected to varying concentrations of seawater.
   (B) protein 1 was affected more by the increasing concentration of seawater than protein 2.
   (C) protein 2 was affected more by the increasing concentration of seawater than protein 1.
   (D) the data could not be analyzed.

9. Regarding the functional implications of the urophysis in osmoregulation, which of the following statements is valid?
   (A) The protein of the urophysis appears to be unaltered by salinity concentration and is not implicated in osmoregulation.
   (B) The protein secretion is active and directly influences osmoregulation by its action on the gills.
   (C) Female fish adapt faster to osmotic stress than male fish.
   (D) None of the above is correct.

An investigator had been studying the interrelationship (cooperation) of various cell types in tissue culture in the immune response to an antigen. The experiments conducted attempted to determine if spleen and mast cells were required for the production of antibody against a pollen. Various donor cells (spleen and mast cells) were injected into recipient rabbits whose immune system had been rendered nonresponsive by whole body X-irradiation. Antibody levels were determined in the serum of the recipients.

	Experimental Groups	Antibody Level
A.	Spleen and pollen	0
B.	Spleen	0
C.	Mast cells and pollen	0
D.	Mast cells	0
E.	Spleen and mast cells and pollen	++
F.	Bone marrow and pollen	++
G.	Thymocytes and pollen	++

The following statements are related to the information presented above. Based on the information given, select:
(A) if the statement is *supported by* the information given.
(B) if the statement is *contradicted by* the information given.
(C) if the statement is *neither supported nor contradicted by* information given.

10. In the system under investigation, spleen and mast cells together are required for antibody production.

11. Spleen cells are probably found in the thymus.

12. Spleen cells or mast cells are essential to the antibody production against pollen.

13. In the intact animal, the mast cells would probably be important as a source of antibody.

14. X-irradiation serves as an important tool in immunological experimentation.

Four groups of rats were maintained under identical conditions. Three of the groups received drugs in their drinking water over a period of five weeks. The day before autopsy each rat received one microcurie of I^{131}. At autopsy the thyroid glands from each group were pooled and weighed. Iodinated intermediates were isolated and their radioactivity determined. Remember iodide is trapped, oxidized, proteinated, and stored as part of the thyroid hormone.

I^{131} CONTENT
(counts/min./100 mg Thyroid Tissue)

Groups	Drug	Iodine Ion	Monoiodo-tyrosine	Triiodo-thyronine	Thyroxine	Av. Thyroid Wt. mg/100 g body wt.
1	None	6,120	10,140	7,520	35,990	14
2	A	55	46	13	62	76
3	B	40,976	10	9	14	88
4	C	1,592	2,025	1,970	8,985	4

15. Which group was treated with thyroxine, an inhibitor of the production of thyroid stimulating hormone by the pituitary gland?
(A) Group 2
(B) Group 3
(C) Group 4
(D) None of the above

16. Which group was treated with thiocyanate, an inhibitor of the iodine pump of the thyroid cells?
(A) Group 2
(B) Group 3
(C) Group 4
(D) None of the above

17. Which group was treated with propylthiouracil, an inhibitor of iodine oxidation?
(A) Group 2
(B) Group 3
(C) Group 4
(D) None of the above

18. In which of the above groups is iodine NOT taken up and therefore almost no radioactivity can be measured by the assay?
(A) Group 1
(B) Group 2
(C) Group 3
(D) Group 4

Many scientists think of the pituitary gland as the master gland responsible for the secretion of many different hormones. A reciprocal relationship operates between the hormones secreted by the pituitary and the hormones produced by the target organs; this delicate control of balance of production of secretory product between the pituitary and the target organs is known as "negative feedback." Among the many hormones produced by the pituitary gland are ACTH, FSH, LH, TSH, and STH. The following experiments were set up to demonstrate the actions of some of the above factors. Twenty-five day-old immature male and female rats were subjected to the following treatment for 10 days: Group 1 was given a 0.5 cc saline injection; Group 2 was given a 0.5 cc FSH injection; and Group 3 was given a 0.5 cc crude pituitary extract injection. The results were recorded in table form.

MALE RATS

Groups	Body Weight grams	Testes mg	Seminal Vesicles mg	Prostate mg	Thyroid mg	Adrenals mg
1	86	3750	18	71	6.0	20
2	82	5310	57	176	6.1	21
3	83	4830	24	163	7.5	27

FEMALE RATS

Groups	Body Weight grams	Ovaries mg	Uterus mg	Thyroid mg	Adrenals mg
1	83	20	25	5.9	22
2	82	43	83	5.7	21
3	84	33	61	7.1	37

The following statements are related to the information presented. Based on the information given, select:

(A) if the statement is *supported by* the information given.
(B) if the statement is *contradicted by* the information given.
(C) if the statement is *neither supported nor contradicted by* information given.

19. From the table it seems as if the crude pituitary extract had a lesser effect on the sex organs than did FSH.

20. Pituitary extract affected every organ under investigation.

21. Hypophysectomy probably would have resulted in a decreased weight of the organs under investigation.

22. The administration of FSH alone to an immature rat will produce follicular growth, but uterine and vaginal configurations will remain infantile since LH is also needed. The experimental data indicate uterine growth, casting doubt on the purity of the FSH preparation.

23. Both FSH and LH are necessary for the production of estrogen.

24. FSH in the male had the greatest effect on the weight of the prostate gland; the tissue is therefore most refractive to it.

25. The adrenal weight probably would drop if the animals were deprived of ACTH.

26. In these experiments none of the hormones in the pituitary extract probably were as effective as a purified fraction of them might have been.

27. FSH has as its target organs the organs of reproduction.

28. As demonstrated in these experiments ACTH and TSH are produced by the pituitary gland.

After growing turkey red wheat for two years on a dry land farm, John Calendar had accumulated enough capital to move his family to a more fertile area. The first crops he planted on the new 1000-acre farm did well. The bar graphs below indicate his production of wheat and corn over the last five years. Bushels are plotted on the abscissa, and the numbers of acres planted in both crops are shown in parentheses.

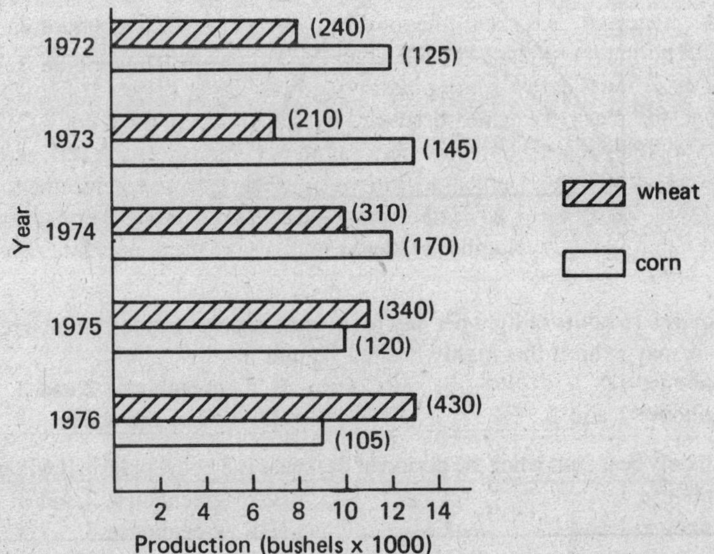

29. What was the average yearly proportion of wheat production to corn production?
(A) 3/2
(B) 7/8
(C) 10/9
(D) 5/7

30. If corn sold for $2.40/bushel in 1973, how many more bushels of wheat at $4.00/bushel would have to be sold to match the income from corn?
(A) 8,800 bushels
(B) 650 bushels
(C) 800 bushels
(D) 1,500 bushels
(E) none of the above

31. How many acres would have to be converted to wheat to obtain a matching output (in bushels) of both crops in 1972?
(A) 94.75 acres
(B) 127.94 acres
(C) 270.25 acres
(D) 30.25 acres
(E) none of the above

32. The average price for wheat and corn in 1976 was $2.90/bushel and $2.40/bushel, respectively. Assuming that the entire farm was planted in these two crops and that an acre of land could grow three times as much corn as wheat, how many acres would be planted in corn to obtain an equal income from both crops?
(A) 327 acres
(B) 287 acres
(C) 204 acres
(D) 275 acres
(E) none of the above

33. Suppose that too great a surplus of wheat was expected in 1977, and the federal government passed a bill to reimburse growers $25 for each acre not planted in that crop, as long as the previous year's income from wheat and corn (in this case, $59,300) was not exceeded. Out of 500 acres, how many could be left unplanted if the remainder were planted in corn which would sell at $2.50/bushel with an average yield of 90 bushels per acre?
(A) 266 acres
(B) 106 acres
(C) 55 acres
(D) 217 acres
(E) none of the above

Three greenhouses were constructed to examine different light cycles and their effects on the growth of several plants.

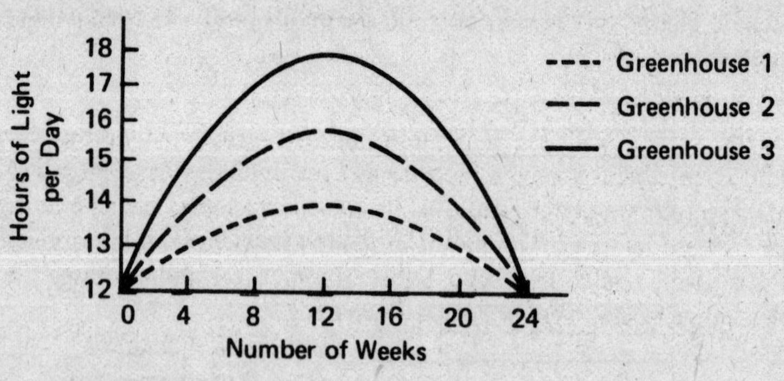

34. Plant X requires 15 hours of light per day for at least three weeks to exhibit a red coloration in its leaves. It may exhibit this highly desired feature in
(A) greenhouse 1.
(B) greenhouse 1 and 2.
(C) greenhouse 2 and 3.
(D) all of the above.

35. Plant Y will only bear fruit when the period of darkness is 8 hours or less. It will not bear fruit in
(A) greenhouse 1.
(B) greenhouse 1 and 2.
(C) greenhouse 2 and 3.
(D) greenhouse 3.

36. Plant Z will only form flowers and seeds when exposed to days of no more than 15 hours in length. It is therefore not native in areas that are simulated by
(A) greenhouse 1.
(B) greenhouse 1 and 2.
(C) greenhouse 2 and 3.
(D) greenhouse 1 and 3.

In order to obtain the results as listed in the table below, golden hamsters were fed 0.05% propylthiouracil (PTU) in their diets. At various times hamsters were sacrificed; the pituitaries were dissected out, fixed in Bouin's solution, dehydrated, embedded in paraffin, and sectioned at a thickness of 6 micra. Sections were stained with a modified Masson trichrome stain. A differential adenohypophyseal cell count was obtained.

PERCENTAGES OF ADENOHYPOPHYSEAL CELLS AFTER ADMINISTRATION OF 0.05% PROPYLTHIOURACIL IN THE DIET

Days of PTU	No. of Animals	Body Wt., grams	Pituitary Wt., mg./100 gr. B.W.	% Cell Types		
				Acidophils	Basophils	Chromophobes
0	10	129	2.40	29	19	51
3	10	117	3.20[1]	26	36[1]	37[1]
6	10	112	3.40	27	36	37
12	10	120	3.10	27	37	36
15	10	130	4.10	26	36	38

[1]Fisher's "T" significant to .001

37. The objective of the experiment was to
(A) show that propylthiouracil induces thyroidal deficiency which is overcome by the increased production of TSH.
(B) see if propylthiouracil would change the weight of the pituitary gland.
(C) see if propylthiouracil would change the proportion of the various cell types of the pituitary.
(D) prove that chromophobes give rise to basophils which secrete TSH.

38. It was found that
(A) pituitary weight is a good indicator of PTU action.
(B) the mitotic rate of the pituitary increased resulting in an increase of pituitary weight.
(C) there was a percentage increase of basophils with a concomitant decrease in chromophobes.
(D) basophils secrete TSH.

39. The investigator started with the hypothesis that the paucity of mitotic divisions in the adenohypophysis precludes a weight increase as a result of new cell formation. It is believed that one cell type (chromophobe) changes; its transformation to become an active basophil results in an increase in secretory material in it and this increase in metabolic and secretory activity in the gland could bring about this observed weight increase. The differential adenohypohyseal cell count supports such an hypothesis.
(A) True
(B) False
(C) Bad hypothesis
(D) Pure speculation

One hundred ml of blood was drawn from a healthy male donor. Following centrifugation (4°C) and removal of the "buffy coat" by aspiration, hemoglobin was extracted from the pelleted red blood cells. The extracted hemoglobin was then divided into equal aliquots and these were treated as follows:

Aliquot 1: Analyzed on the day of extraction by polyacrylamide gel electrophoresis, followed by densitometer scanning of the stained gel

Aliquot 2: Stored for 30 days at room temperature

Aliquot 3: Stored for 30 days at 4°C

Aliquot 4: Stored for 30 days as a 50% solution (V/V) in glycerol at −20°C

At the end of the 30-day storage period each of the aliquots was analyzed in the same way as aliquot 1. The following densitometer tracings were obtained:

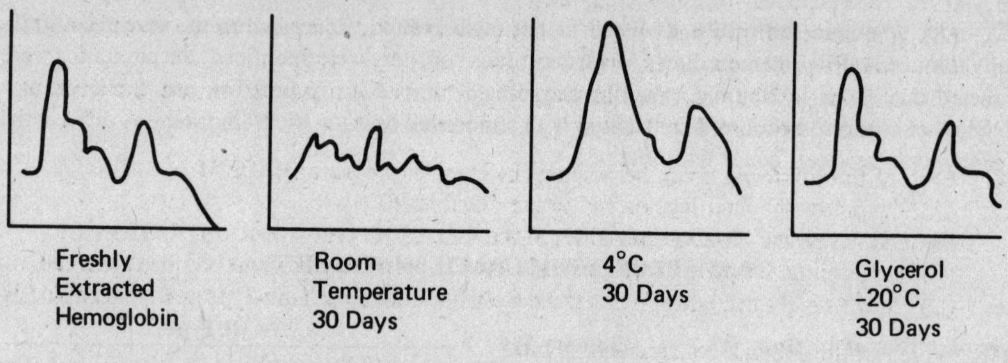

40. The purpose of this experiment was to test the effect of
(A) polyacrylamide gel on hemoglobin concentration.
(B) removing the buffy coat on red blood cell inability.
(C) glycerol on hemoglobin concentration.
(D) different storage conditions on hemoglobin polypeptide composition as revealed by gel electrophoresis.

41. From these data it is clear that
(A) none of the storage conditions were able to maintain hemoglobin in an unchanged state.
(B) hemoglobin peptides are strongly affected by heating.
(C) hemoglobin contains peroxidase activity.
(D) hemoglobin coupled with oxygen has a longer shelf-life than hemoglobin coupled with CO_2.

42. It may also be seen that
(A) there are remarkable sex differences in hemoglobin polypeptide patterns.
(B) centrifugation in the cold may alter oxygen affinity curves for hemoglobin.
(C) of all the storage methods tried, storage at −20°C in glycerol allowed the least change from the fresh configuration.
(D) hemoglobin is useful for species identification.

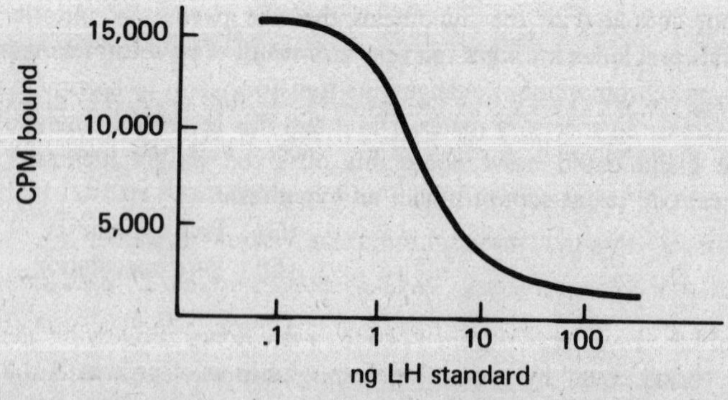

Blood samples from 10 female rats were withdrawn at 5 PM on the day of proestrus, when LH levels in the blood should be high if ovulation were to occur that night. The blood was assayed by double-antibody radioimmunoassay for LH. An antibody specific for LH is allowed to bind with the LH in the sample, then is partially displaced by radio-labeled LH whose binding to the limited amount of anti-LH is inversely proportional to the amount of unlabeled LH present (see standard curve). The antigen-antibody complex is precipitated with an antibody to the anti-LH, and the number of counts per minute bound in the precipitate is determined after the supernatant containing the unbound labeled LH has been poured off. The blood samples from 5 untreated rats (which ovulated) had cpm of 4000, 3000, 5000, 4000 and 3000, whereas those from 5 drug-treated animals had 5000, 13,000, 15,000, 3,000, 13,000.

43. It can be concluded from this study that
(A) the untreated rats had very little LH in their blood compared to the treated group.
(B) the drug does not block ovulation.
(C) the dose of the drug used in this study inhibits LH release in most of the animals.
(D) ovulation occurred in 3 out of 5 of the treated rats.

44. Each of the following could be a source of error in the assay EXCEPT
(A) trapping unbound labeled LH in the precipitate.
(B) the presence of other hormones in the blood.
(C) separating the bound from free labeled LH before equilibrium had been reached.
(D) using an LH standard which reacted with the antibody differently from the unknown LH.

45. Which of the following statements is true?
(A) The antibody cannot be saturated with hormone.
(B) The antigen-antibody reaction is not reversible.
(C) Counting error and decay have no effect.
(D) Only the middle portion of the standard curve is usable.

Selective protein transport from the maternal circulation to the rat fetus is thought to occur via the visceral yolk sac. The maternal proteins are transferred to the yolk sac cavity and then must pass through the visceral endoderm, the visceral basement membrane (VBM), and the vitelline capillary endothelium to reach the fetal blood. Proteins X, Y, and Z were injected into a pregnant rat on day 12 of gestation and then were localized in the layers of the visceral yolk sac at 2 minutes, 6 hours, and 12 hours following injection. The results below demonstrate where each protein was localized at the three postinjection intervals.

Protein	Visceral Endoderm	VBM	Vitelline Endothelium	Fetal Blood
X	2 min.	6 hrs.	12 hrs.	—
Y	2 min., 6 hrs., & 12 hrs.	—	—	—
Z	2 min.	6 hrs.	12 hrs.	12 hrs.

The following statements are related to the information presented above. Based on the information given, select:
(A) if the statement is *supported by* the information given.
(B) if the statement is *contradicted by* the information given.
(C) if the statement is *neither supported nor contradicted by* information given.

46. All three proteins were absorbed at the same rate by the visceral endoderm.

47. The transport of protein X is blocked by the visceral basement membrane.

48. The visceral endoderm appears to block the transport of protein Y.

49. Protein X appears to be transported through the visceral endoderm.

50. Only proteins with a low molecular weight, such as protein Z, pass into the fetal blood.

51. Proteins X and Z are transported at the same rate through the visceral endoderm.

52. The vitelline endothelium appears to block the transport of protein X into the fetal blood.

53. Protein Y is not transported into the fetal circulation because of its large molecular weight.

54. All proteins are transported into the fetal circulation by the visceral yolk sac placenta.

55. Proteins X and Z are absorbed and transported to the vitelline endothelium by the same transport mechanism.

56. Proteins X and Z are transported at the same rate into the vitelline endothelium.

57. Protein transport in the rat occurs only on day 12 of gestation.

The following graph represents an experiment designed to measure the rate of collagen synthesis in developing chondrocytes. Chondrocytes were isolated from developing sterna of chick embryos and incubated in culture media containing proline ^3H, a precursor of collagen. Specimens were fixed after various time intervals and prepared for autoradiography. The graph represents number of silver grains counted (μm/square of organelle).

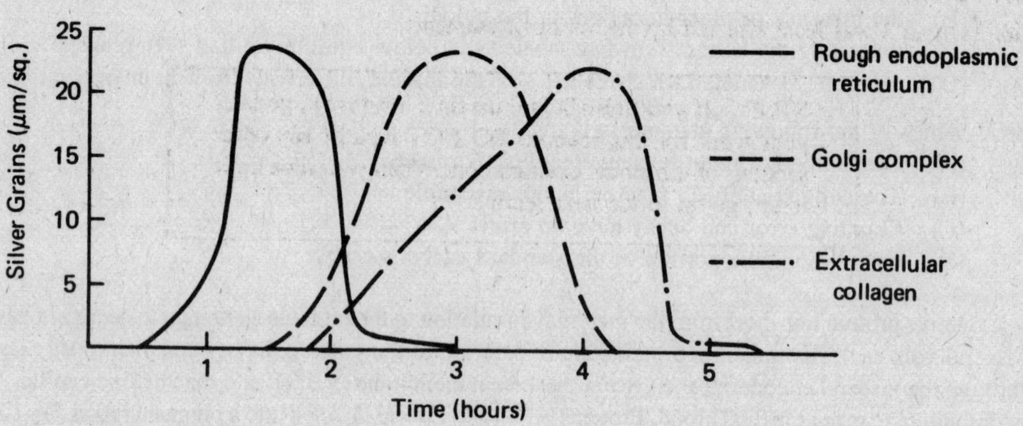

The following statements are related to the information presented. Based on this information, select:

(A) if the statement is *supported by* the information given.
(B) if the statement is *contradicted by* the information given.
(C) if the statement is *neither supported nor contradicted by* information given.

58. The radioactive label found in the rough endoplasmic reticulum is transferred directly into the extracellular collagen without passing through the Golgi complex.

59. Radioactive isotope is incorporated into the extracellular collagen within 2 hours.

60. Collagen is a highly stable molecule and is not degraded.

61. The amount of rough endoplasmic reticulum in the cell increases during collagen synthesis.

EFFECT OF VARIOUS TREATMENTS ON ORGAN WEIGHTS

Treatments	No. of Animals	Body Weight Grams	Organ Weight (mg/100 g Body Weight) Organ 1	Organ 2	Organ 3
Control	8	70	1509 ± 34	223 ± 20	22 ± 0.8
Drug A	8	66	1044 ± 30	87 ± 14	23 ± 1.0
Drug B	8	73	1432 ± 51	224 ± 24	26 ± 0.9
Drug A + B	8	71	1586 ± 68	208 ± 28	25 ± 1.2
Drug C	8	73	1383 ± 80	146 ± 19	31 ± 1.3
Drug B + C	8	65	954 ± 50	61 ± 3	26 ± 2.0

The following statements are related to the table above. Based on the information given, select:

(A) if the statement is *supported by* the information in the table.
(B) if the statement is *contradicted by* the information in the table.
(C) if the statement is *neither supported nor contradicted by* information in the table.

62. Casual evaluation of the results leads one to believe that treatment resulted in significant effects.

63. Drugs B and C seem to have acted in an additive manner.

64. The experimenters should have paid closer attention to body weights.

65. Drug C affected all parameters under investigation.

66. Significant microscopic changes were detected in the organs under investigation.

67. Drugs A and B countered (offset) each other.

68. Organ 3 was least affected by the various treatments.

STOP. If you finish before the time limit is up, go over your work for this section. DO NOT look at any other sections of the model examination. When your time limit is up, go on to the next section.

Model Test C Answers*

SCIENCE KNOWLEDGE

Biology

1. D	9. A	17. A	25. A	33. C
2. A	10. C	18. E	26. E	34. C
3. C	11. D	19. C	27. A	35. D
4. B	12. A	20. C	28. A	36. D
5. B	13. C	21. C	29. E	37. D
6. D	14. D	22. B	30. E	38. D
7. B	15. B	23. C	31. A	
8. A	16. A	24. B	32. C	

Chemistry

1. C	11. E	21. D	31. D	41. B
2. A	12. C	22. C	32. D	42. C
3. D	13. D	23. D	33. D	43. B
4. A	14. B	24. A	34. D	44. D
5. B	15. C	25. A	35. A	45. D
6. A	16. C	26. B	36. C	46. D
7. B	17. C	27. C	37. B	47. B
8. A	18. D	28. A	38. A	48. D
9. C	19. D	29. C	39. B	49. B
10. B	20. A	30. B	40. C	

Physics

1. D	9. E	17. C	25. E	33. C
2. B	10. D	18. D	26. E	34. D
3. E	11. B	19. D	27. A	35. E
4. D	12. E	20. B	28. C	36. A
5. C	13. A	21. C	29. D	37. C
6. A	14. B	22. A	30. B	38. D
7. B	15. A	23. E	31. E	
8. B	16. E	24. D	32. A	

*Explanations for science answers can be found on p. 255.

SCIENCE PROBLEMS

1. E
2. D
3. A
4. E
5. A
6. B
7. C
8. D
9. C
10. C
11. D
12. A
13. B
14. B
15. C
16. D
17. E
18. B
19. C
20. E
21. B
22. E
23. C
24. D
25. A
26. D
27. C
28. E
29. E
30. E
31. A
32. B
33. D
34. B
35. E
36. C
37. B
38. C
39. B
40. D
41. B
42. E
43. C
44. A
45. D
46. D
47. B
48. D
49. E
50. B
51. D
52. B
53. A
54. C
55. D
56. B
57. C
58. C
59. B
60. C
61. C
62. C
63. B
64. A
65. C
66. C

SKILLS ANALYSIS: READING

1. B
2. C
3. A
4. B
5. C
6. C
7. C
8. A
9. A
10. C
11. C
12. B
13. B
14. A
15. A
16. C
17. A
18. C
19. B
20. B
21. A
22. C
23. A
24. B
25. B
26. C
27. B
28. B
29. A
30. B
31. C
32. A
33. C
34. C
35. C
36. B
37. B
38. B
39. A
40. C
41. B
42. B
43. B
44. A
45. B
46. A
47. C
48. A
49. C
50. B
51. D
52. C
53. D
54. C
55. A
56. A
57. B
58. C
59. B
60. A
61. E
62. C
63. B
64. A
65. B
66. C
67. A
68. B

SKILLS ANALYSIS: QUANTITATIVE

1. B
2. A
3. D
4. B
5. C
6. A
7. C
8. C
9. D
10. A
11. A
12. B
13. C
14. A
15. C
16. A
17. B
18. B
19. A
20. A
21. A
22. A
23. C
24. B
25. A
26. C
27. A
28. A
29. B
30. C
31. D
32. B
33. A
34. C
35. A
36. C
37. C
38. C
39. A
40. D
41. A
42. C
43. C
44. B
45. D
46. A
47. B
48. A
49. A
50. C
51. A
52. A
53. C
54. B
55. C
56. A
57. C
58. B
59. A
60. B
61. C
62. A
63. A
64. B
65. A
66. C
67. A
68. A

Explanation of Answers for Science Questions-Model Test C

SCIENCE KNOWLEDGE

Biology

1. **(D)** Mitochondria are the biochemical powerplants of the cell. They recover energy from foodstuffs (via Krebs cycle and respiratory chain) and convert it (via phosphorylation) into ATP (adenosine triphosphate). In this manner they produce the energy necessary for the metabolic processes.

2. **(A)** Lysosomes contain acid phosphatase and other hydrolytic enzymes. These enzymes are enclosed by a membrane and are released when needed into phagocytic vesicles, etc.

3. **(C)** The Golgi complex is prominent in glandular cells and is thought to function in the production, concentration, packaging, and transportation of secretory material.

4. **(B)** Ribosomes are attached to the membranes of the endoplasmic reticulum which is designed as rough ER. Ribosomes are responsible for synthesis of proteins.

5. **(B)** It is believed by some that parathyroid hormone acts upon bone eliciting changes in calcium and phosphorus. Osteoclasts are the cells stimulated by parathyroid hormone to facilitate the resorption of calcium and phosphorus from bone. Administration of parathyroid hormone to animals without parathyroids results in an increase of phosphorus excretion in the urine, a fall in serum inorganic phosphorus levels, an increase in serum calcium, and an increase of calcium excretion in the urine.

6. **(D)** The function of the adrenal cortex is to secrete: a. sex hormones—androgens, estrogens, and progesterone b. corticosteroids—glucocorticoids and mineralocorticoids. These are all steroid hormones. The functional aspects of mineral and carbohydrate control by the adrenal are far more important than the influence it has on the reproductive organs (reproduction).

7. **(B)** Tetany is a state of increased neuromuscular excitability caused by a decrease in serum calcium. This can exhibit itself by numbness, cramps, spasms, loss of consciousness, convulsions, and possible death.

8. **(A)** Symptoms of hyperthyroidism can be listed as loss of weight, nervousness, irritability, rapid pulse, sweating, protrusion of the eyeballs (exophthalamus), and goiter.

9. **(A)** Hypothyroidism results in sluggish mental and physical behavior. Pulse rate is down and skin appears dry.

10. **(C)** Lymphocytes which participate in such immunologic activities as delayed hypersensitivity reactions and graft rejection are able to do so because of the influence of the thymus. Stem cells for this population are thought to pass through the thymus, and having come under its influence seed more peripheral lymphoid organs with their progeny. Removal of the thymus from newborn animals seriously impairs their immunologic system because of the lack of thymic influences.

11. **(D)** Chymotrypsinogen is the precursor in pancreatic juice of the enzyme chymotrypsin. Trypsin is active in this conversion. Chymotrypsin acts with trypsin to hydrolyze proteins and protein products to polypeptides and amino acids.

12. **(A)** Pepsin is a proteinase of gastric juice (derived from its precursor pepsinogen) which is secreted by the chief cells of the gastric mucosa. The pH of the stomach varies around 1.5.

13. **(C)** Pancreatic juice contains proteolytic, lipolytic, and amylolytic enzymes. Pancreatic amylase is an enzyme which hydrolyzes starch to maltose.

14. **(D)** See explanation for question 11.

15. **(B)** Budding as in hydra involves the multiplication of cells in one region of the organism and the organization of these cells into a new individual. Binary fission or mitosis is a division of a cell into two equal parts and in this respect two new organisms (cells). Parthenogenesis involves a mechanism in which a single cell is set apart for the purpose of reproduction. This cell has the capability to develop into a new organism.

16. **(A)** The term "limey," as applied to British individuals, refers to the early dietary approach (i.e., providing limes and/or lime juice) of the prevention of scurvy in the British navy while they were on extended absence from access to fresh vegetables and fruits.

17. **(A)** From the right ventricle blood is sent to the lungs via the pulmonary arteries; this blood is rich in carbaminohemoglobin and the CO_2 will be exchanged for O_2. Blood returns from the lungs to the left auricle via the pulmonary veins; this blood has been oxygenated and is rich in oxyhemoglobin. Blood then passes to the left ventricle and then out via the aorta to supply the tissues of the body.

18. **(E)** The uterus is prepared every month via the phases of the menstrual cycle for reception of the fertilized egg. If fertilization does not occur, the endometrium sloughs off (menstruation), is then repaired, and awaits the fertilized egg again. FSH and LH are the gonadotrophins and estrogen and progesterone the hormones responsible for the cyclic changes.

19. **(C)** The heart has its own rhythmicity. The rate of contraction and force of contraction, however, are modified by the sympathetic and parasympathetic influences. The SA node is considered the pacemaker and initiates heart beat; the AV node will take over at a slower rate and its own cardiac rhythmicity will keep the heart beating at a slower rate for some time in this experiment.

20. **(C)** The whole activity is controlled by its genetic components which are located in the nucleus.

21. **(C)** Excretion concerns itself with the elimination of water (fluid) while egestion is the process of eliminating undigested food materials. Catabolism is the chemical breakdown of molecules.

22. **(B)** Immuno-assays are the most sensitive of methods available for the detection of many substances.

23. **(C)** Several gonadotropins occur during pregnancy; they are not of pituitary origin. Chorionic gonadotropin (CG) is of placental origin, appears in the urine during pregnancy, resembles LH in some of its actions, and is the basis of most pregnancy tests.

24. **(B)** This is basically a definition. The blooming of plants is influenced by the length of exposure to darkness and is a prime example of photoperiodism.

25. **(A)** Dendrites function in receiving information and conducting it toward the cell body. Axons carry that information away from the cell body and will synapse on dendrites of another neuron.

26. **(E)** A male carries a XY and a female a XX complement of chromosomes. If a male embryo were to result, in our example the sperm that fertilized the egg would have to possess a Y chromosome.

27. **(A)** Umbilical arteries carry deoxygenated blood from the fetus to the placenta for exchange and umbilical veins bring oxygenated blood back to the fetus. Foramen ovale is located between the right and left atria, and in this manner most pulmonary circulation is bypassed. The ductus arteriosus is a communication between the left pulmonary artery and the arch of the aorta through which blood is shunted into the aorta. The ductus venosus is a bypass of the liver in the fetus. All close after birth.

28. **(A)** The cuticle of *Ascaris* protects it from the enzymes that are produced in the intestinal tract of the host.

29. **(E)** Virchow, who was a German physician, is known for his statement that all cells originate from preexisting cells.

30. **(E)** The sympathetic component of the autonomic nervous system mobilizes the body's reserves in case of emergencies.

31. **(A)** Homologous structures exhibit a structural similarity which is attributable to a common genetic and embryologic origin.

32. **(C)** Basic genetic knowledge is applied.
rough — R (dominant)
smooth — r (recessive)
brown — B (dominant)
gray — b (recessive)

The male is crossed to several smooth gray females; they had to be homozygous recessive genotype. Since all four combinations appeared, we can assume that the male was genotypically heterozygous even though he appeared phenotypically dominant. If first we crossed this heterozygous male RrBb × rrbb, the result would be RrBb; rrBb; rrbb; Rrbb; in other words the four combinations given. Now let us cross the RrBb male × RrBb female; the following combinations would have to be considered in both male and female: RB; Rb; rB; rb. If these are crossed, we find 3 out of 16 possess rough gray coats (namely RRbb; Rrbb and Rrbb).

33. **(C)** Epidermis or, broadly speaking, skin functions in protection against trauma, etc.; it is also important in the regulation of body temperature

which it accomplishes by insulation and sweating. Skin possess receptors that make the organism aware of his or her immediate surroundings and it is a depot for glycogen, cholesterol, and water.

34. **(C)** Skeletal (striated) muscle is under voluntary control. The autonomic nervous system innervates cardiac muscle, smooth muscle, and glands. Arrector pili musculature is associated with skin and is smooth musculature.

35. **(D)** Apical meristems are responsible for the extension in length, while cambium meristems are responsible for the increase in thickness. The capacity for division is lost by the main mass of the plant body.

36. **(D)** In general the major derivatives of the germ layers are as follows: *Mesoderm* gives rise to connective tissue, bone, and cartilage; both striated and smooth muscle; blood and lymph cells and the walls of the vascular channels; kidneys; gonads and spleen.

37. **(D)** *Ectoderm* gives rise to the epidermis, the hypophysis, the central and peripheral nervous system, the epithelium of the sense organs, and the epithelial lining of some other organs.

38. **(D)** *Endoderm* gives rise to tonsils, thyroid, parathyroids, thymus, liver, and pancreas; epithelial lining of gut; respiratory tract, and urinary bladder.

Chemistry

1. **(C)** Substrate(s) or reactant(s) react(s) with the enzyme to form an enzyme-substrate complex. This complex breaks down into product(s) and frees enzymes ready for formation of a new enzyme-substrate complex.

2. **(A)** See explanation for question 1.

3. **(D)** See explanation for question 1.

4. **(A)** This is a definition of an ionic bond.

5. **(B)** This is a definition of a covalent bond.

6. **(A)** Potassium donates the single electron in the outer shell to fluorine (previously one electron deficient in the outer shell).

7. **(B)** This is a covalent bond involving the sharing of electrons between two atoms. A hydrogen bond (sometimes called a proton bond) results when a proton is attracted almost equally by two atoms (particularly fluorine, oxygen or nitrogen).

8. **(A)** The development of our solar system is thought to have proceeded from the condensation of gases composed primarily of hydrogen, the simplest element.

9. **(C)** Most enzymes are named to indicate the reaction they catalyze and have the suffix *-ase* (e.g., lipase, carboxypeptidase, and amylase).

10. **(B)** We have described conditions for the formation of a diazonium salt and then replacement of the diazonium salt by Br to produce monobromobenzene. (The replacement is known as the Sandmeyer reaction). The intermediate diazonium salt is often unstable at room temperature, so a lower temperature is used.

11. **(E)** See explanation for question 10.

12. **(C)** See explanation for question 10.

13. **(D)** Enzymes and other proteins are primarily composed of L-amino acids, and they may be hydrolyzed to produce free amino acids. Enzymes are proteins and may be considered as such chemically and physically.

14. **(B)** Sharing of a pair of electrons between two atoms results in a covalent bond. This type of bond may occur in organic, inorganic, or organometallic compounds.

15. **(C)** Production of glucose and fructose from sucrose and production of fatty acids and glycerol from triglycerides are both simple hydrolytic reactions in which essentially no energy is gained or lost. Production of steroids from acetate (as is true with most synthetic reactions) requires energy input. Production of CO_2 and water from fatty acids yields large amounts of energy.

16. **(C)** In pure H_2O at 25°C, $(H^+) = (OH^-) = \sqrt{1 \times 10^{-14}} = 1 \times 10^{-7}$ mole/liter. A neutral solution is one in which $(H^+) = (OH^-) = 1 \times 10^{-7}$ mole/liter. In an acid solution (H^+) is greater than 10^{-7} mole/liter, and (OH^-) is less than 10^{-7} mole/liter. In a basic solution (H^+) is less than 10^{-7} mole/liter and (OH^-) is greater than 10^{-7} mole/liter.

17. **(C)** A molecule having NH_2 and COOH groups is an amino acid. Naturally occurring amino acids ordinarily have the NH_2 group on the alpha carbon and are of the L-configuration. Proteins are high molecular weight polymers of amino acids. In proteins one amino acid is attached to the adjacent one by dehydration to form the peptide bond. In proteins there are very few free amino or carboxyl groups because most are in the peptide bonds.

18. **(D)** $CO_2 + H_2O \rightarrow H_2CO_3$ (i.e., carbonic acid). This reaction occurs nonenzymatically, but it occurs *faster* in the presence of the enzyme, carbonic anhydrase.

19. **(D)** Carbon, oxygen, and hydrogen are the most common elements in protoplasm. These three elements are found in most of the molecules. Only these three plus nitrogen, calcium, and (possibly) phosphorus are in a concentration exceeding 1%.

20. **(A)** The nucleus contains DNA which directs the production of messenger RNA in the nucleus. Messenger RNA leaves the nucleus to influence transfer RNA and eventual production of proteins.

21. **(D)** A colloid is composed of submicroscopic particles which in solution or suspension do not settle out. If such a solution is subjected to spinning in a centrifuge which creates gravitational forces much greater than normally experienced, one can, of course, precipitate colloidal particles.

22. **(C)** Remember that the aldol condensation cannot occur in a compound without alpha-hydrogen. Instead the Cannizarro reaction occurs, resulting in oxidation of one aldehyde molecule and reduction in another. In this case oxidation produces benzoic acid, and reduction produces benzyl alcohol.

23. **(D)** The Lambert-Beer law relates absorption of light (at a particular wavelength) to solution concentration and light path: $\log\left(\frac{I_i}{I_t}\right) - a\ b\ c$ where I_i = intensity of incident light, I_t = intensity of transmitted light, a = extinction coefficient (a proportionality constant that depends on wavelength and the units of the other variables), b = light path, and c = concentration of the solution.

24. **(A)** Phenol, like many organic compounds, is most soluble in aqueous medium in the ionized form. Phenol will not react with $NaHCO_3$, but it will react with a stronger base (such as NaOH) to form the more highly ionized salt, sodium phenolate.

25. **(A)** In general the metabolism of fats (triglycerides) produces about 9 calories per gram as compared with about 4 calories per gram for carbohydrates (e.g., fructose or glucose) or protein.

26. **(B)** A conjugated diene is a compound in which there are double bonds adjacent to a single bond on both sides (e.g., 1,3-butadiene) while a cumulative diene is one in which the double bonds are adjacent to each other (e.g., 1,2-butadiene). An isolated diene is a diene that is neither conjugated nor cumulative (e.g., 1,4-pentadiene).

27. **(C)** Optical isomers that are not mirror images are called diastereomers. In the resolution of racemic lactic acid, we may wish to use L-strychnine to make a salt. The L-strychnine salt of L-lactic acid is a diastereomer of the L-strychnine salt of D-lactic acid. Diastereomers differ somewhat in such physical properties as solubility and may be separated. It is then necessary only that we break down the salt and recover the resolved lactic acid isomers from the L-strychnine.

28. **(A)** DNA is made up of adenine, guanine, thymine, and cytosine; in RNA cytosine is replaced by uracil. These are the nitrogenous bases of the compounds.

29. **(C)** The base-catalyzed reaction of urea with 2,2-diethylmalonic acid (or more likely its diethyl ester) results in a condensation to produce barbital (diethylbarbituric acid).

30. **(B)** See explanation for question 1.

31. **(D)** DNA possesses a deoxyribose while RNA possesses a ribose sugar. For a discussion of their nitrogenous bases see answer to question 28.

32. **(D)** Charge, solubility, and molecular size determine the rate at which molecules enter and leave a cell.

33. **(D)** The compound shown is an unsaturated aldehyde.

34. **(D)** The elements listed are referred to as noble gases. They tend to be unreactive and they are ordinarily found in uncombined monoatomic form.

35. **(A)** Hydrolysis of sucrose produces one molecule each of glucose and fructose for each molecule of sucrose.

36. **(C)** Remember that cycloalkanes and unbranched alkenes have the formula C_nH_{2n}. Thus cyclopropane would be C_3H_6.

37. **(B)** Dacron is a polymer of a dicarboxylic acid and a diol; thus it is a polyester. Nylon is a polyamide.

38. **(A)** Most home units for softening water utilize a zeolite with exchangeable sodium ions. The sodium ions exchange for ions such as calcium that are in the untreated water.

39. **(B)** The Hall process produces metallic aluminum by electrolysis of alumina in molten cryolite.

40. **(C)** Electrolysis of brine (sodium chloride solution) produces chlorine and sodium hydroxide respectively at the two electrodes.

41. **(B)** The metabolism of sugar by yeast provides carbon dioxide. This carbon dioxide gas is responsible for the rising of bread.

42. **(C)** The major component of permanent-type antifreeze for automobile cooling systems is ethylene glycol. It is suitable because it is water-soluble, high-boiling, stable, and noncorrosive to the system.

43. **(B)** Although many compounds evolve heat as they dissolve (e.g., NaOH), others (e.g., NH_4Cl) are endothermic and thus utilize heat in dissolving.

44. **(D)** Hydrolysis is a necessary step before macromolecules can be absorbed by the intestines.

45. **(D)** To accomplish the conversion of carbohydrates into CO_2, H_2O, and ATP, the Krebs cycle must operate and in addition oxygen and electron transport reactions must be present.

46. **(D)** Self-explanatory.

47. **(B)** The basicity of the aromatic amine is decreased by electrophilic substituents such as $-NO_2$ and increased by nucleophilic substituents such as -methyl and -methoxy.

48. **(D)** Fats and carbohydrates contain little or no nitrogen, but proteins contain about 16% nitrogen. Some carbohydrates do contain small amounts of nitrogen. Some *lipids* contain small amounts of nitrogen, but these are not strictly fats (triglycerides).

49. **(B)** Reaction of an alkyl alcohol with PCl_3 or PCl_5 produces a good yield of the corresponding alkyl chloride. The reaction with HCl is an equilibrium reaction and thus not so good.

Physics

1. **(D)** Average speed is the speed at which the car would travel the given distance in the given time.

$$S_1 = \frac{d_1}{t_1} \qquad S_2 = \frac{d_2}{t_2}$$

$$t_1 = \frac{d_1}{S_1} \qquad t_2 = \frac{d_2}{S_2}$$

$$t_1 = \frac{15}{30} = \frac{1}{2} \qquad t_2 = \frac{30}{60} = \frac{1}{2}$$

$$t_{tot} = t_1 + t_2 = (\frac{1}{2}) + (\frac{1}{2}) = 1$$

$$S_{ave} = d_{tot}/t_{tot} = \frac{45}{1} = 45 \text{ km/hr.}$$

2. **(B)** This is a statement of uniform acceleration implying that the body will increase its velocity at 9.8 m/sec./sec. of free fall.

3. **(E)** The ideal gas law states that $\frac{PV}{T} = \frac{P_0V_0}{T_0}$ with temperature and pressure in absolute units. Given: $P_0 = 1, V_0 = 2m^3, T_0 = 293°K, P = 4, V = 3m^3$, and $T = ?$

$$T = (\frac{PV}{P_0V_0})\,T_0 = \frac{(4)(3)}{(1)(2)}\,293°$$

$$T = 1758°K$$

4. **(D)** During an exothermal reaction, chemical energy is converted to heat energy and therefore the components are heated up.

5. **(C)** Number C is the true statement since isotopes have different mass numbers, that is, different numbers of nucleons in the nucleus.

6. **(A)** Density (P) equals mass (m) per unit volume (V), therefore: $P = \frac{m}{V}$ when $P = 7.8$ gm/cm^3, $m = ?$, and $V = 2 \times 3 \times 5 = 30$ m^3.

$$m = PV = (7.8 \text{ gm/cm}^3)(30 \text{ m}^3)$$

convert m^3 to cm^3

$$m = (7.8)(30)(10^6) \text{ gm}$$

$$m = 234 \times 10^6 \text{ gm}$$

7. **(B)** $KE = \frac{mv^2}{2}$ when $m = 100$ gm $= .1$ kg and $v = 60$ m/sec.

$$KE = (.1)(3600)/2 \text{ kg m}^2/\text{sec.}^2$$

$$KE = 180 \text{ kg m}^2/\text{sec.}^2 = 180 \text{ joules}$$

8. **(B)** One newton is, by definition, the amount of force that will give 1 kg of mass an acceleration of 1 m/sec.^{2}.

9. **(E)** The force changing the course of a body from a straight line to a circular motion is known as centripetal force.

10. **(D)** Work = force × distance when force = 5 kg × 9.8 n and *distance* = 10 m.
Work = (5)(9.8)(10) in joules
Work = 490 joules

11. **(B)** $x_1 = 3m$
$y_1 = 2m$
$x_2 = 15m$
$y_2 = ?$

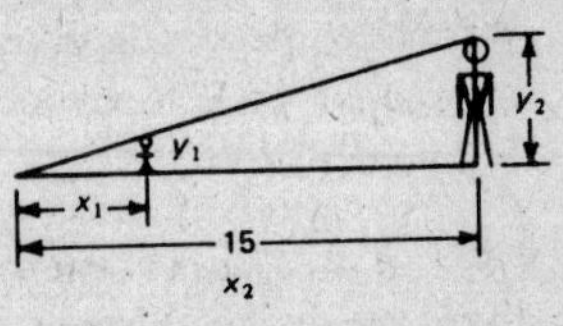

$$\frac{x_1}{y_1} = \frac{x_2}{y_2}$$

$$\frac{3}{2} = \frac{15}{y_2}$$

$$y_2 = \frac{30}{3} = 10 \text{ m}$$

12. **(E)** Refraction can be defined as a change in direction of waves due to a change in their velocity.

13. **(A)** $V = IR$ and $P = I^2R$ when R_0 = original resistance, I_0 = original current, V_0 = voltage (constant), and $3R_0$ = new resistance.

$$V_0 = I_0R_0 = 3R_0\frac{I_0}{3}$$

$$P_0 = \left(\frac{I_0}{3}\right)^2(3R_0) = \frac{I_0^2R_0}{3}$$

14-18. **(14-B) (15-A) (16-E) (17-C) (18-D)** The answers to questions *14-18* are self-explanatory.

19. **(D)** A body is said to be in unstable equilibrium when it does not return to its original equilibrium position when slightly displaced but moves to another position after displacement.

20. **(B)** A body entirely or partially submerged in a fluid is forced upward in a fluid by a force equal to the weight of the fluid displacement.

21. **(C)** $E = h^2$; when h is doubled
$E = (2h)^2$
$E = 4h^2$, therefore E is quadrupled.

22. **(A)** A vector has both magnitude and direction. The illustration gives a 3, 4, 5 triangle, therefore the angles are 37° and 63°. The resultant vector is 5 cm at 37°.

23. **(E)** Use $v = v_0 + at$ when v = 2690 cm/sec., v_0 = 1340 cm/sec., t = 15 seconds, and $at = v - v_0$.

$$a = \frac{v - v_0}{t}$$

$$a = \frac{2690 - 1340}{15} = \frac{1350}{15}$$

a = 90 cm/sec.^{2}

24. **(D)** $\tan\theta = \frac{v^2}{ra}$ when v = 2500 cm/sec., a = 980 cm/sec.^{2}, r = ?, and $\tan\theta = 1$.

$$r = \frac{v^2}{(\tan\theta)a} = \frac{v^2}{a}$$

$$r = \frac{(2500 \text{ cm/sec.})^2}{980 \text{ cm/sec.}^2}$$

r = 6378 cm
r = 63.78 m = 64 m

25. **(E)** All of the above.

26. **(E)** The process is called sublimation.

27. **(A)** The velocity of sound through an ideal gas is proportional to the square root of the absolute temperature. Therefore, $v/v_0 = (T/T_0)^{1/2}$ when v_0 = 332 m/sec., T_0 = 273°K, and T = 293°K.
$v = v_0(T/T_0)^{1/2}$
$v = (332)(293/273)^{1/2}$
v = 344 m/sec.

28. **(C)** The velocity (C) of a wave is directly proportional to its wavelength (L) and inversely proportional to its period (T). $C = L/T = fL$ and C = 1435 m/sec. and f = 410 cycles/sec.
$L = C/f$
L = 1435/410 = 3.5 m

29. **(D)** Reflection of an object from a plane mirror has an image that is the same size as the object.

30-34. **(30-B) (31-E) (32-A) (33-C) (34-D)** The answers to questions *30-34* are self-explanatory.

35. **(E)** The fraction of the element left after 80 years is given by:

$$F = \left(\frac{1}{2}\right)^{\frac{80}{10}} = \frac{1}{2}^8 = \frac{1}{512}$$

Another way of arriving at the above is that $\frac{1}{2}$ of the element disintegrates every 10 years or

$$\left(\frac{1}{2}\right)\left(\frac{1}{2}\right)\left(\frac{1}{2}\right)\left(\frac{1}{2}\right)\left(\frac{1}{2}\right)\left(\frac{1}{2}\right)\left(\frac{1}{2}\right)\left(\frac{1}{2}\right)$$ is the amount of original sample at the end of 80 years.

36. **(A)** Boron is an element.

37. **(C)** That part of radiant power in the visible range is known as luminous flux.

38. **(D)** Charging a body without making contact with the body is known as charging by induction.

SCIENCE PROBLEMS

1. **(E)** Knowing that α = 10 radians/sec.^{2}, $w_0 = 0$, t = 4 seconds, and w = ? Use $w = w_0 + \alpha t$
$w = 0 + (10)(4)$
w = 40 radians/sec.

2. **(D)** Calculate for the values above by using

$$\theta = w_0t + \frac{1}{2}\alpha t^2$$

$$\theta = 0 + \frac{1}{2}(10)(16)(\text{rad/sec.}^2)(\text{sec.}^2)$$

θ = 80 radians
To convert radians to revolutions, multiply

$$80 \text{ radians} \times \frac{1 \text{ revolution}}{2 \text{ radians}} = \frac{80}{2} \text{ revolutions} =$$

12.7 revolutions

3. **(A)** The magnitude of the angular acceleration changes to 5 radians/sec./sec. Use $w = w_0 + \alpha t$, where w_0 = 40 radians/sec., α = ?, t = 4 seconds,

$w = 60$ radians/sec., and sec = sec + rad/sec. α.
$60 = 40 + 4\alpha$
$\alpha = 5$ radians/sec.^{2}
(In other words, it slows down.)

4. **(E)** Most insoluble at pH 5.2. The protein is least soluble at the isoelectric point.

5. **(A)** The protein at its isoelectric point has a net zero charge which is why it is least soluble.

6. **(B)** Positive since there will be more $\overset{\overset{\displaystyle O}{\|}}{C}-O^-$ protonated; thus the charge on the protein will be due to $-NH_3^{\oplus}$.

7. **(C)** $4H + O_2 \rightarrow 2H_2O$

$\frac{X}{4} = \frac{0.145}{36}$ $X = 0.0161$ g H/0.100 g compound

$\frac{0.0161}{1} = 0.0161$ g H/0.100 g compound

$C + O_2 \rightarrow CO_2$

$\frac{X}{12} = \frac{0.142}{44}$ $X = 0.0387$ g C/0.100 g compound

$\frac{0.0387}{12} = 0.0032$ g C/0.100 g compound

$0.100\text{ g} \times 0.452 = 0.0452$ g N/0.100 g compound

$\frac{0.0452}{14} = 0.0032$ g N/0.100 g compound

$\frac{0.0161}{0.0032} = 5$ atoms H/atom C

$\frac{0.0032}{0.0032} = 1$ atom N/atom C

Empirical formula is CH_5N.

8. **(D)** The compound could only be an amine.

9. **(C)** CH_5N could be written as $C_2H_{10}N_2$.

10-15. **(10-C) (11-D) (12-A) (13-B) (14-B) (15-C)** The experiments demonstrated basic biological principles. The absorption of water by colloidal substances, such as starch and cellulose, and their subsequent swelling can be defined as inbibition. When the test tubes were placed in the beakers and, as you observed, only solvent or water molecules passed the semipermeable membrane, we speak in terms of osmosis; but when both the solvent and solute pass from a place of higher concentration to one of lower concentration, the principle of diffusion is illustrated. Both processes are related. The test tubes were placed into a hypotonic solution. The following definitions must be considered: (1) isotonic—solutions exhibiting the same osmotic pressure; (2) hypotonic—a solution that possesses a lesser osmotic pressure; and (3) hypertonic—a solution that possesses a greater osmotic pressure.

16. **(D)** The number of molecules in a mole is 6.02×10^{23} (Avogadro's number).

17. **(E)** Pressure has no effect on the number of molecules in a mole.

18. **(B)** One mole contains 6.02×10^{23} molecules. The number given in the question, 3.01×10^{23}, represents 0.5 mole. One mole of gas at STP occupies a volume of 22.4 liters; 0.5 mole occupies a volume of 22.4×0.5 or 11.2 l.

19. **(C)** $Na + Bu—OH \rightarrow Bu—ONa + 0.5\ H_2$ (Remember to balance equations.)

20. **(E)** See answer to previous question. Only one mole of butyl alcohol is required to consume all the sodium.

21. **(B)** Since 1 mole equals 22.4 liters, 0.5 mole equals 11.2 liters.

22. **(E)** 1 liter V_o and 5 liters V_n are combined to make the total V_m equal to 6 liters. To calculate the pressure of oxygen in the new mixture, use Boyle's law: $P_1V_1 = P_2V_2$ where $P_1 = 4$ atm, $v_1 = 1$ liter, $P_2 = ?$, and $V_2 = 6$ liters.

$(4)(1) = (P)(6)$
$P_2 = 0.67$ atm after mixing

23. **(C)** The total pressure of the new mixture = P_oP_n after mixing. $P_o = 0.67$ atm, calculate P_n and add to P_o for P_t.

original after mixing
$P_1V_1 = P_2V_2$
$(5)(2) = (P_2)(6)$
$1.67 = P_n$ after mixing
$P_o + P_n = 0.67 + 1.67 = 2.34$ atm

24. **(D)** What is the volume if the pressure on the container is 5 atm?

$P_1V_1 = P_2V_2$
$(2.34)(6) = (5)(V_2)$
$2.8 \text{ liters} = V_2$

By subjecting the mixture of 5 atm pressure, the volume is reduced to 2.8 liters.

25. **(A)** Triglycerides, which are esters of glycerol, show a net increase in liver tissue following alcohol ingestion.

26. **(D)** An increase in liver lipids due to net increase in liver triglyceride caused by carbon tetrachloride. Lipids are soluble in organic solvents.

27. **(C)** Note that the lipid has increased from 25 μg to 50 μg in the hydrazine treated liver showing an increased secretion into the blood. Data on A and B is not given and hydrazine is a known factor in fatty liver formation.

28. (E) $CO_2 + Ca(OH)_2 \rightarrow CaCO_3 + H_2O$. The $CaCO_3$ precipitates.

29. (E) Carbon dioxide will not ignite; thus the gas must be a mixture.

30. (E) If the gas will not support combustion, it does not contain a high concentration of O_2.

31. (A) Cations migrate to the cathode, and anions migrate to the anode. Anode $2\ Cl^- \rightarrow Cl_2 + 2$ electrons.

32. (B) Electrolysis of the fused salt allows the collection of sodium at the cathode.

33. (D) Electrolysis of the aqueous salt does not allow sodium production. Instead, hydrogen gas and sodium hydroxide may be collected at the cathode (provided diffusion of the sodium hydroxide is prevented).

34. (B) The parallel resistors in A can be expressed as:
$$\frac{1}{R_A} = \frac{1}{R_1} + \frac{1}{R_2}$$

35. (E) If one resistor were to replace the entire group of resistors (R_S) it would be equal to the sum of the resistance in each part of the circuit or:
$R_S = R_A + R_B + R_C$

36. (C) If $I = 2$ amp and $R = 60$ ohms the relationship between potential difference, current and resistance can be used and it states that:
$V = IR$
$V = (2)(60)$
$V = 120$ volts

37. (B) The cohesiveness of blood by itself causes an increase in viscosity and if there is an increase, a concomitant loss of speed of flow and pressure is observed.

38. (C) As the stream becomes more compact, the radius decreases and the layers of blood are brought closer to one another. This results in an increase in viscosity and a decrease in pressure, speed and flow.

39. (B) $\frac{1}{2} \times \frac{1}{2} \times \frac{1}{2} \times \frac{1}{2} = \frac{1}{16}$

40. (D) An equilibrium shift to the right would be favored by decreased temperature (since it is exothermic) and increased pressure (since the volume is greater on the left side) according to the principle of LeChatelier.

41. (B) The equilibrium is favored toward the left by increased temperature and decreased pressure. Decreased pressure is the best choice presented in the question.

42. (E) The changes in temperature and pressure would have effects in opposing directions whose total effect could not be predicted from the information given.

43. (C) Use $F = \left(\frac{1}{2}\right)^{t/T}$ where T = half-life = 10; t = time = 90
$$F = \left(\frac{1}{2}\right)^{90/10} = \left(\frac{1}{2}\right)^9$$
$$F = \frac{1}{512}$$
$$\left(\frac{1}{512}\right)(10^9) = \text{atoms remaining} = 2 \times 10^6 \text{ atoms}$$

44. (A) To calculate the % of disintegration use 100% − % remaining = % disintegrated.
$$\% \text{ remaining} = \frac{\text{no. of atoms remaining}}{\text{no. of atoms at start}} \times 100$$
$$= \frac{2 \times 10^6}{1 \times 10^9} \times 100 = 2 \times 10^{-3} \times 10^2$$
$$= 2 \times 10^{-1} = 0.2\%$$
$$\% \text{ disintegrated} = 100 - 0.2 = 99.8\%$$

45. (D) The answer to the question is self-explanatory.

46. (D) All the statements are true.

47. (B) Use $F = G\frac{M_1 M_2}{d^2}$, where $M_1 = 1$ kg, $M_2 = 5$ kg, $d = 20$ m and $G = 6.67 \times 10^{-11} \frac{N \cdot M^2}{kg^2}$.
$$F = \frac{(6.67)(1)(5) \times 10^{-11} \frac{N \cdot M^2}{kg^2} \cdot kg^2}{(20)^2 \quad M^2}$$
F = Newtons = correct unit
$$F = \frac{33.35 \times 10^{-11}}{400} \text{ Newtons}$$
$F = 0.08 \times 10^{-11}$ Newtons
$F = 8 \times 10^{-13}$

48. (D) $F = \frac{4}{3}\pi G M_1 r D$. Since G, D, $\frac{4}{3}\pi$ are constant $M_E r_E = M_p r_p$ where E = earth and p = other planet; $M_E = 70$ kg, $r_E = 6380\ K_m$; $M_p = ?$, $r_p = (\frac{1}{4})(6380)$ = object's weight + on planet = (70)(4) = 280 kg.

49. (E) $k\,[A]\,[B]^2$

50. (B) Doubling A would double the reaction rate; doubling B would have a fourfold effect on the reaction rate. Doubling C or D would have no effect on the reaction rate as shown, but this would increase the reaction rate of a possible reverse reaction.

51. (D) Doubling A doubles the rate; doubling C has no effect.

52. **(B)** ml × N = ml × N
(20) (0.5) = ml × 1 = 10

53. **(A)** 120 × 0.5 = 60 milliequivalents
120 × 1 = 120 milliequivalents

54. **(C)** 1 M solution of H_2X is 2 N. 1 M solution of ZOH is 1 N.

55. **(D)** Specific gravity $= \frac{\rho \text{ substance}}{\rho \text{ water}}$

ρ water in gm/cm³ = 1.0

$(11.3)\frac{\text{gm}}{\text{cm}^3} = \rho \text{ lead}$

56. **(B)** $\rho = \frac{M}{\text{Vol.}}$ = 11.3 g/cm = density, Vol. = ?, and Mass = 600 kg then Mass = 600×10^3.

$11.3\ V = M$

$V = \frac{M}{11.3} = \frac{600 \times 10^3 \text{ gm}}{11.3 \text{ gm/cm}^3}$

$V = 53.1 \times 10^3 \text{ cm}^3$

57. **(C)** $11.3 = \frac{\rho \text{ lead}}{\rho \text{ water}} = \frac{\rho \text{ lead}}{62.5 \text{ lb./ft.}^3}$

ρ lead = (11.3) (62.5) lb./ft.³

ρ lead = 786.25 lb./ft.³

58. **(C)** Water dissociates to give equal concentrations of H_3O^+ and OH^-, although the concentrations are very small, only 1×10^{-7} moles/liter of each.

59. **(B)** Solving, $K_w = [H_3O^+][OH^-]$

$10^{-14} = 10^{-7}[OH^-]$

$[OH^-] = \frac{10^{-14}}{10^{-7}}$

$[OH^-] = 10^{-7}$

60. **(C)** An increase in OH^- must have a decrease in H_3O^+. The decrease is controlled through the special equilibrium constant K_w.

$K_w = 10^{-4} = [10^{-4}][H_3O^+]$ and

$[H_3O^+] = 10^{-10}$

61. **(C)** The combined vapor pressure must equal atmospheric pressure (760 torr in this case).
760 − 526 = 234 torr.

62. **(C)** Compound Z is highly sensitive to elevated temperatures.

63. **(B)** Remember that the liquids are essentially immiscible.

64-66. **(64-A) (65-C) (66-C)** The answers to these questions are easily deduced from the experimental design.

Answer Sheet–Model Test D

SCIENCE KNOWLEDGE

Biology

1. Ⓐ Ⓑ Ⓒ Ⓓ Ⓔ
2. Ⓐ Ⓑ Ⓒ Ⓓ Ⓔ
3. Ⓐ Ⓑ Ⓒ Ⓓ Ⓔ
4. Ⓐ Ⓑ Ⓒ Ⓓ Ⓔ
5. Ⓐ Ⓑ Ⓒ Ⓓ Ⓔ
6. Ⓐ Ⓑ Ⓒ Ⓓ Ⓔ
7. Ⓐ Ⓑ Ⓒ Ⓓ Ⓔ
8. Ⓐ Ⓑ Ⓒ Ⓓ Ⓔ
9. Ⓐ Ⓑ Ⓒ Ⓓ Ⓔ
10. Ⓐ Ⓑ Ⓒ Ⓓ Ⓔ
11. Ⓐ Ⓑ Ⓒ Ⓓ Ⓔ
12. Ⓐ Ⓑ Ⓒ Ⓓ Ⓔ
13. Ⓐ Ⓑ Ⓒ Ⓓ Ⓔ
14. Ⓐ Ⓑ Ⓒ Ⓓ Ⓔ
15. Ⓐ Ⓑ Ⓒ Ⓓ Ⓔ
16. Ⓐ Ⓑ Ⓒ Ⓓ Ⓔ
17. Ⓐ Ⓑ Ⓒ Ⓓ Ⓔ
18. Ⓐ Ⓑ Ⓒ Ⓓ Ⓔ
19. Ⓐ Ⓑ Ⓒ Ⓓ Ⓔ
20. Ⓐ Ⓑ Ⓒ Ⓓ Ⓔ
21. Ⓐ Ⓑ Ⓒ Ⓓ Ⓔ
22. Ⓐ Ⓑ Ⓒ Ⓓ Ⓔ
23. Ⓐ Ⓑ Ⓒ Ⓓ Ⓔ
24. Ⓐ Ⓑ Ⓒ Ⓓ Ⓔ
25. Ⓐ Ⓑ Ⓒ Ⓓ Ⓔ
26. Ⓐ Ⓑ Ⓒ Ⓓ Ⓔ
27. Ⓐ Ⓑ Ⓒ Ⓓ Ⓔ
28. Ⓐ Ⓑ Ⓒ Ⓓ Ⓔ
29. Ⓐ Ⓑ Ⓒ Ⓓ Ⓔ
30. Ⓐ Ⓑ Ⓒ Ⓓ Ⓔ
31. Ⓐ Ⓑ Ⓒ Ⓓ Ⓔ
32. Ⓐ Ⓑ Ⓒ Ⓓ Ⓔ
33. Ⓐ Ⓑ Ⓒ Ⓓ Ⓔ
34. Ⓐ Ⓑ Ⓒ Ⓓ Ⓔ
35. Ⓐ Ⓑ Ⓒ Ⓓ Ⓔ
36. Ⓐ Ⓑ Ⓒ Ⓓ Ⓔ
37. Ⓐ Ⓑ Ⓒ Ⓓ Ⓔ
38. Ⓐ Ⓑ Ⓒ Ⓓ Ⓔ

Chemistry

1. Ⓐ Ⓑ Ⓒ Ⓓ Ⓔ
2. Ⓐ Ⓑ Ⓒ Ⓓ Ⓔ
3. Ⓐ Ⓑ Ⓒ Ⓓ Ⓔ
4. Ⓐ Ⓑ Ⓒ Ⓓ Ⓔ
5. Ⓐ Ⓑ Ⓒ Ⓓ Ⓔ
6. Ⓐ Ⓑ Ⓒ Ⓓ Ⓔ
7. Ⓐ Ⓑ Ⓒ Ⓓ Ⓔ
8. Ⓐ Ⓑ Ⓒ Ⓓ Ⓔ
9. Ⓐ Ⓑ Ⓒ Ⓓ Ⓔ
10. Ⓐ Ⓑ Ⓒ Ⓓ Ⓔ
11. Ⓐ Ⓑ Ⓒ Ⓓ Ⓔ
12. Ⓐ Ⓑ Ⓒ Ⓓ Ⓔ
13. Ⓐ Ⓑ Ⓒ Ⓓ Ⓔ
14. Ⓐ Ⓑ Ⓒ Ⓓ Ⓔ
15. Ⓐ Ⓑ Ⓒ Ⓓ Ⓔ
16. Ⓐ Ⓑ Ⓒ Ⓓ Ⓔ
17. Ⓐ Ⓑ Ⓒ Ⓓ Ⓔ
18. Ⓐ Ⓑ Ⓒ Ⓓ Ⓔ
19. Ⓐ Ⓑ Ⓒ Ⓓ Ⓔ
20. Ⓐ Ⓑ Ⓒ Ⓓ Ⓔ
21. Ⓐ Ⓑ Ⓒ Ⓓ Ⓔ
22. Ⓐ Ⓑ Ⓒ Ⓓ Ⓔ
23. Ⓐ Ⓑ Ⓒ Ⓓ Ⓔ
24. Ⓐ Ⓑ Ⓒ Ⓓ Ⓔ
25. Ⓐ Ⓑ Ⓒ Ⓓ Ⓔ
26. Ⓐ Ⓑ Ⓒ Ⓓ Ⓔ
27. Ⓐ Ⓑ Ⓒ Ⓓ Ⓔ
28. Ⓐ Ⓑ Ⓒ Ⓓ Ⓔ
29. Ⓐ Ⓑ Ⓒ Ⓓ Ⓔ
30. Ⓐ Ⓑ Ⓒ Ⓓ Ⓔ
31. Ⓐ Ⓑ Ⓒ Ⓓ Ⓔ
32. Ⓐ Ⓑ Ⓒ Ⓓ Ⓔ
33. Ⓐ Ⓑ Ⓒ Ⓓ Ⓔ
34. Ⓐ Ⓑ Ⓒ Ⓓ Ⓔ
35. Ⓐ Ⓑ Ⓒ Ⓓ Ⓔ
36. Ⓐ Ⓑ Ⓒ Ⓓ Ⓔ
37. Ⓐ Ⓑ Ⓒ Ⓓ Ⓔ
38. Ⓐ Ⓑ Ⓒ Ⓓ Ⓔ
39. Ⓐ Ⓑ Ⓒ Ⓓ Ⓔ
40. Ⓐ Ⓑ Ⓒ Ⓓ Ⓔ
41. Ⓐ Ⓑ Ⓒ Ⓓ Ⓔ
42. Ⓐ Ⓑ Ⓒ Ⓓ Ⓔ
43. Ⓐ Ⓑ Ⓒ Ⓓ Ⓔ
44. Ⓐ Ⓑ Ⓒ Ⓓ Ⓔ
45. Ⓐ Ⓑ Ⓒ Ⓓ Ⓔ
46. Ⓐ Ⓑ Ⓒ Ⓓ Ⓔ
47. Ⓐ Ⓑ Ⓒ Ⓓ Ⓔ
48. Ⓐ Ⓑ Ⓒ Ⓓ Ⓔ
49. Ⓐ Ⓑ Ⓒ Ⓓ Ⓔ

Physics

1. Ⓐ Ⓑ Ⓒ Ⓓ Ⓔ
2. Ⓐ Ⓑ Ⓒ Ⓓ Ⓔ
3. Ⓐ Ⓑ Ⓒ Ⓓ Ⓔ
4. Ⓐ Ⓑ Ⓒ Ⓓ Ⓔ
5. Ⓐ Ⓑ Ⓒ Ⓓ Ⓔ
6. Ⓐ Ⓑ Ⓒ Ⓓ Ⓔ
7. Ⓐ Ⓑ Ⓒ Ⓓ Ⓔ
8. Ⓐ Ⓑ Ⓒ Ⓓ Ⓔ
9. Ⓐ Ⓑ Ⓒ Ⓓ Ⓔ
10. Ⓐ Ⓑ Ⓒ Ⓓ Ⓔ
11. Ⓐ Ⓑ Ⓒ Ⓓ Ⓔ
12. Ⓐ Ⓑ Ⓒ Ⓓ Ⓔ
13. Ⓐ Ⓑ Ⓒ Ⓓ Ⓔ
14. Ⓐ Ⓑ Ⓒ Ⓓ Ⓔ
15. Ⓐ Ⓑ Ⓒ Ⓓ Ⓔ
16. Ⓐ Ⓑ Ⓒ Ⓓ Ⓔ
17. Ⓐ Ⓑ Ⓒ Ⓓ Ⓔ
18. Ⓐ Ⓑ Ⓒ Ⓓ Ⓔ
19. Ⓐ Ⓑ Ⓒ Ⓓ Ⓔ
20. Ⓐ Ⓑ Ⓒ Ⓓ Ⓔ
21. Ⓐ Ⓑ Ⓒ Ⓓ Ⓔ
22. Ⓐ Ⓑ Ⓒ Ⓓ Ⓔ
23. Ⓐ Ⓑ Ⓒ Ⓓ Ⓔ
24. Ⓐ Ⓑ Ⓒ Ⓓ Ⓔ
25. Ⓐ Ⓑ Ⓒ Ⓓ Ⓔ
26. Ⓐ Ⓑ Ⓒ Ⓓ Ⓔ
27. Ⓐ Ⓑ Ⓒ Ⓓ Ⓔ
28. Ⓐ Ⓑ Ⓒ Ⓓ Ⓔ
29. Ⓐ Ⓑ Ⓒ Ⓓ Ⓔ
30. Ⓐ Ⓑ Ⓒ Ⓓ Ⓔ
31. Ⓐ Ⓑ Ⓒ Ⓓ Ⓔ
32. Ⓐ Ⓑ Ⓒ Ⓓ Ⓔ
33. Ⓐ Ⓑ Ⓒ Ⓓ Ⓔ
34. Ⓐ Ⓑ Ⓒ Ⓓ Ⓔ
35. Ⓐ Ⓑ Ⓒ Ⓓ Ⓔ
36. Ⓐ Ⓑ Ⓒ Ⓓ Ⓔ
37. Ⓐ Ⓑ Ⓒ Ⓓ Ⓔ
38. Ⓐ Ⓑ Ⓒ Ⓓ Ⓔ

SCIENCE PROBLEMS

1. Ⓐ Ⓑ Ⓒ Ⓓ Ⓔ
2. Ⓐ Ⓑ Ⓒ Ⓓ
3. Ⓐ Ⓑ Ⓒ Ⓓ Ⓔ
4. Ⓐ Ⓑ Ⓒ Ⓓ Ⓔ
5. Ⓐ Ⓑ Ⓒ Ⓓ Ⓔ
6. Ⓐ Ⓑ Ⓒ Ⓓ Ⓔ
7. Ⓐ Ⓑ Ⓒ Ⓓ Ⓔ
8. Ⓐ Ⓑ Ⓒ Ⓓ Ⓔ
9. Ⓐ Ⓑ Ⓒ Ⓓ Ⓔ
10. Ⓐ Ⓑ Ⓒ Ⓓ Ⓔ
11. Ⓐ Ⓑ Ⓒ Ⓓ Ⓔ
12. Ⓐ Ⓑ Ⓒ Ⓓ Ⓔ
13. Ⓐ Ⓑ Ⓒ Ⓓ Ⓔ
14. Ⓐ Ⓑ Ⓒ Ⓓ Ⓔ
15. Ⓐ Ⓑ Ⓒ Ⓓ Ⓔ
16. Ⓐ Ⓑ Ⓒ Ⓓ Ⓔ
17. Ⓐ Ⓑ Ⓒ Ⓓ Ⓔ
18. Ⓐ Ⓑ Ⓒ Ⓓ Ⓔ
19. Ⓐ Ⓑ Ⓒ Ⓓ Ⓔ
20. Ⓐ Ⓑ Ⓒ Ⓓ Ⓔ
21. Ⓐ Ⓑ Ⓒ Ⓓ Ⓔ
22. Ⓐ Ⓑ Ⓒ Ⓓ Ⓔ
23. Ⓐ Ⓑ Ⓒ Ⓓ Ⓔ
24. Ⓐ Ⓑ Ⓒ Ⓓ Ⓔ
25. Ⓐ Ⓑ Ⓒ Ⓓ Ⓔ
26. Ⓐ Ⓑ Ⓒ Ⓓ Ⓔ
27. Ⓐ Ⓑ Ⓒ Ⓓ Ⓔ
28. Ⓐ Ⓑ Ⓒ Ⓓ Ⓔ
29. Ⓐ Ⓑ Ⓒ Ⓓ Ⓔ
30. Ⓐ Ⓑ Ⓒ Ⓓ Ⓔ
31. Ⓐ Ⓑ Ⓒ Ⓓ Ⓔ
32. Ⓐ Ⓑ Ⓒ Ⓓ Ⓔ
33. Ⓐ Ⓑ Ⓒ Ⓓ Ⓔ
34. Ⓐ Ⓑ Ⓒ Ⓓ Ⓔ
35. Ⓐ Ⓑ Ⓒ Ⓓ Ⓔ
36. Ⓐ Ⓑ Ⓒ Ⓓ Ⓔ
37. Ⓐ Ⓑ Ⓒ Ⓓ Ⓔ
38. Ⓐ Ⓑ Ⓒ Ⓓ Ⓔ
39. Ⓐ Ⓑ Ⓒ Ⓓ Ⓔ
40. Ⓐ Ⓑ Ⓒ Ⓓ Ⓔ
41. Ⓐ Ⓑ Ⓒ Ⓓ Ⓔ
42. Ⓐ Ⓑ Ⓒ Ⓓ Ⓔ
43. Ⓐ Ⓑ Ⓒ Ⓓ Ⓔ
44. Ⓐ Ⓑ Ⓒ Ⓓ Ⓔ
45. Ⓐ Ⓑ Ⓒ Ⓓ Ⓔ
46. Ⓐ Ⓑ Ⓒ Ⓓ Ⓔ
47. Ⓐ Ⓑ Ⓒ Ⓓ Ⓔ
48. Ⓐ Ⓑ Ⓒ Ⓓ Ⓔ
49. Ⓐ Ⓑ Ⓒ Ⓓ Ⓔ
50. Ⓐ Ⓑ Ⓒ Ⓓ Ⓔ
51. Ⓐ Ⓑ Ⓒ Ⓓ Ⓔ
52. Ⓐ Ⓑ Ⓒ Ⓓ Ⓔ
53. Ⓐ Ⓑ Ⓒ Ⓓ Ⓔ
54. Ⓐ Ⓑ Ⓒ Ⓓ Ⓔ
55. Ⓐ Ⓑ Ⓒ Ⓓ Ⓔ
56. Ⓐ Ⓑ Ⓒ Ⓓ Ⓔ
57. Ⓐ Ⓑ Ⓒ Ⓓ Ⓔ
58. Ⓐ Ⓑ Ⓒ Ⓓ Ⓔ
59. Ⓐ Ⓑ Ⓒ Ⓓ Ⓔ
60. Ⓐ Ⓑ Ⓒ Ⓓ Ⓔ
61. Ⓐ Ⓑ Ⓒ Ⓓ Ⓔ
62. Ⓐ Ⓑ Ⓒ Ⓓ Ⓔ
63. Ⓐ Ⓑ Ⓒ Ⓓ Ⓔ
64. Ⓐ Ⓑ Ⓒ Ⓓ Ⓔ
65. Ⓐ Ⓑ Ⓒ Ⓓ Ⓔ
66. Ⓐ Ⓑ Ⓒ Ⓓ Ⓔ

SKILLS ANALYSIS: READING

1. Ⓐ Ⓑ Ⓒ
2. Ⓐ Ⓑ Ⓒ
3. Ⓐ Ⓑ Ⓒ
4. Ⓐ Ⓑ Ⓒ
5. Ⓐ Ⓑ Ⓒ
6. Ⓐ Ⓑ Ⓒ
7. Ⓐ Ⓑ Ⓒ
8. Ⓐ Ⓑ Ⓒ
9. Ⓐ Ⓑ Ⓒ
10. Ⓐ Ⓑ Ⓒ
11. Ⓐ Ⓑ Ⓒ
12. Ⓐ Ⓑ Ⓒ
13. Ⓐ Ⓑ Ⓒ
14. Ⓐ Ⓑ Ⓒ
15. Ⓐ Ⓑ Ⓒ
16. Ⓐ Ⓑ Ⓒ
17. Ⓐ Ⓑ Ⓒ
18. Ⓐ Ⓑ Ⓒ
19. Ⓐ Ⓑ Ⓒ
20. Ⓐ Ⓑ Ⓒ
21. Ⓐ Ⓑ Ⓒ
22. Ⓐ Ⓑ Ⓒ
23. Ⓐ Ⓑ Ⓒ
24. Ⓐ Ⓑ Ⓒ
25. Ⓐ Ⓑ Ⓒ
26. Ⓐ Ⓑ Ⓒ
27. Ⓐ Ⓑ Ⓒ
28. Ⓐ Ⓑ Ⓒ
29. Ⓐ Ⓑ Ⓒ
30. Ⓐ Ⓑ Ⓒ
31. Ⓐ Ⓑ Ⓒ
32. Ⓐ Ⓑ Ⓒ
33. Ⓐ Ⓑ Ⓒ
34. Ⓐ Ⓑ Ⓒ
35. Ⓐ Ⓑ Ⓒ
36. Ⓐ Ⓑ Ⓒ
37. Ⓐ Ⓑ Ⓒ
38. Ⓐ Ⓑ Ⓒ
39. Ⓐ Ⓑ Ⓒ
40. Ⓐ Ⓑ Ⓒ
41. Ⓐ Ⓑ Ⓒ
42. Ⓐ Ⓑ Ⓒ
43. Ⓐ Ⓑ Ⓒ
44. Ⓐ Ⓑ Ⓒ
45. Ⓐ Ⓑ Ⓒ
46. Ⓐ Ⓑ Ⓒ
47. Ⓐ Ⓑ Ⓒ
48. Ⓐ Ⓑ Ⓒ
49. Ⓐ Ⓑ Ⓒ
50. Ⓐ Ⓑ Ⓒ
51. Ⓐ Ⓑ Ⓒ
52. Ⓐ Ⓑ Ⓒ
53. Ⓐ Ⓑ Ⓒ
54. Ⓐ Ⓑ Ⓒ
55. Ⓐ Ⓑ Ⓒ
56. Ⓐ Ⓑ Ⓒ
57. Ⓐ Ⓑ Ⓒ
58. Ⓐ Ⓑ Ⓒ
59. Ⓐ Ⓑ Ⓒ
60. Ⓐ Ⓑ Ⓒ
61. Ⓐ Ⓑ Ⓒ
62. Ⓐ Ⓑ Ⓒ
63. Ⓐ Ⓑ Ⓒ
64. Ⓐ Ⓑ Ⓒ
65. Ⓐ Ⓑ Ⓒ
66. Ⓐ Ⓑ Ⓒ
67. Ⓐ Ⓑ Ⓒ
68. Ⓐ Ⓑ Ⓒ

SKILLS ANALYSIS: QUANTITATIVE

1. Ⓐ Ⓑ Ⓒ Ⓓ
2. Ⓐ Ⓑ Ⓒ Ⓓ
3. Ⓐ Ⓑ Ⓒ Ⓓ
4. Ⓐ Ⓑ Ⓒ Ⓓ
5. Ⓐ Ⓑ Ⓒ Ⓓ
6. Ⓐ Ⓑ Ⓒ Ⓓ
7. Ⓐ Ⓑ Ⓒ Ⓓ
8. Ⓐ Ⓑ Ⓒ Ⓓ
9. Ⓐ Ⓑ Ⓒ Ⓓ
10. Ⓐ Ⓑ Ⓒ Ⓓ
11. Ⓐ Ⓑ Ⓒ Ⓓ
12. Ⓐ Ⓑ Ⓒ
13. Ⓐ Ⓑ Ⓒ
14. Ⓐ Ⓑ Ⓒ
15. Ⓐ Ⓑ Ⓒ
16. Ⓐ Ⓑ Ⓒ
17. Ⓐ Ⓑ Ⓒ
18. Ⓐ Ⓑ Ⓒ
19. Ⓐ Ⓑ Ⓒ
20. Ⓐ Ⓑ Ⓒ
21. Ⓐ Ⓑ Ⓒ
22. Ⓐ Ⓑ Ⓒ
23. Ⓐ Ⓑ Ⓒ
24. Ⓐ Ⓑ Ⓒ
25. Ⓐ Ⓑ Ⓒ
26. Ⓐ Ⓑ Ⓒ
27. Ⓐ Ⓑ Ⓒ
28. Ⓐ Ⓑ Ⓒ
29. Ⓐ Ⓑ Ⓒ
30. Ⓐ Ⓑ Ⓒ
31. Ⓐ Ⓑ Ⓒ
32. Ⓐ Ⓑ Ⓒ
33. Ⓐ Ⓑ Ⓒ
34. Ⓐ Ⓑ Ⓒ
35. Ⓐ Ⓑ Ⓒ
36. Ⓐ Ⓑ Ⓒ
37. Ⓐ Ⓑ Ⓒ Ⓓ
38. Ⓐ Ⓑ Ⓒ Ⓓ
39. Ⓐ Ⓑ Ⓒ Ⓓ
40. Ⓐ Ⓑ Ⓒ Ⓓ
41. Ⓐ Ⓑ Ⓒ Ⓓ
42. Ⓐ Ⓑ Ⓒ Ⓓ
43. Ⓐ Ⓑ Ⓒ Ⓓ
44. Ⓐ Ⓑ Ⓒ Ⓓ
45. Ⓐ Ⓑ Ⓒ
46. Ⓐ Ⓑ Ⓒ
47. Ⓐ Ⓑ Ⓒ
48. Ⓐ Ⓑ Ⓒ
49. Ⓐ Ⓑ Ⓒ
50. Ⓐ Ⓑ Ⓒ
51. Ⓐ Ⓑ Ⓒ
52. Ⓐ Ⓑ Ⓒ Ⓓ
53. Ⓐ Ⓑ Ⓒ Ⓓ
54. Ⓐ Ⓑ Ⓒ Ⓓ
55. Ⓐ Ⓑ Ⓒ
56. Ⓐ Ⓑ Ⓒ
57. Ⓐ Ⓑ Ⓒ
58. Ⓐ Ⓑ Ⓒ
59. Ⓐ Ⓑ Ⓒ
60. Ⓐ Ⓑ Ⓒ
61. Ⓐ Ⓑ Ⓒ
62. Ⓐ Ⓑ Ⓒ
63. Ⓐ Ⓑ Ⓒ
64. Ⓐ Ⓑ Ⓒ
65. Ⓐ Ⓑ Ⓒ
66. Ⓐ Ⓑ Ⓒ
67. Ⓐ Ⓑ Ⓒ
68. Ⓐ Ⓑ Ⓒ

The New MCAT Model Examination D*

SCIENCE KNOWLEDGE

135 MINUTES
125 QUESTIONS

The following questions are varied; therefore, you are advised to pay careful attention to the instructions for each portion.

Biology

DIRECTIONS: Each of the statements or questions is followed by four or five suggested completions or answers. Choose the one that best completes the statement or answers the question, and mark the letter of your choice on the answer sheet.

1. Sperm utilize the substance ______________ to penetrate the corona radiata of the egg in fertilization.
(A) spermatase
(B) chondroitin sulfatase
(C) hyaluronidase
(D) deoxyribonuclease
(E) ribonuclease

2. During gamete production in the human female, the cell which undergoes the reduction divisions (meiosis) eventually produces ______________ functional egg(s).
(A) four
(B) around three hundred
(C) eight
(D) one
(E) around one hundred

3. A patient has suffered a cerebral hemorrhage that has caused injury and nonfunctioning of the primary motor area of his left cerebral cortex. As a result,
(A) he cannot voluntarily move his right arm or hand nor his right leg or foot.
(B) he feels no sensation on the left side of his body.
(C) reflexes cannot be elicited on the left side of his body.
(D) he cannot voluntarily move his right arm nor his left leg.
(E) he feels no sensation on the right side of his body.

4. The pituitary (master) gland releases a gonadotrophic hormone which stimulates the production of testosterone by
(A) spermatogonia.
(B) interstitial cells of Leydig.
(C) Sertoli cells.
(D) epididymis.
(E) ductus deferens.

5. The structure(s) responsible for the production of progesterone is (are)
(A) ovarian follicle.
(B) corpus albicans.
(C) corpus luteum.
(D) corpus spongiosum.
(E) corpus cavernosum.

*Explanations for science answers can be found on p. 314.

6. The sperm count of a normal 25-year-old male would be
   (A) one milion/ml.
   (B) one hundred million/ml.
   (C) one hundred thousand/ml.
   (D) four million/ml.
   (E) ten thousand/ml.

7. Each of the following is under control of the adenohypophysis EXCEPT the
   (A) thyroid.
   (B) adrenal medulla.
   (C) testis.
   (D) adrenal cortex.
   (E) ovary.

8. Mutations
   (A) are changes that take place and will always be passed on to the next generation.
   (B) are influenced by use and disuse of body parts.
   (C) occur spontaneously and cannot be produced experimentally.
   (D) are mainly due to diseases associated with development.
   (E) occur spontaneously and can also be produced by experimental means.

9. The functional unit of a striated muscle is known as the sarcomere. A sarcomere on an electron micrograph is the region between
   (A) two A bands.
   (B) two I bands.
   (C) two H bands.
   (D) two Z bands.

10. Bacteriophages are
    (A) quite dangerous to humans.
    (B) grown by innoculation of sterile broth.
    (C) reproduced only in living cells.
    (D) used as a source of vaccine against many bacterial diseases.
    (E) used in the production of vaccine against specific viral agents.

11. The czarinas of Russia and the queens of England popularized the disease hemophilia. These normal women produced sons suffering from hemophilia, a disease that is caused by a sex-linked recessive gene, h. The more common dominant gene, H, produces normal blood clotting. Genotypically these women must have carried
    (A) HH.
    (B) Hh.
    (C) hh.
    (D) none of the above.

12. Phenotype may be defined as
    (A) genetic make up of an individual.
    (B) hidden traits of an individual.
    (C) unrelated characteristics.
    (D) visible expression of genotype.
    (E) genetic material carried on the Y chromosome only.

13. Among the defense mechanisms available to humans to ward off their destruction by the environment is (are)
    (A) skin.
    (B) white blood corpuscles.
    (C) antibodies.
    (D) sebaceous secretions.
    (E) all of the above.

14. Alleles are genes which
    (A) arise during the cross-over process.
    (B) are linked to one chromosome only.
    (C) are always sex-linked and are transmitted from mothers to their sons.
    (D) occupy corresponding positions on homologous chromosomes.
    (E) are sex-linked and are transmitted from fathers to their daughters.

15. The neurotransmitter acetylcholine is released by
(A) axon terminals.
(B) dendrite terminals.
(C) Golgi apparatus of neuron cell bodies.
(D) Schwann cells.
(E) node of Ranvier.

16. Two people are planning to have a family. The woman has blood type A/A and the man B/B. Their children might have the following
(A) A and B.
(B) B only.
(C) A/B only.
(D) A and B and A/B.

17. A man with blood cell genotype B/O marries a woman with type A/B. Their offspring could have any of the following
(A) A/B, B/B, A/O, B/O.
(B) A/B and B/O only.
(C) A/O and B/B only.
(D) none of the combinations above.

18. Of the pairs below which one is mismatched?
(A) lymphatics: contain amino acids, salt, water, but no blood corpuscles
(B) hepatic portal vein: drains the intestinal tract and carries nutrients
(C) inferior vena cava: carries oxygenated blood and has a low blood pressure
(D) hypothalamus: secretes releasing factors that influence pituitary-target organ relationships
(E) pulmonary veins: carry oxygenated blood

19. A lack of iodine in the diet usually is associated with which disorder?
(A) acromegaly
(B) goiter
(C) rickets
(D) skin rash
(E) tetanus

20. One enzyme that is important in protein digestion is
(A) ptyalin.
(B) trypsin.
(C) maltose.
(D) pancreatic lipase.
(E) rennin.

21. If we examine the three types of muscles in respect to their characteristics, which of the series below is false?

	Characteristic	Cardiac	Skeletal	Smooth
(A)	No. of Nuclei	Several	Several	One
(B)	Position of Nuclei	Central	Central	Central
(C)	Striations	Present	Present	Absent
(D)	Control	Autonomic	Voluntary	Autonomic

22. Twinning is an interesting biological phenomenon. Identical twins usually result from fertilization of
(A) two eggs by one sperm.
(B) one egg by two sperms.
(C) one egg by one sperm and separation of cells during the early cleavage division.
(D) one egg and one polar body.
(E) two eggs by two sperms.

23. The basic scientific finding that finally led to the development of the oral contraceptive (pill) used by many females in our society was that the preovulatory surge of LH can be prevented by the administration of
(A) FSH.
(B) estrogen.
(C) progesterone.
(D) ICSH.
(E) androgen.

24. Dialysis (as is used for the treatment of chronic kidney ailments) differs from the process of osmosis in the respect that
(A) both solvent and solute pass through the membrane.
(B) solute selectively passes through the membrane only.
(C) solvent selectively passes through the membrane only.
(D) gases are the only substances that pass the membrane and blood is cleansed.

25. A foreign protein, when introduced into the body, is recognized and elicits an immunologic response; this substance is known as a (an)
(A) antigen.
(B) antibody.
(C) complement.
(D) vitamin.
(E) enzyme.

26. Vasectomy is becoming a fashionable form of birth control in our society. In a vasectomy the ______________ is (are) cut, a portion is removed, and the stumps are sutured.
(A) epididymis
(B) spermatic cords
(C) oviducts
(D) urethra
(E) seminal vesicles

27. Sweating is a mechanism of temperature regulation by the body. This mechanism is usually far less effective in cooling the organism if the person is in an environment where the
(A) wind is of hurricane proportion.
(B) humidity is at least 0°.
(C) humidity is almost 0°.
(D) all of the above.
(E) none of the above.

28. Hypersecretion of the hormone ______________ will result in acromegaly (giantism).
(A) TSH—thyroid stimulating hormone
(B) STH—somatotropin (growth hormone)
(C) ACTH—adrenocorticotrophic hormone
(D) thyroxin
(E) adrenalin

29. Conservation of body heat is aided by
(A) constriction of the capillaries of the skin.
(B) decreased respiratory activity.
(C) decreased heart rate.
(D) decreased sweating.
(E) all of the above.

30. Testosterone is produced by
(A) spermatogonia of the testes.
(B) interstitial cells of the testes (Leydig cells).
(C) the glans penis.
(D) the prostate gland.
(E) Sertoli cells.

31. Glucagon, which is produced by the pancreas, and epinephrine, which is produced by the adrenal glands, are hormones which
(A) raise blood sugar level.
(B) lower blood sugar level.
(C) do not affect blood sugar markedly.
(D) markedly increase liver glycogen.

32. Abnormal blood clots (thrombi) occur more frequently in people with
(A) prothrombin deficiency.
(B) impeded venous blood flow.
(C) vitamin K deficiency.
(D) platelet deficiency.
(E) none of the above.

33. Growth hormone releasing factor is
(A) a precursor of growth hormone.
(B) the same as growth hormone (somatotropin).
(C) a hypothalamic releasing factor.
(D) a dietary stimulant regulating positive nitrogen balance.
(E) an enzyme.

34. The large intestine functions mainly in
(A) absorption of water.
(B) excretion of water.
(C) absorption of sodium and potassium.
(D) finishing the digestive process.
(E) excretion of digestive enzymes.

35. Blood pH is influenced by respiration; experimental hyperventilation in a physiology laboratory will result in the student's blood pH being
(A) lowered.
(B) raised.
(C) unaffected.
(D) raised to pH6.

36. Heart beat is initiated by the
(A) vagus nerve.
(B) sympathetic nervous system.
(C) A-V (atrio-ventricular) node.
(D) Purkinje system.
(E) S-A (sino-atrial) node.

37. Resolution may be defined as ability to discriminate between two points that are close together; resolution depends on the wavelength and the numerical aperture of the objective lens used. Which of the following are incorrectly paired?
(A) human eye: resolves 100 μ
(B) light microscope: resolves 0.2 μ
(C) transmission electron microscope: resolves 3-5 Å
(D) ophthalmoscope: resolves 1 μ
(E) scanning electron microscope: resolves 70-100 Å

38. A patient is awaiting surgery and routine blood tests are conducted. It is found that problems may arise due to the patient's abnormally long clotting time. This patient may be deficient in

(A) vitamin K.
(B) platelets.
(C) prothrombin.
(D) any or all of the above.

STOP. If you finish before the time limit is up, go over your work for this section. DO NOT look at any other sections of the model examination. When your time limit is up, go on to the next section.

Chemistry

DIRECTIONS: Each of the statements or questions is followed by four or five suggested completions or answers. Choose the one that best completes the statement or answers the question, and mark the letter of your choice on the answer sheet.

1. The basic building block of proteins is (are)
(A) nitrogenous bases.
(B) amino acids.
(C) ammonia.
(D) transfer RNA.
(E) messenger RNA.

2. Catalytic hydrogenation of phenyl diazonium bromide produces
(A) bromobenzene.
(B) phenylhydrazine.
(C) benzene.
(D) phenylamine.

3. In transcription of RNA from DNA, thymine will form a base pair only with
(A) adenine.
(B) guanine.
(C) cytosine.
(D) uracil.
(E) thymine.

4. Calcium carbide reacts with water to produce
(A) carbon dioxide.
(B) methane.
(C) carbohydrate.
(D) acetylene.
(E) ethylene.

5. Addition of water to metallic sodium produces
(A) oxygen and sodium hydride.
(B) hydrogen and sodium hydroxide.
(C) sodium hydrate.
(D) nitrogen and sodium hydride.
(E) no reaction.

6. The common lead storage battery produces electricity by two hall cell reactions, one of which is (written in the direction of production of electricity)
(A) $PbSO_2 + 2H_2O \rightarrow PbO_2 + 4H^+ + SO_4^= + 2e^-$
(B) $PbSO_4 + 2e^- \rightarrow Pb + SO_4^=$
(C) $Pb + SO_4^= \rightarrow PbSO_4 + 2e^-$
(D) none of the above

7. If one wished to remove substantially all of the chloride ions from an aqueous solution, this could be done by the addition of an aqueous solution of
(A) KNO_3.
(B) Na_2SO_4.
(C) $AgNO_3$.
(D) starch.
(E) gelatin.

8. Methyl iodide and n-propyl iodide may be reacted with sodium metal to produce ______________ organic products.
(A) 2
(B) 3
(C) 4
(D) 6
(E) 8

9. In the previous question the compound listed below that would be produced in greatest yield is
(A) n-hexane.
(B) sodium propane.
(C) hexyl iodide.
(D) n-butane.
(E) none of the above.

10. If it is known that H_2S is a weak acid that ionizes to form $2H^+$ and $S^=$, lowering the pH of a solution of H_2S by adding HCl should
(A) raise the $S^=$ concentration.
(B) lower the $S^=$ concentration.
(C) have no effect on $S^=$ concentration.
(D) not be possible.

11. Which of the following aqueous solutions will have the lowest freezing point?
(A) 1 M NaCl
(B) 0.3 M Na_2SO_4
(C) 1.5 M glucose
(D) 0.5 M $BaSO_4$
(E) H_2O

12. Consider this reaction $Fe^{++} \rightleftharpoons Fe^{+++} + e^-$
(A) The reaction toward the right is an oxidation.
(B) The reaction toward the right is a reduction.
(C) The reaction toward the left is a reduction.
(D) A and C are correct.
(E) None of the above is correct.

13. A negative iodoform test (i.e., no yellow precipitate) will be the result when NaOH + I_2 is reacted with
(A) 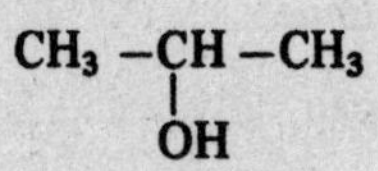
(B) 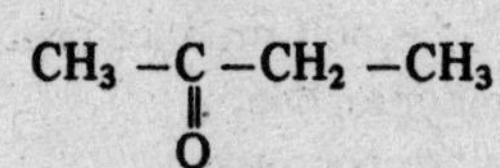
(C) 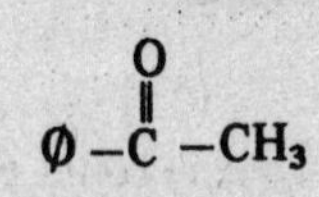
(D) 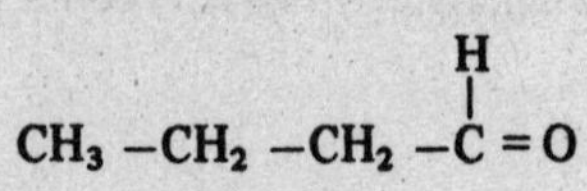

14. The hydronium ion is
(A) a protonated water molecule.
(B) formed by removal of H^- from a water molecule.
(C) really a free radial rather than an ion.
(D) an ion with the formula of H_2O^+.
(E) an uranium byproduct.

15. The alpha helix in a protein is classified as the
(A) primary structure.
(B) secondary structure.
(C) tertiary structure.
(D) quaternary structure.
(E) permanent structure.

16. The neutralization of 50 ml of 0.25 N H_2SO_4 will require ________ ml of 0.50 N NaOH.
(A) 25
(B) 50
(C) 0.25
(D) 2.5
(E) none of the above

17. The smallest organic ring compound that may be synthesized contains ________ carbon atoms.
(A) 3
(B) 4
(C) 5
(D) 6
(E) 7

18. Factor(s) that influence(s) enzymatic activity is (are)
(A) temperature.
(B) pH.
(C) concentration, substrate, cofactors
(D) enzyme poisons.
(E) all of the above.

19. A zwitterion is a molecule containing
(A) both cationic and anionic functions.
(B) more than one cationic or anionic function.
(C) polar and nonpolar groups.
(D) a Z^+ charge.
(E) none of the above.

20. Prolonged boiling of animal fat with lye is called
(A) ecology.
(B) stain removal.
(C) saponification.
(D) alchemy of glyceridization.
(E) conjugation.

21. Without considering stereoisomers the number of possible dibromobutane isomers is
(A) 3.
(B) 4.
(C) 5.
(D) 6.
(E) 8.

22. The reaction of HBr with 1-propene in the presence of peroxides will produce primarily
(A) 1-bromopropane.
(B) 2-bromopropane.
(C) 1,2-dibromopropane.
(D) 2-bromopropene.
(E) 1,3-dibromopropane.

23. Theoretically, the ring monobromination of 4-bromo-1,2-diisopropylbenzene could produce ______________ isomers.
(A) 1
(B) 2
(C) 3
(D) 4
(E) 5

24. In a titration of iodine with sodium thiosulfate, the formation of a blue color on the addition of colorless starch solution indicates that
(A) all of the iodine has not been oxidized.
(B) the glassware has not been washed sufficiently.
(C) all of the iodine has not been reduced.
(D) a blue complex of starch, iodine, and sodium thiosulfate has been produced.
(E) the temperature is above 50°C.

25. Of the compounds listed below which has the greatest affinity for combining with hemoglobin?
(A) nitrogen, N_2
(B) carbon dioxide, CO_2
(C) oxygen, O_2
(D) helium
(E) carbon monoxide, CO

26. Use of helium is preferred over use of hydrogen in airships (e.g., blimps) because
(A) helium has a lower density.
(B) helium is chemically less reactive.
(C) both of the above.
(D) none of the above.

27. Nucleotides are composed of two types of sugars:
(A) glucose and maltose.
(B) glucose and ribose.
(C) maltose and deoxyribose.
(D) ribose and deoxyribose.
(E) none of the above.

28. The process of fermentation can be considered to be
(A) oxidation.
(B) dehydration.
(C) aerobic respiration.
(D) anaerobic respiration.
(E) hydrolytic.

29. Low molecular weight mercaptans are often added to natural gas to
(A) increase the flammability.
(B) slightly retard the burning.
(C) produce a pleasant deodorant during burning.
(D) provide a stench which is helpful in the detection of gas leaks.
(E) prevent corrosion of the pipelines.

30. In the reaction sequence used in breakdown of glycogen in the liver or muscle—glycogen → glucose-1-phosphate → glucose-6-phosphate → glucose—the first step is
(A) catalyzed by phosphorylase.
(B) catalyzed by pepsin.
(C) catalyzed by pancreatic amylase.
(D) nonenzymatic.
(E) catalyzed by trypsin.

31. An inorganic cation has been precipitated from water by the addition of NaOH. When we find that the precipitate may be redissolved upon the addition of NaOH or dilute HNO_3, we may conclude that the precipitate was
(A) colloidal.
(B) amphoteric.
(C) anthromorphic.
(D) amorphous.
(E) crystalline.

32. The inorganic cation in the question above could be
(A) silver.
(B) ferric.
(C) aluminum.
(D) nickel.
(E) barium.

33. Transuranium elements are
(A) found on earth as a result of bombardment by particles from the planet Uranus.
(B) found naturally in abundance greater than that of uranium isotopes.
(C) man-made elements with more than 92 protons in the nucleus.
(D) elements that have been postulated but not found naturally or produced artificially.

34. The particles which spin around the nucleus of an atom and are negatively charged are the
(A) neutrons.
(B) positrons.
(C) protons.
(D) electrons.
(E) ions.

35. Below are listed the major differences between compounds and mixtures. Which one is an incorrect pairing?

	Mixture	Compound
(A)	Physical union	Chemical union
(B)	No new substances are formed	New substances are formed
(C)	Can be separated by physical means	Can be separated by physical means
(D)	Elements form no definite proportions	Elements form definite proportions

36. 2,4-D (2,4-dichlorophenoxyacetic acid) is a potent stimulator of plant metabolism. Most sensitive to it is (are)
(A) monocotyledons.
(B) dicotyledons.
(C) phytoplankton.
(D) Kentucky blue grass.
(E) Kentucky fescue grass.

37. Solids
(A) are rigid and have a definite form.
(B) possess molecules which vibrate very slowly in a fixed position.
(C) possess molecules which are close together.
(D) have all of the above characteristics.
(E) have none of the above characteristics.

38. Which of the following reactions is a decomposition reaction?
(A) $CO_2 + H_2O \rightarrow H_2CO_3$
(B) $2HgO \xrightarrow{\Delta} 2Hg + O_2$
(C) $Zn + CuSO_4 \rightarrow ZnSO_4 + Cu$
(D) $HCl + NaOH \rightarrow NaCl + H_2O$
(E) $2H_2 + O_2 \rightarrow 2H_2O$

39. Which of the following is an incorrect statement?
(A) Ions have a charge equal to the number of electrons gained or lost.
(B) The fewer ions formed, the greater the electric current carried by an electrolyte.
(C) Atoms and ions of the same element have different properties.
(D) Certain substances break up into ions when dissolved in water.
(E) All of the above.

40. Which of the following structural formulas is not properly identified?
(A) Methane
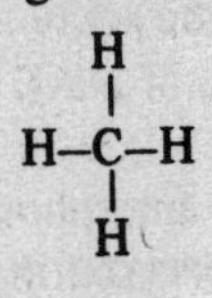
(B) Ethane
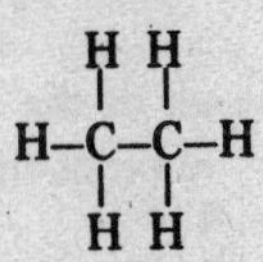
(C) Propane
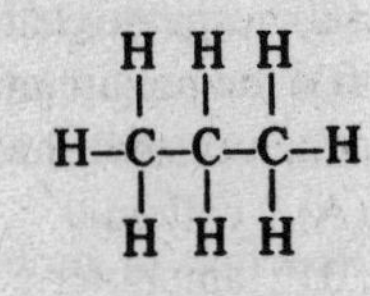
(D) Pentane
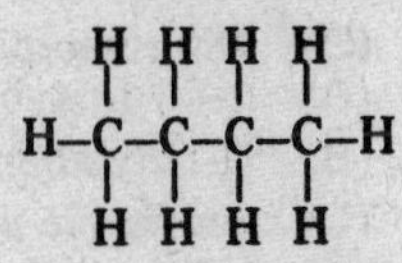

41. The pH of a weak solution of ammonium hydroxide has been measured. If ammonium chloride is now added
(A) the pH will increase.
(B) the pOH will decrease.
(C) the acidity will decrease.
(D) the pH will decrease.
(E) no pH change is observed.

42. Black and white photographic film is based on the light-catalyzed chemical reaction
(A) $gelatin_c \rightarrow gelatin_B + H_2O$.
(B) $Cd^{++}He \rightarrow Cd^{+}$.
(C) $quinone_1 \rightarrow quinone_2 \rightarrow hydroquinone$.
(D) $Ag^{+}He \rightarrow Ag^{o}$.
(E) none of the above.

43. According to the principle of LeChatelier, a higher pressure applied to the reversible reaction $N_2 + 3H_2 \rightleftarrows 2NH_3$ would be expected to result in
(A) shifting the equilibrium to the left.
(B) shifting the equilibrium to the right.
(C) no change in the equilibrium.
(D) increased percentages of NH_3 and H_2.
(E) increased N_2 and decreased H_2.

44. The neutron was discovered by
(A) Marie and Pierre Curie.
(B) Ernest Rutherford.
(C) James Chadwick.
(D) Enrico Fermi.
(E) Albert Einstein.

45. Reaction of acetic anhydride with toluene (methylbenzene) in the presence of $AlCl_3$ produces
(A) an aromatic ester.
(B) an aromatic acid.
(C) an aromatic ketone.
(D) an aromatic anhydride.
(E) an aromatic lipid.

46. In order to produce polyvinyl alcohol we would expect to
(A) polymerize the monomer, vinyl alcohol.
(B) polymerize another vinyl monomer and convert the polymer to polyvinyl alcohol.
(C) hydroxylate polyethylene.
(D) ask for another task. This one has not been done successfully.

47. Acetaldehyde, in the presence of NaOH, will
(A) not react.
(B) be converted to acetic acid.
(C) produce 3-hydroxybutanal.
(D) produce ethyl acetate.
(E) do none of the above.

48. Treatment of aniline with $NaNO_2$ and HCl followed by the addition of phenol will produce primarily
(A) conversion of aniline to phenol.
(B) conversion of aniline to toluene.
(C) diphenylether.
(D) an azo compound containing two aromatic rings.
(E) chlorobenzene.

49. Reaction of propanal with HCN followed by acid hydrolysis of the reaction product will produce
(A) α-hydroxybutanoic acid.
(B) 1-butylamine.
(C) propanoic acid.
(D) all of the above.
(E) none of the above.

STOP. If you finish before the time limit is up, go over your work for this section. DO NOT look at any other sections of the model examination. When your time limit is up, go on to the next section.

Physics

DIRECTIONS: Each of the statements or questions is followed by five suggested completions or answers. Choose the one that best completes the statement or answers the question, and mark the letter of your choice on the answer sheet.

1. If the uniform acceleration near the surface of the earth is about 9.8 m/sec.^{2} for a free-fall, what is the velocity at the end of 2 seconds of fall (neglect friction)?
(A) 19.6 m/sec.
(B) 17.0 m/sec.
(C) 14.6 m/sec.
(D) 12.2 m/sec.
(E) 9.8 m/sec.

2. The amount of heat measured in calories needed to raise the temperature of 1 gram of substance by 1 degree Celsius is known as
(A) coefficient of expansion.
(B) specific heat.
(C) heat of fusion.
(D) mechanical equivalent of heat.
(E) latent heat.

3. If a force of 30.6 kg acts on a 60 kg mass, calculate the resulting acceleration. (1 kg of force = 9.8 newtons)
(A) 0.5 m/sec.^{2}
(B) 2 m/sec.^{2}
(C) 5 m/sec.^{2}
(D) 6 m/sec.^{2}
(E) 9.8 m/sec.^{2}

4. If an object is moving with a constant acceleration, the net force acting on that body is
(A) constant.
(B) increasing.
(C) decreasing.
(D) zero.
(E) none of the above.

5. What is the potential energy of a 10 kg steel ball which has been raised vertically 9 m above the floor?
(A) 90 joules
(B) 98 joules
(C) 441 joules
(D) 882 joules
(E) 1938 joules

6. If the mass of a moving projectile is tripled and its velocity is doubled, the kinetic energy will be multiplied by
(A) 2.
(B) 6.
(C) 8.
(D) 12.
(E) 16.

7. The direction of the force exerted on a surface by a liquid at rest is
(A) tangential to the surface.
(B) parallel to the surface.
(C) normal to the surface.
(D) 45° to the surface.
(E) 30° to the surface.

8. The volume of a confined gas varies inversely with the absolute pressure provided that the temperature remains unchanged. This statement is known as
(A) Avogadro's law.
(B) Bernoulli's law.
(C) the gas law.
(D) Dalton's law.
(E) Boyle's law.

9. Which ratio below best defines the efficiency of simple machines?
(A) $\frac{\text{useful work output}}{\text{work input}} \times 100\%$
(B) $\frac{\text{work input}}{\text{work output}} \times 100\%$
(C) $\frac{\text{theoretical mechanical advantage}}{\text{actual mechanical advantage}} \times 100\%$
(D) $\frac{\text{centrifugal force}}{\text{centripetal force}} \times 100\%$
(E) $\frac{\text{useful work input}}{\text{useful work output}} \times 100\%$

10. You are standing 1000 m from the point where a steel block strikes the sidewalk. How long will it take the sound to reach your ears if the speed of sound in air at 0°C is about 333 m/sec.?
(A) 1 second
(B) 2 seconds
(C) 3 seconds
(D) 4 seconds
(E) 5 seconds

11. In simplest terms, the energy of a wave is directly proportional to the square of its
(A) period.
(B) length.
(C) reflection.
(D) refraction.
(E) height.

12. Shadows consist of two portions, the umbra and the penumbra. Which statement below applies ONLY to the umbra?
(A) It is circular in shape.
(B) It is always the longest portion.
(C) It is a partial shadow.
(D) It receives no light from any part of the source.
(E) It receives light from part of the source.

13. What is the work done in joules if a 100-kg ball is raised to 3 m above the floor in 1 second?
(A) 300 joules
(B) 980 joules
(C) 1960 joules
(D) 2940 joules
(E) 3240 joules

DIRECTIONS: Below are listed five basic unit names and five phrases of definition for these units. Match the correct definition with the correct unit name.

Questions 14-18:

(A) The work done when a force of 1 newton is extended through a distance of 1 meter.
(B) The quantity of heat needed to raise the temperature of 1 gm of water 1°C.
(C) The amount of force that will give 1 kg of mass an acceleration of 1 m/sec.^{2}.
(D) The resistance of a device in which heat is generated at 1 watt by a current of 1 ampere.
(E) The magnetic flux through a surface.

14. newton
15. joule
16. ohm
17. calorie
18. weber

19. Which of the statements below is correct?
(A) If a road is properly banked for the speed of the vehicle, the resultant force on the vehicle is a horizontal centripetal force.
(B) The resultant force action on a vehicle will be that which maintains it in a circular path.
(C) There is no tendency for the vehicle to skid if a road is banked for the speed at which the vehicle is moving.
(D) The angle of bank for a road is obtained from a consideration of the centripetal force required.
(E) All of the above statements are correct.

20. How far will a body free-fall in 1 second if released from rest?
(A) 0.0 m
(B) 4.9 m
(C) 9.8 m
(D) 14.7 m
(E) 19.6 m

21. A resultant force of 45 kg is acting on a body whose acceleration is 10 m/sec.². Calculate the mass of the body.
(A) 4.5 kg
(B) 44.1 kg
(C) 450 kg
(D) 980 kg
(E) 1960 kg

22. $F = Gm_1m_2/d_2$ is the equation representing Newton's law of universal gravitation. Which of the statements below is true?
(A) G is called the gravitation constant.
(B) The law can be used to calculate the mass of an object on another planet if the mass and radius of that planet are known.
(C) Knowing the value of G, one can easily calculate the mass of the earth.
(D) The force of attraction of the earth for a body is equal to the force of attraction of the body for the earth.
(E) All of the above are true.

23. Two forces of 45 kg-*f* and 40 kg-*f* act on a body in opposite directions. What is the resultant force?
(A) 5 kg-*f*
(B) 40 kg-*f*
(C) 45 kg-*f*
(D) 85 kg-*f*
(E) 90 kg-*f*

24. A good floor lamp has a wide heavy base to increase its stability through
(A) raising the center of gravity.
(B) lowering the center of gravity.
(C) banking.
(D) neutral equilibrium.
(E) none of the above.

25. When analyzed, most complicated machines are found to consist of a combination of various simple machines. Which machine below is NOT a simple machine?
(A) wheel-and-axle
(B) pulley
(C) lever
(D) electric motor
(E) inclined plane

26. Calculate the velocity of a test sled that is propelled by a device that has 2500 joules of available energy to propel a sled of 50 kg mass.
(A) 50 m/sec.
(B) 25 m/sec.
(C) 10 m/sec.
(D) 5 m/sec.
(E) 1 m/sec.

27. Using the figure below as a reference, identify the true statement. The large tank is full of water and is exposed to the atmosphere.

d_1 = diameter of opening
v_1 = velocity at d_1
v_2 = velocity at d_2

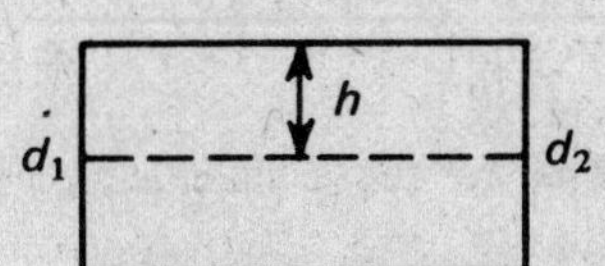

(A) $v_1 > v_2$
(B) $v_2 > v_1$
(C) $v_1/v_2 = 1$
(D) $(v_1)(v_2) = (d_1)(d_2)$
(E) none of the above

28. If the density of a given body is 10 gm/cm³, what is its specific gravity?
(A) 0.01 gm/cm³
(B) 1.0 gm
(C) 0.01
(D) 10.0
(E) 1.0

29. The amount of a liquid's cohesive force per unit of length is called
(A) apparent weight.
(B) adhesion.
(C) depression.
(D) surface tension.
(E) capillary rise.

30. When light is reflected from a surface it can be either regular reflection or diffuse reflection. The essential difference between regularly and diffusely reflecting surfaces is that
(A) the regularly reflecting surface is coarser than the diffusely reflecting surface.
(B) only mirrors reflect in a regular manner, every other surface reflects diffusely.
(C) regularly reflecting surfaces are smoother than diffusely reglecting surfaces.
(D) light can not be reflected from a diffusely reflecting surface.
(E) all of the above are essential differences between regularly and diffusely reflecting surfaces.

31. If a color disc composed of red, orange, yellow, green, blue, indigo, and violet pie-shaped sections is rapidly rotated, which color will your eye see?
(A) black
(B) brown
(C) red
(D) white
(E) blue

DIRECTIONS: Given below are some fundamentals of electricity, followed by phrases defining these fundamentals or equations symbolically representing these characteristics. Match the fundamental with the correct identifying item.

Questions 32-36:

(A) Ratio of charge to potential difference
(B) Ratio of work done to unit charge in moving the charge from point 1 to point 2 (voltage)
(C) $V = I$ or $V = IR$
(D) $F = \frac{KQ_1Q_2}{d^2}$
(E) $P = I^2$ or $P = IR$

32. Ohm's law
33. Joule's law
34. capacitance
35. potential difference
36. Coulomb's law

37. Radium (^{236}Ra) has a half-life of 1590 years. How much of the original amount of ^{236}Ra would remain after 6360 years?

(A) $\frac{1}{2}$

(B) $\frac{1}{4}$

(C) $\frac{1}{8}$

(D) $\frac{1}{16}$

(E) $\frac{1}{32}$

38. A ball is located in a semicircular trough. The ball is moved slightly to one side and returns to its original location. The ball is said to be in

(A) stable equilibrium.

(B) unstable equilibrium.

(C) neutral equilibrium.

(D) coupled equilibrium.

(E) all of the above.

STOP. If you finish before the time limit is up, go over your work for this section. DO NOT look at any other sections of the model examination. When your time limit is up, go on to the next section.

SCIENCE PROBLEMS

85 MINUTES
66 QUESTIONS

The following questions require you to use your knowledge of science to solve problems.

DIRECTIONS: The following questions are in groups. Preceding each series of questions is a paragraph or short explanatory statement, a formula or set of formulas, or a definition. Read the written material and then answer the questions. Eliminate those choices that you think to be incorrect and mark the letter of your choice on the answer sheet.

In uniformly accelerated motion the following equations hold:

$$V = V_0 + at$$
$$X = V_0t + \frac{1}{2}at^2$$

when X = displacement, V = velocity at time t, V_0 = initial velocity, t = time, and a = acceleration. A ball is projected directly upward at a velocity of 15 m/sec.

1. What is the distance above the ground after 3 seconds?
(A) 0 m
(B) 0.9 m
(C) 1.8 m
(D) 2.7 m
(E) 3.6 m

2. What is its velocity at that point?
(A) 14.4 m/sec. upward
(B) 14.4 m/sec. downward
(C) 29.4 m/sec. upward
(D) 29.4 m/sec. downward

3. What is the highest point this ball will reach?
(A) 9.80 m
(B) 11.48 m
(C) 38.66 m
(D) 22.95 m
(E) 1.53 m

In the dark, bromine adds to double bonds to produce dibromo additional compounds. The addition of bromine to conjugated dienes can produce 1,2-dibromo-3-alkenes or 1,4-dibromo-2-alkenes.

4. The reaction of 1 mole of 1,3-butadiene with 1 mole of bromine would be expected to result in production of
(A) 1,4-dibromo-3-butene.
(B) 1,4-dibromobutane.
(C) 1,2-dibromo-2-butene.
(D) 1,3-dibromo-2-butene.
(E) none of the above.

5. Another example of the reaction of bromine with conjugated dienes is that in which bromine reacts with
(A) acetylene.
(B) allene (propadiene).
(C) 1,4-pentadiene.
(D) B and C.
(E) none of the above.

6. The formation of 1,4-addition products with conjugated dienes is evidence of
(A) ionic mechanism.
(B) free radical mechanism.
(C) radiant energy.
(D) A and B.
(E) none of the above.

The solubility of compound R in water is 5 gm/100 ml. The distribution coefficient between water and ether, $K_{H_2O/ether}$, is 2 at room temperature.

7. Extraction of 50 ml of water containing 1.0 g of compound R with 50 ml of ether will result in ______________ of compound R being in the ether phase.
(A) 1.0 g
(B) 0.5 g
(C) 0.33 g
(D) 0.1 g
(E) 0.05 g

8. A second extraction of the remaining aqueous solution by another 50 ml of ether would result in the extraction of an additional
(A) 0.1 g.
(B) 0.2 g.
(C) 0.3 g.
(D) 0.5 g.
(E) 0.55 g.

9. In order to remove 0.8 g in the first extraction it would be necessary to use ______________ of ether.
(A) less than 150 ml
(B) 200 ml
(C) 300 ml
(D) 400 ml
(E) more than 475 ml

Assume that the membrane of a neuron is unimolecular, and that an impulse travelling along the nerve involves the same type of ions regardless of location along the fiber. While examining with the oscilloscope the nature of an impulse traveling along the sciatic nerve of a test animal, an unusually large spike is visualized and seems out of phase.

10. One can assume that the unusually large spike height visualized is
(A) typical of a repeated nerve impulse.
(B) an artifact.
(C) not typical of a nerve impulse but definitely a result of the nerve's physiology.
(D) all of the above.
(E) none of the above.

11. The usual wave function seen while studying neural impulses is an example of
(A) an all or none response.
(B) a gradient response.
(C) subthreshold transmission.
(D) all of the above.
(E) none of the above.

12. The spike height of the wave can be altered by
(A) external application of a saline solution to the nerve.
(B) injecting a saline solution into the nerve fiber.
(C) increasing the voltage of the applied stimulus.
(D) all of the above.
(E) none of the above.

A block weighing 1 kg = 1000 grams is totally submerged in a liquid whose specific gravity is 1.25. The apparent weight of this body in the liquid is 800 grams.

13. What is the buoyant force?
(A) 125 gm
(B) 200 gm
(C) 800 gm
(D) 1000 gm
(E) 1800 gm

14. What is the volume of the body or that of the displaced liquid?
(A) 50 cm^3
(B) 160 cm^3
(C) 250 cm^3
(D) 350 cm^3
(E) 450 cm^3

15. Calculate the density of the body.
(A) 1 gm/cm^3
(B) 2 gm/cm^3
(C) 3 gm/cm^3
(D) 6.25 gm/cm^3.
(E) 5 gm/cm^3

Use the following graph to answer questions 16-18:

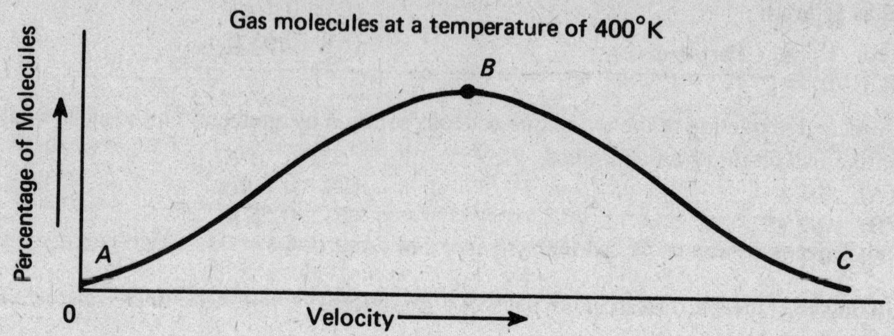

16. In the graph above, point B is
(A) the escape velocity.
(B) the average velocity.
(C) the most probable velocity.
(D) the maximum velocity.
(E) B and C

17. Point C indicates
(A) cessation of motion.
(B) escape velocity.
(C) maximum velocity.
(D) an improbable velocity under these conditions.
(E) an impossible velocity under these conditions.

18. If the above velocity plot were changed to 500°K, the peak of the curve would
(A) be displaced to the right.
(B) remain unchanged.
(C) be displaced to the left.
(D) have three maxima.
(E) be flattened to such an extent that no maximum could be observed.

The equilibrium constant for the reaction $C + D \rightleftharpoons E + 2F$ may be represented by the equation:

$$K_{eq} = \frac{[E]\,[F]^2}{[C]\,[D]}$$

19. Doubling the concentration of C will
(A) double the equilibrium constant.
(B) halve the equilibrium constant.
(C) increase the equilibrium constant by a factor of 3.
(D) increase the equilibrium constant by a factor of 4.
(E) do none of the above.

20. Doubling the concentration of D would result in
(A) an increase in the concentration of E.
(B) an increase in the concentration of F.
(C) a decrease in the concentration of C.
(D) all of the above.
(E) none of the above.

21. The greatest change in the equilibrium constant would be noted upon
(A) doubling the concentration of A.
(B) doubling the concentration of B.
(C) doubling the concentration of C.
(D) doubling the concentration of D.
(E) none of the above.

The A B O blood grouping system is explained on the basis of a single triallelic system with genes A, B, and O operating at a single genetic locus. Phenotypic and genotypic characteristics may be expressed as follows:

Phenotype	Genotype
A	A/A; A/O
B	B/B; B/O
O	O/O
AB	A/B

The A and B genes appear to be codominant; they are dominant over O, which is recessive.

22. Utilizing this system, transfusions have become relatively safe. The universal recipient is considered to be type
(A) A.
(B) B.
(C) O.
(D) AB.
(E) Rh.

23. These individuals carry on their red blood cells the following agglutinogens
(A) A.
(B) B.
(C) O.
(D) A,B.
(E) None.

24. A person of blood type A can receive blood of type(s)
(A) A.
(B) B; A.
(C) O.
(D) A; O.
(E) A; AB.

The equation of Snell's law is $\frac{\text{Sin } \theta_i}{\text{Sin } \theta_r} = \frac{N_r}{N_i}$ where θ_i = angle of incidence, θ_r = angle of refraction, N_r = index of refraction of pass through medium, and N_i = index of refraction of incident medium.

A beam of light is traveling through air and strikes a medium whose index of refraction is 1.414 at 45° with a normal to the glass.

25. The ray of light as it enters will
(A) bend toward the normal.
(B) bend away from the normal.
(C) be totally reflected.
(D) travel along the normal.
(E) do none of the above.

26. The index of refraction can be defined as the velocity of light in a vacuum divided by the velocity in the medium ($N = \frac{C}{S}$). If this is the case, another valid expression for Snell's law is
(A) $\frac{S_i}{S_r} = \frac{N_r}{N_i}$
(B) $\frac{\text{Sin } \theta_i}{\text{Sin } \theta_r} = \frac{C_i}{S_i}$
(C) $\frac{\text{Sin } \theta_i}{\text{Sin } \theta_r} = \frac{C_r}{S_r}$
(D) $\frac{\text{Sin } \theta_i}{\text{Sin } \theta_r} = \frac{S_i}{S_r}$
(E) $\frac{\text{Sin } \theta_i}{\text{Sin } \theta_r} = \frac{S_r}{S_i}$

27. What is the velocity of the light in the medium if Sin θ_i = 0.707, Sin θ_r = 0.500, and the velocity of light in a vacuum is 3.0×10^8 m/sec.?
(A) 1.4×10^8 m/sec.
(B) 2.1×10^8 m/sec.
(C) 2.8×10^8 m/sec.
(D) 3.5×10^8 m/sec.
(E) 4.2×10^8 m/sec.

Two containers of equal volume are filled with helium gas at different temperatures and pressures.

28. If container X is at 760 torr and 0°C while container Y is at 137°C and 1140 torr, then container X (compared to container Y) has
(A) fewer atoms of gas and a higher average velocity.
(B) more atoms of gas and a lower average velocity.
(C) an equal number of atoms of gas and an equal average velocity.
(D) fewer atoms of gas and a lower average velocity.
(E) none of the above.

29. Increasing the number of atoms in container X while retaining the volume constant would result in
(A) increased pressure.
(B) decreased pressure.
(C) increased temperature.
(D) decreased temperature.
(E) Choices A and C.

30. If containers X and Y (above) had been at the temperatures and pressures given but container Y had contained argon rather than helium, then container X (compared to container Y) would be observed to have
(A) fewer atoms of gas and a higher average velocity.
(B) more atoms of gas and lower average velocity.
(C) an equal number of atoms of gas with an equal average velocity.
(D) an equal number of atoms of gas with an unknown average velocity.
(E) none of the above.

A muscle fiber is a single muscle cell. Each fiber is composed of numerous cylindrical fibrils running the entire length of the fiber. The fibril exhibits light and dark bands—the I and A bands respectively. The I band is bisected by the M line. There is a somewhat lighter band within the A band that is called the H band. These striations are produced by the arrangement within the fibril of myofilaments; myosin is the thick myofilament while actin is considered the thin myofilament.

31. A sarcomere is the area between
(A) two A bands.
(B) two H bands.
(C) two I bands.
(D) two Z bands.
(E) two M bands.

32. During contraction the lengths of the thick and thin myofilaments
(A) increase.
(B) decrease.
(C) remain the same.

33. If we could imagine observing a contraction under a light microscope we would see the narrowing of the
(A) H and I bands.
(B) A bands.
(C) Z bands.
(D) H bands only.
(E) I bands only.

Given the circuit diagram below:

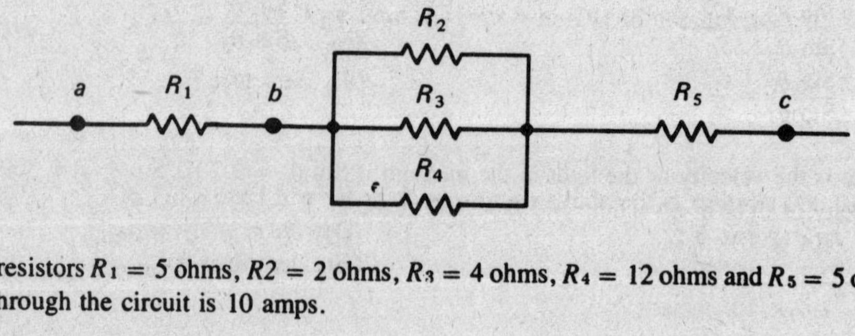

with the resistors R_1 = 5 ohms, $R2$ = 2 ohms, R_3 = 4 ohms, R_4 = 12 ohms and R_5 = 5 ohms. The current through the circuit is 10 amps.

34. Calculate the potential differences across R_1.
(A) 10 volts
(B) 20 volts
(C) 30 volts
(D) 40 volts
(E) 50 volts

35. Calculate the resistance in the parallel resistors.
(A) 1.2 ohms
(B) 5.6 ohms
(C) 6.0 ohms
(D) 18 ohms
(E) 28 ohms

36. Calculate the potential difference across the parallel resistors.
(A) 12 volts
(B) 60 volts
(C) 120 volts
(D) 180 volts
(E) none of the above

An unknown organic compound is observed to react with phenylhydrazine to form a crystalline derivative. Mild oxidation produces one or more acidic compounds.

37. The compound could be
(A) acetone.
(B) 1,3-butadiene.
(C) ethylene glycol.
(D) butanol.
(E) all of the above.

38. Another compound fulfilling the requirements would be
(A) glycerol.
(B) ethanol.
(C) acetic acid.
(D) aniline.
(E) none of the above.

39. If oxidation with permanganate and then oxidation with periodic acid is performed prior to the reactions with phenylhydrazine and the mild oxidation (treatment and results mentioned above), the compound could be
(A) 2-butene.
(B) acetone.
(C) 2-butanone.
(D) butane.
(E) 2-butanol.

Strong acids such as HCl are considered to be completely ionized unless they are at very high concentrations.

40. A 1×10^{-4} *M* solution of HCl in water will have a pH of
(A) 11.
(B) 7.
(C) 9.
(D) 4.
(E) less than 3.

41. A 1:10,000 dilution of the above solution with water will have a pH of
(A) greater than 8.5.
(B) 8.
(C) 7.
(D) 6.
(E) less than 5.6.

42. A mixture of 10 ml of 1×10^{-4} *M* HCl with 90 ml of the diluted solution of the previous question will have a pH of

(A) 0.4.
(B) 3.1.
(C) 4.
(D) 5.
(E) greater than 6.2.

The diagram illustrates a typical single neuron; the basic unit of the nervous system. Neurons connect with each other and in that manner an impulse is conducted and transmitted throughout the body. Two types of cell processes are indicated.

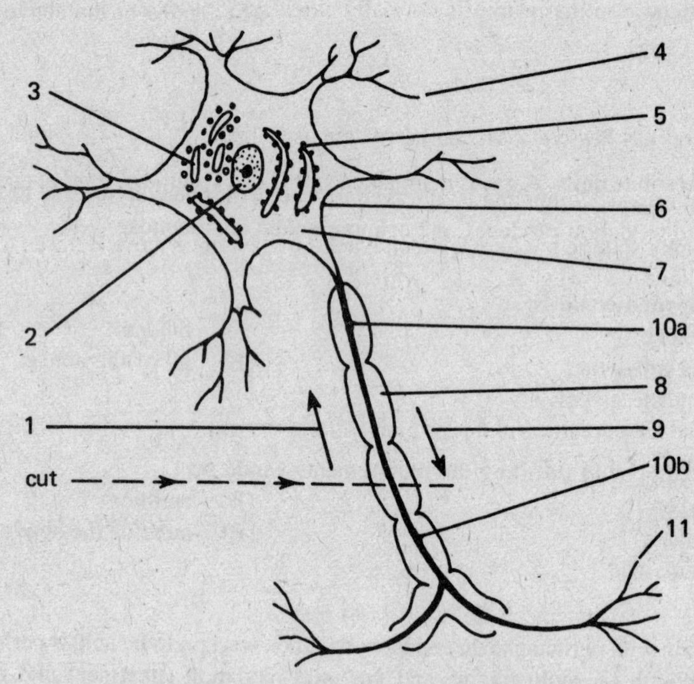

43. An impulse on the skin will be picked up by

(A) 4.
(B) 6.
(C) 7.
(D) 10.
(E) 11.

44. The genetic material of the cell is located in

(A) 2.
(B) 3.
(C) 5.
(D) 7.
(E) 9.

45. Protein synthesis is carried out under the direction of

(A) 3 in 5.
(B) 2 in 3.
(C) 2 in 5.
(D) 2 in 7.
(E) 5 in 2.

A person has been in an accident and the physician is conducting a neurological examination. Sensation is lost over several fingers and the examiner fears that a nerve has been cut. Note the cut indication on the diagram.

46. Which process would completely degenerate?
(A) 4
(B) 8
(C) 10a
(D) 10b
(E) 11

47. Retrograde degeneration would be visible in
(A) 2.
(B) 3.
(C) 6.
(D) 10b.
(E) 11.

48. The impulse in the neuron is normally conducted in which direction?
(A) 9
(B) 1

The general gas law equation can be written as follows: $\frac{PV}{T} = \frac{P_0V_0}{T_0}$ with the temperature and pressure in absolute units. A gas is maintained at 0°C in a volume of 5 m³ at atmospheric pressure.

49. If the atmospheric pressure is maintained, but the temperature is raised to 20°C, what will be its volume?
(A) 2.50 m^3
(B) 3.75 m^3
(C) 4.65 m^3
(D) 5.36 m^3
(E) 6.65 m^3

50. At what temperature will this original volume of gas occupy 2.5 m^3 at 4 atmospheres absolute pressure?
(A) 273°K
(B) 373°K
(C) 456°K
(D) 546°K
(E) 679°K

51. Which of the statements below is (are) true?
(A) $\frac{P}{P_0} = \frac{T}{T_0}$
(B) $\frac{V}{V_0} = \frac{T}{T_0}$
(C) $PV = P_0V_0$
(D) $\frac{PV}{T} = \frac{P_0V_0}{T_0}$
(E) all of the above

On the Celsius scale (°C) the freezing point of water is 0° and the boiling point is 100°. On the Fahrenheit scale (°F) they are respectively 32° and 212°. The absolute Kelvin scale lists as absolute zero a temperature of −273°, and therefore the Kelvin and Celsius scales differ only in the choice of point zero. Kelvin temperature is, therefore, 273 plus the Celsius temperature. For calculations the following formula may be utilized:

$$\text{Celsius equals } \frac{5}{9} \times (\text{Fahrenheit} - 32)$$

52. 104°F is _______________ degrees on the Kelvin scale.
(A) 40
(B) 377
(C) 169
(D) 113
(E) 313

53. 45°C will equal ____________ degrees F.
(A) 145
(B) 318
(C) 313
(D) 113
(E) 90

54. The normal body temperature for human beings on the Celsius scale is
(A) 98.6°
(B) 40°
(C) 30°
(D) 37°
(E) 32°

A newly synthesized, weakly ionized acid is being studied. It is found to have an ionization constant of 1×10^{-7}.

55. A 0.1 *N* solution of the acid will have a pH of
(A) 4.
(B) 5.5.
(C) 6.1.
(D) 6.9.
(E) none of the above.

56. A tenfold dilution of the above solution with water will have a pH between
(A) 3.5 and 4.5.
(B) 4.6 and 5.5.
(C) 5.6 and 6.7.
(D) 6.75 and 7.1.
(E) none of the above.

57. Assuming the acid is highly soluble in water, prediction of pH at very high concentrations might be in error because of
(A) higher temperatures in the solution.
(B) errors in that area of logarithm tables.
(C) decreased ionization at higher concentrations.
(D) all of the above.
(E) none of the above.

Compound *V* is known to contain only carbon, hydrogen, and oxygen. Elemental analysis reveals 40.0% carbon and 6.67% hydrogen.

58. The empirical formula of compound *V* is
(A) CH_2O.
(B) CH_3O.
(C) CH_4O.
(D) none of the above.
(E) not possible to determine with the data given.

59. If the molecular weight of the compound is twice the molecular weight of the empirical formula, then the molecular formula is
(A) $C_2H_4O_2$.
(B) $C_2H_6O_2$.
(C) $C_2H_8O_2$.
(D) none of the above.
(E) not possible to determine with the information from this question and the previous one.

60. With the information from the two previous questions, compound V could be
(A) methanol.
(B) methyl ether.
(C) formaldehyde.
(D) glucose.
(E) none of the above.

For the base pyridinium hydroxide the K_b is 1×10^{-9}

$$\text{PyrOH} \rightleftharpoons \text{Pyr}^+ + \text{OH}^-$$

$$K_b = \frac{[\text{Pyr}^+][\text{OH}^-]}{[\text{Pry OH}]}$$

61. The pH of a 0.1 M solution of PyrOH would be
(A) 4.
(B) 5.
(C) 6.
(D) 7.5.
(E) greater than 8.5.

62. A hundredfold dilution with water would produce a solution with a pH
(A) greater than 10.
(B) between 8.5 and 9.5.
(C) between 7.5 and 8.5.
(D) between 6.5 and 7.5.
(E) less than 6.3.

63. The terms pH and pOH are always related in the following manner:
(A) pH/pOH = 1.
(B) pH/pOH = k.
(C) pH + pOH = 100.
(D) pH + 1/pOH = 14.
(E) none of the above.

Using the illustration below when both surfaces 1 and 2 are exposed to the atmosphere, P_1 and P_2 are gauge pressure, and h_1 and h_2 are heights. The Bernoulli equation for this situation is

$$h_1 + \frac{P_1}{W} + \frac{V_1^2}{2a} = h_2 + \frac{P_2}{W} + \frac{V_2^2}{2a}$$

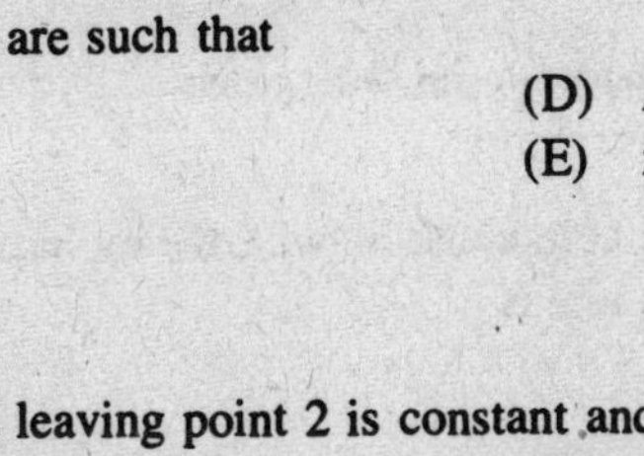

64. The values of P_1 and P_2 are such that
(A) $P_1 = P_2 = 0$.
(B) $P_1 > P_2$.
(C) $P_2 < P_1$.
(D) $P_1/P_2 = 0$.
(E) $P_2/P_1 = 0$.

65. The velocity of the fluid leaving point 2 is constant and can be expressed as
(A) $V_2 = [(h_1 - h_2)(2a)]^{1/2}$
(B) $V_2 = (P_1/P_2)ah$.
(C) $V_2 = (P_1/P_2)V_1$.
(D) $V_2 = V_1$.
(E) none of the above.

66. If an identical outlet were placed at exactly the same point on the left side of the container, the velocity would be
(A) computable.
(B) zero.
(C) ½ V_2.
(D) 2 V_2.
(E) none of the above.

STOP. If you finish before the time limit is up, go over your work for this section. DO NOT look at any other sections of the model examination. When your time limit is up, go on to the next section.

SKILLS ANALYSIS: READING

85 MINUTES
68 QUESTIONS

The following questions are to be answered based on your careful reading of selections from scientific writings.

DIRECTIONS: Read each passage carefully, then answer the questions following it. Consider only the material within the passage in answering the questions. Eliminate those choices that you think to be incorrect and mark the letter of your choice on the answer sheet.

The origin of the ovarian follicle has long been a subject of confusion. It is generally recognized that germ cells arise extragonadally during fetal development and migrate to the prospective gonadal region. There is still confusion, however, concerning the manner by which these germ cells enter the gonad and become enveloped by the follicular epithelium.

In their study of ovarian development in mice, Doctors Odor and Blandau suggested that stromal cells within the ovary surround the germ cells which have migrated into this region. The stromal cells thus become the follicular epithelium. Observations of previous investigators, however, suggest that the situation in the primate may be different. Witschi in 1948 described the migration of germ cells in humans. He stated that these cells were present in the endoderm (the epithelium of the presumptive gut), the mesothelium (an epithelium lining the body cavity) adjacent to the gut, and the mesenchymal tissue (which lies between these two epithelia). According to Dr. Witschi, the cells within the endoderm leave this epithelium and migrate through the mesenchymal tissue to the presumptive gonadal region which is a thickening of the mesenchyme of the body wall covered by a continuation of the same mesothelium found in proximity to the gut. In another investigation, Dr. Gillman described the presence of cords of cells within the fetal ovary. These cords were continuous with the mesothelium of the ovary. Initially these cords were devoid of germ cells; however, in the later stage of development the germ cells which had been seen in the stroma were incorporated into the cords. These cords subsequently split up into follicles. More recently, Dr. Merchant has reexamined ovarian development in the rat. By injecting a mitotic poison into a pregnant female at the time of germ cell migration, he has produced offspring which are lacking germ cells. In these animals follicles are absent but epithelial cell cords which are continuous with the ovarian mesothelium are present. Other investigators have also noted the presence of cords in the ovaries of normal laboratory animals.

Studies of human ovaries during the early stages of development are difficult because of technical as well as legal and medical problems. Nevertheless, observations by this investigator of ovaries from human and monkey fetuses after germ cell migration, confirm Gillman's observation that germ cells are present in the epithelial cords and that from these cords follicles are produced. However, this investigator is not in agreement with the proposed method by which the germ cells become incorporated into the cords. We have observed germ cells in the ovarian mesothelium which is in continuity with the epithelial cords. At the points of continuity, dividing cells within the mesothelium are oriented so that their mitotic spindles are perpendicular to the plane of the mesothelium. One daughter cell from such a division would be retained in the mesothelium, while the other would become part of the underlying cord. These observations suggest that the germ cell-containing cords arise from inward growth of a germ cell containing mesothelium. An extension of this conclusion would be that it is the germ cells which are found in the mesothelium in the region of the gut rather than those in the gut itself which are the cells that populate the gonad; and that this region of the mesothelium because of differential growth is, at a later time, positioned over the stroma of the presumptive gonad where the inward growth takes place.

The following statements are related to the passage above. Based on the information given, select:

(A) if the statement is *supported by* the information in the passage.
(B) if the statement is *contradicted by* the information in the passage.
(C) if the statement is *neither supported nor contradicted by* information in the passage.

1. The manner by which the germ cells are enveloped by follicle cells is generally agreed on.
2. Germ cells arise within the ovary by differentiation of ovarian stromal cells.
3. In primates follicles arise by splitting off of ovarian cords.
4. Ovarian cords grow from the ovarian mesothelium.
5. Germ cells are moved by ciliary action.
6. The author believes that germ cells move independently of surrounding cells.
7. Due to less rigid abortion laws, studies on humans will increase and allow for the solution of the problem.

Does the order of a child's birth in a family have a bearing on his or her personality and on the type of adult he or she will grow up to be, or is the entire theory of ordinal position simply a bag of tricks that makes for interesting cocktail party conversation but little else?

While it has been the highlight of numerous debates and most certainly the subject of various studies, ordinal position remains a little-understood personality variable.

Consider the oldest child in a family of three children. Parents often claim that their first-born has a solid head on his or her shoulders, behaves in a mature manner, and is capable of getting along with adults. This important family member often exhibits a quiet front, yet is able to take the lead, care for his or her siblings and act like a miniature adult. Parents view the first-born as an intelligent individual who will grow up to be a pillar of the community.

What on earth happened to the second-born (again in a family of three children) to make him or her so different from the eldest? This child is much more lively, less willing to take orders, does not show the same interest in adults, and often has difficulty communicating with them. He or she may even become a "problem" child in school. Teachers have been heard to complain that "B— is not in the least like A— was. . . ." Could it be that the second-born is striking out in an attempt to find his or her own place? The problems of the second child in a family seem to intensify even more when the "baby" comes along and moves him or her into the "middle-child" position. Now he or she has to contend not only with a successful older brother or sister, but also with the youngest who seems to be the favorite. The youngest, on the other hand appears not to feel the need to measure up to anyone and goes along his or her own way to develop into an often exuberant, well-rounded individual. Because he or she is the baby, the mother doesn't expect this third sibling to function like a miniature adult, and she considers "cute" a great number of the actions that were viewed as unsatisfactory in the case of the other children.

Surely the questions related to ordinal position will provide research material for years to come. The problem is much like that of the chicken and the egg in that it is difficult to tell whether the numerical place a child occupies in a family *or* the attitudes which parents have developed in connection to child-rearing through years of trial and error, have the greatest effect on his or her personality.

The following statements are related to the information presented above. Based on the information given, select:

(A) if the statement is *supported by* the information in the passage.
(B) if the statement is *contradicted by* the information in the passage.
(C) if the statement is *neither supported nor contradicted by* information in the passage.

8. It is a proven fact that the first-born always grows up to be a responsible citizen.
9. Ordinal position has been the topic of research for many years.
10. Parents often claim that first-born children behave in a more mature manner than later-born.
11. To date, ordinal position is a little-understood personality variable.
12. Second-born children who later move into the "middle-child" position achieve on a higher plane in school than do second-born who remain in the same position.
13. Comparison to older siblings, by teachers and other adults is the best method for stimulating the middle child to work harder.

14. By the time the third child comes along, mothers no longer seem to put the same emphasis on certain aspects of behavior that they did when raising their first-born.

15. The best place to discuss ordinal position is at a cocktail party, because it is such an interesting topic of conversation.

16. The youngest child is most adversely affected by his or her family position because he or she has more than one sibling to live up to.

17. The "baby" of the family is often a child with an outgoing personality.

Two systems modulate, integrate, and control the activities of the body; they are the nervous and endocrine systems. The response in nervous control is rapid while control via the endocrine system is fairly slow and longer lasting. The endocrine glands are ductless glands and secrete their products called hormones into the capillaries (bloodstream). Hormones are substances that are secreted into the bloodstream and travel to their target organs to elicit their effects. The product of the target organ may also feed back upon the organ that stimulated its activity and production; and manipulate in this respect its cycle of function. It may shut off the supply of stimulating hormone; this activity is called a negative feedback. The controlling mechanism can be though of as a neuro-endocrine-somatic tissue relationship, or the brain affecting the pituitary gland, which in turn affects the target organs, which then elicit their effect upon the body tissues and cells. Hormones cannot be classified into one chemical class; they are, however, all organic substances and may be proteins, peptides, amino acids (or amino acid derivatives), and steroids, or prostaglandins (derivatives of essential fatty acids). Generally the glands which produce protein hormones embryologically originate from the alimentary tract; they are the anterior pituitary, thyroid, parathyroids, and pancreas. Glands which produce steroid products are derived from the celomic mesothelium and are the testes, ovaries, and adrenal cortex. Glands whose products are small molécular weight amines arise from cells of nervous tissue derivation and are the neurohypophysis and the adrenal medulla.

The following statements are related to the information presented above. Based on the information given, select:

(A) if the statement is *supported by* the information in the passage.
(B) if the statement is *contradicted by* the information in the passage.
(C) if the statement is *neither supported nor contradicted by* information in the passage.

18. Nervous impulses are conducted quickly and produce long-acting effects.

19. The endocrine system achieves its functions via the bloodstream.

20. Releasing factors produced by the hypothalamus affect the pituitary gland.

21. Hormones are similar in nature.

22. The pancreas produces hormones that are proteins.

23. Steroids are produced by the reproductive organs.

24. The cells of the adrenal medulla may be thought of as postganglionic sympathetic cells.

Contraction in a skeletal muscle is triggered by the generation of an action protential in the muscle membrane. Each motor neuron upon entering a skeletal muscle loses its myelin sheath and divides into branches with each branch innervating a single muscle fiber, forming a neuromuscular junction. Each fiber normally has one neuromuscular junction which is located near the center of the fiber. A motor unit consists of a single motor neuron and all the muscle fibers innervated by it. The motor end plate is the specialized part of the muscle fiber's membrane lying under the nerve.

The impulse arriving at the end of the motor neuron causes liberation of acetylcholine from vesicles in the nerve terminal. The acetylcholine acts at specific sites normally found only on the motor end plate section of the fiber membrane and increases the permeability of the motor end plate. The resulting $Na+$ influx produces a depolarizing potential called the end plate potential. This in turn depolarizes adjacent areas of the fiber membrane, triggering an action potential which is propagated in both directions from the central neuromuscular junction toward the fiber ends. Normally the magnitude of the endplate potential is sufficient to discharge the muscle membrane, so that each impulse in the nerve ending produces a response in the muscle. The acetylcholine is rapidly destroyed by the enzyme acetylcholinesterase which is found in high concentrations at the neuromuscular junction.

The following statements are related to the information presented. Based on the information given, select:

(A) if the statement is *supported by* in the passage.
(B) if the statement is *contradicted by* the information in the passage.
(C) if the statement is *neither supported nor contradicted by* information in the passage.

25. The contraction of skeletal muscle is quicker and of shorter duration than the activation of smooth muscle.

26. Acetylcholinesterase is released at the motor end plate.

27. Motor neurons are myelinated.

28. Acetylcholine is produced by muscle.

29. While there is a sodium ion influx, potassium ions leave the cell.

30. Sodium ion influx plays a role in the conduction of a nerve impulse.

31. Magnitude of the end plate potential is of critical importance.

Primogeniture was the custom of allowing the oldest member of a family, in most situations this meant the oldest male member, to inherit all lands and possessions of his parents, to the exclusion of his siblings.

The ordinal position of being the first-born male therefore carried much power, as the first-born was considered to be intelligent, level-headed, and capable of taking over as family protector and landlord once the father died. Theoretically the oldest would be unselfish and see to the care of the younger family members, but in actuality this was often not the case.

The custom of primogeniture was particularly popular during the federal period and was practiced in many countries of Europe, especially in France and England where, for example, a fief descended intact to the oldest son. One European country where this custom was not in force during the Middle Ages was Germany.

Outlawed in the United States and no longer the mode of inheritance in Europe for today's population as a whole, primogeniture was in evidence as late as the 1920s and can still be seen in degree with some of Europe's royal families.

The following statements are related to the information presented above. Based on the information given, select:

(A) if the statement is *supported by* the information in the passage.
(B) if the statement is *contradicted by* the information in the passage.
(C) if the statement is *neither supported nor contradicted by* information in the passage.

32. Countries in Europe that have royal families still practice the custom of primogeniture

33. Ordinal position was of utmost importance in medieval Europe

34. In Germany during the federal period the oldest son could be certain of inheriting his father's fief intact.

35. In the United States each sibling recieves the same amount of inheritance.

36. Modern society often calls upon the first-born male to be the executor of his parents' will.

37. The first-born male was thought to be the most intelligent level-headed sibling and therefore considered the proper landlord of his parents' holdings.

38. Under the primogeniture custom, younger brothers and sisters were granted their fair share.

39. France and England were two of the countries where primogeniture was practiced during the federal period.

40. Today the royal family of England carries on this custom.

41. The oldest child—whether male or female—*always* inherited everything.

A term that has been very much in vogue over the past five years or so is that of behavior modification or the changing of a subject's behavior from an unacceptable to an acceptable pattern.

While it may be argued that behavior is continually being altered and modified, the term as used here refers to a very structured approach by which the undesirable behavior is identified and specific monitored steps are undertaken to modify and move it into the path of becoming acceptable. A token system is included so that progress in the correct direction can be rewarded immediately.

This type of management system has been widely used by educators, especially at the elementary level, so that when children come home on any given afternoon with scores of M&M's in their pockets, mothers realize that teachers are busily modifying some aspect of behavior and that the candy is the reward system. Education does not, however, have a monopoly on behavior modification techniques. They have proven to be successful in certain scientific areas as well as many other fields.

Consider the person who has a weight problem yet claims to consume very little at meal time. Often this frustrated soul will eat next to nothing morning, noon, and evening, thus convinced that he or she is starving, but will forget to account for the 20 sidetrips to the refrigerator.

Such a person would be wise to use behavior modification techniques. Two charts are called for in this case. The first to cover every waking hour for one week with a check to indicate the times when something was eaten. The second could be identical except that the subject would now make a conscious effort to reduce the checks and give a token each time this happens. Thus, for instance, for each check missing a dime could be thrown in a kitty and saved for a nonfood splurge later on. Hopefully the subject would eventually alter his or her previous habit without the need for charting.

The following statements are related to the information presented above. Based on the information given, select:

(A) if the statement is *supported by* the information in the passage.
(B) if the statement is *contradicted by* the information in the passage.
(C) if the statement is *neither supported nor contradicted by* information in the passage.

42. The only way behavior can be altered is through use of a token system.

43. Doctors should suggest behavior modification to their overweight patients.

44. One area where this technique is used frequently is in elementary education.

45. Overweight people often eat too many carbohydrates and too little proteins.

46. Behavior modification can be classified as a type of management system.

47. In order to be successful, a person using behavior modification must first identify the undesirable behavior and then plan specific structured steps to change it.

48. Problem identification is an important facet of the behavior modification process.

49. Just because they are in vogue does not mean that behavior modification techniques are reliable.

50. Charting a specific behavior is often one way of pinpointing the undesirable action.

51. Once the problem has been spotted behavior modification will always eliminate it.

The major structural and functional cellular unit of nervous tissue is the neuron. The neuronal cell body or soma, like all cells, contains a distinct nucleus and nucleolus and a cytoplasm rich in organelles.

Prominent among these organelles are mitochondria, the Golgi apparatus, and profiles of rough-surfaced endoplasmic reticulum. Extending from the neuronal cell bodies are numerous appendages which are characterized as either axons or dendrites. The dendrites are generally multiple in number and from their primary shafts secondary, tertiary, and higher order branches arise.

Frequently, extending from the dendritic surfaces are numerous spines or gemmules which are reminiscent of thorns extending along the branches of a rose bush. The dendrites and their associated spines provide a greatly increased neuronal surface area which ultimately allows for increased interaction with other neuronal elements. Unlike their dendritic counterparts, the axons are usually singular and generally are quite long and thin. Many axons are encompassed by a lipoprotein sheath known as myelin and this myelin sheath displays periodic discontinuities referred to as the Nodes of Ranvier. At terminal points these axons transmit impulses to the dendrites of other neurons and such sites of contacts between individual neurons are called synapses. In the human nervous system there are approximately 8 billion neurons, all of which display great variability in both size and form. Also, in addition to these 8 billion neurons, there exist 80 billion supportive elements known as glial cells. In view of both the number and complexity of the neurons and their supportive elements, it is readily apparent as to why our present understanding of nervous tissue interaction and function is quite limited.

The following statements are related to the passage. Based on the information given, select:
(A) if the statement is *supported by* the information in the passage.
(B) if the statement is *contradicted by* information in the passage.
(C) if the statement is *neither supported nor contradicted by* information in the passage.

52. Axons and dendrites are appendages of neuronal cell bodies and as such are structurally and functionally the same.

53. It is apparent from the passage that dendrites greatly increase the neuronal surface area.

54. It can be deduced from this article that the neurons and glial cells are structurally and functionally comparable.

55. The site of functional contact between two individual neurons constitutes a synapse.

56. It is clear from the preceding passage that the precise nature of nervous tissue interaction has been completely elucidated.

Local anesthetics are frequently used and because of this widespread clinical use, knowledge concerning the effects of these drugs at the cellular level is desirable. Most local anesthetics produce a cytotoxic effect; tissues that are affected usually degenerate, and the fragments are phagocytised. This process is followed by a phase of regeneration. There is evidence that the severity of the effect—recognized by the size of the lesion produced—varied with the potency of the anesthetic, the concentration of the anesthetic, the route of administration, and the sequence of injections. The significance of potency—that is, the variability of effect produced by different local anesthetics at the same concentration—was clearly demonstrated when tetracaine produced more severe lesions than lidocaine which in turn produced more severe lesions than procaine. The severity of the lesion increased as the concentration increased. Differences in route of injection were apparent as more severe lesions were produced following intramuscular injection of the anesthetic when compared with subcutaneous injection. Muscle degeneration and subsequent regeneration is found irrespective of the sequence of injection (as for example, one large dose or two smaller doses). No muscular damage has been found following an injection when the same volume of physiologic saline, instead of the anesthetic, is administered. Limited information is available concerning the effect of local anesthetics on enzyme activity in the highly ordered metabolic machinery of the cell.

The following statements are related to the passage above. Based on the information given, select:
(A) if the statement is *supported by* the information in the passage.
(B) if the statement is *contradicted by* the information in the passage.
(C) if the statement is *neither supported nor contradicted by* information in the passage.

57. All local anesthetics are alike.

58. Local anesthetics are used more often by dentists than physicians.

59. Potency and concentration may be considered one and the same.

60. Severity of lesion and concentration show a direct relationship.

61. Physiologic saline can be substituted for an anesthetic.

62. General anesthesia does not result in any damage.

63. Tissues are sensitive to local anesthetics.

The blood vessels of the mammalian brain normally provide a barrier that blocks the passage of certain molecules which readily permeate other body tissues. This unique property of the brain vasculature is referred to as the blood-brain barrier and in normal functional states this property prevents the entrance of numerous intravascular probes such as horseradish peroxidase into the substance of the brain. However, in experimental studies of brain dysfunction, such as seen in mechanical brain injury, a disruption of the blood-brain barrier occurs, and experimental probes such as horseradish peroxidase now enter the brain's substance. The mechanism of this blood-brain barrier dysfunction in brain injury is poorly understood. Some contend that the mechanical stress of the injury physically disrupts the vessels and allows for peroxidase leakage through defects in the vascular walls. However, others argue that brain injury activates cellular mechanisms which allow the blood vessels to rapidly uptake substances such as horseradish peroxidase and then to both deposit them within and ultimately flood the substance of the brain tissue.

To date few substantive experimental data have been advanced to support any of the above-stated theories of blood-brain barrier dysfunction in instances of mechanical brain injury. However, research continues, for medical scientists realize that any rational therapeutic treatment of brain-injured patients, is totally dependent upon the elucidation of those mechanisms involved in blood-brain barrier dysfunction.

The following statements are related to the passage. Based on the information given, select:

(A) if the statement is *supported by* the information in the passage.

(B) if the statement is *contradicted by* the information in the passage.

(C) if the statement is *neither supported nor contradicted by* information in the passage.

64. The blood-brain barrier is a structural rather than a physiological barrier.

65. The mechanisms responsible for blood-brain barrier dysfunction in brain injury have been identified and it is apparent that blood-brain barrier dysfunction is related to vasogenic shock.

66. This passage implies that the appropriate therapeutic management of the head-injured patient awaits the elucidation of the those mechanisms responsible for blood-brain barrier dysfunction in brain trauma.

67. The blood vessels of the human brain normally provide a barrier which blocks the passage of certain substances which readily permeate the body tissues.

68. Mechanical brain injury may physically disrupt the integrity of the brain's vasculature.

> STOP. If you finish before the time limit is up, go over your work for this section. DO NOT look at any other sections of the model examination. When your time limit is up, go on to the next section.

SKILLS ANALYSIS: QUANTITATIVE

85 MINUTES
68 QUESTIONS

The following questions are to be answered based on your knowledge of basic mathematical principles and relationships.

DIRECTIONS: Read each passage carefully, study each table or chart, then answer the questions following it. Consider only the material presented in answering the questions. Eliminate those choices that you think to be incorrect and mark the letter of your choice on the answer sheet.

Diet	Losing Weight	Mortality
Balanced Diet	4%	2%
Diet A	90%	74%
Diet A + Vitamin C	84%	72%
Diet A + Vitamin B	4%	2%
Diet A + Vitamin A	88%	76%

Groups of 50 mice were fed the diets listed in the table, and the percentage losing more than 10% of their initial body weight and the percentage mortality after 30 days were recorded.

1. The study was designed to determine
(A) what vitamins are missing from a balanced diet.
(B) what vitamins aid in losing weight.
(C) what vitamins were missing from diet A.
(D) what mice need that humans do not.

2. The best conclusion to be drawn from this study is that
(A) diet A is a good reducing diet.
(B) diet A lacks B vitamins.
(C) vitamin C is not necessary for life.
(D) vitamin A is necessary for life.

3. The difference between percentage losing weight and percentage mortality within each group is best explained by
(A) individual variation among mice within each group.
(B) variations in importance of the different vitamins.
(C) the fact that the effectiveness of vitamins is reduced by purification and later addition to food.
(D) the fact that some mice were overweight and therefore were not resistant.

The epiphyseal cartilage plate is very sensitive to somatotrophin (growth hormone) and, therefore, can be used as an assay for this compound. Species variations exist and other hormones such as estrogen, thyroxine, and several antibiotics also have an effect upon cartilage growth. The assay must be carried out on hypophysectomized animals.

The following experiments were conducted as can be seen from the table:

Test Groups	No. of Animals	Cartilage Growth in μ: 1 Injection Daily	Cartilage Growth in μ: 2 Injections/Day (½ amount each time)
Control (normal) (saline)	20 (10/injecting group)	100	100
Hypophysectomized (saline)	20	60	60
Hypox + 100 mg STH	20	150	160
Hypox + 300 mg STH	20	180	195
Stressed normal animals (saline)	20	175	190
Hypox & stressed (saline)	20	50	50
Stressed normal + 100 mg STH	20	200	210
Hypox, stressed + 100 mg STH	20	110	120

4. The reason the assay must be carried out on hypophysectomized rats is
   (A) just to add another sophisticated method to the experiment.
   (B) because the pituitary produces its own growth hormone and it might interfere with the assay.
   (C) to study the pituitary composition of growth hormone.
   (D) to obtain the animals' own growth hormone.

5. These experiments show
   (A) the route of administration was critical.
   (B) the route of administration made no difference.
   (C) the route should be adjusted from procedure to procedure.
   (D) none of the above.

6. Twice daily administration proved to be
   (A) less effective in eliciting a response.
   (B) more effective in eliciting a response.
   (C) of no great consequence in the experiment.
   (D) none of the above.

7. Stressed animals
   (A) do not need growth hormone.
   (B) produce substances that act like growth hormone.
   (C) produce growth hormone that has an additive affect upon stress factors.
   (D) both B and C.

The following experimental protocol was carried out. Bean seeds were picked for their uniformity and 20 were planted/pot. One hundred percent germination was observed; and when the seedlings were 9 days old, the seedlings of uniform growth were selected for treatment with X-rays. Four hundred r units/minute were applied at a distance of 30 cm from the object. Seedlings were exposed up to 60 minutes with up to 24,000 r. After exposure, seedlings were placed in a greenhouse and kept at uniform light, temperature, and moisture conditions. Seedlings were measured as indicated in the table.

CODE

	I		II
1	From ground to cotyledon (a mark was made on the seedling near the ground with india ink)	A	0 minutes — control
		B	7.5 minutes — 3,000 r
2	Cotyledon to 1st node	C	15 minutes — 6,000 r
3	Petiole length of 1st leaf	D	30 minutes — 12,000 r
4	Midrib of 1st leaf	E	60 minutes — 24,000 r
5	From 1st node to tip of the plant (when included).		

EXPERIMENTAL RESULTS

	10 Days					17 Days					33 Days				
	A	B	C	D	E	A	B	C	D	E	A	B	C	D	E
1	6.20	6.58	7.30	5.45	4.43	7.08	6.73	8.00	6.99	5.82	7.21	6.73	8.00	7.00	6.05
2	2.17	2.16	2.30	1.15	.76	8.06	7.11	5.36	2.50	1.63	8.07	7.11	5.48	2.65	1.65
3	.87	1.11	1.10	0.65	.53	4.12	4.50	4.15	2.13	1.70	4.33	4.61	4.86	2.30	1.90
4	3.00	3.23	3.02	2.03	1.86	5.44	5.27	5.68	5.33	4.97	5.50	5.50	6.13	5.91	5.25
5											12.56	11.38	5.27		

8. The purpose of this experiment was
(A) to observe the germination rate.
(B) to check for uniform growth rate.
(C) test output and scatter of the X-ray machine.
(D) observe X-ray effect on growth.

9. The control plants reached a height at the termination of the experiment of ________ cm and little stunting could be observed in the plants that received 3000 r units. They were only 2.66 cm shorter than the controls.
(A) 25.11
(B) 27.84
(C) 37.67
(D) 18.06

10. When 12,000 r units were employed, plant growth did not go beyond the first node and these plants were 18.19 cm shorter than the controls. Growth from the mark on the stem to the cotyledon is comparable to control plants but growth beyond the cotyledon is greatly diminished.
(A) This cannot be determined from the data given.
(B) These statements are absolutely correct.
(C) Too many assumptions are made.
(D) All of the above are confusing statements.

11. As seen from the table, the plants exposed to 24,000 r units show a marked effect. Growth from the cotyledon to the first node is greatly decreased. This was the part most affected; the midrib lengths were not affected.
(A) The statements are unfounded.
(B) The statements are partly true.
(C) The statements are correct.
(D) Too many assumptions are made.

Both sexes carry a complete complement of sex-linked genes. A female, however, with the XX arrangement will only exhibit a recessive gene if she has received it from both parents (a rare event if we are dealing with an uncommon gene of the population); while in the male with the XY arrangement the recessive gene cannot be masked since there is no partner X chromosome and, therefore, a larger number of recessive genes are expressed (examples are hemophilia and color blindness). A man receives his X chromosome from his mother and passes it on to his daughters not his sons. His daughters in this respect are the carriers of his sex-linked traits and their sons will be the affected ones. Let us illustrate with an example. The normal czarinas of Russia produced sons suffering from hemophilia, a disease that is caused by a sex-linked recessive gene, h. The more dominant gene, H, produces normal blood clotting. Genotypically, these women must have carried Hh (X_H and X_h). A daughter, depending on the father (X_HY or X_hY), could have carried X_HX_h or X_HX_H while a son could have been born either with an X_HY or a X_hY (hemophilic) chromosomal complement.

The following statements are related to the information presented above. Based on the information given, select:
(A) if the statement is *supported by* the information given.
(B) if the statement is *contradicted by* the information given.
(C) if the statement is *neither supported nor contradicted by* information given.

12. A cattle breeder has in a herd a Y-linked trait. A male calf sired by a bull carrying this trait is born. The chances of the inheritance of the trait are 50%.
13. A female calf was born; the chances of exhibiting the trait are zero.
14. If the sex in the above cross is known, there is no doubt about whether a calf has the trait.
15. All males would exhibit the trait.
16. Females in this case would not be the carriers of this trait.

Melanoma tumors were implanted into three strains of mice. Experiments were then performed to determine the types and amounts of host serum antibodies produced against the lipid components of the virus contained in the melanoma cells. The results are summarized in the table below.

Host	Ag A Phenotype	Mg Equivalent Day 40 Post Implant	Antilipid Antibody Day 60 Post Implant
Strain 1	3/3	4.5 ± 0.3	6.3 ± 1.7
Strain 2	1/3	3.4 ± 0.4	5.5 ± 1.3
Strain 3	1/1	1.3 ± 0.1	1.3 ± 0.3

The following statements are related to the information presented above. Based on the information given, select:

(A) if the statement is *supported by* the information given.
(B) if the statement is *contradicted by* the information given.
(C) if the statement is *neither supported nor contradicted by* information given.

17. Strain 1 produced less antilipid antibody at both time periods measured than the other two hosts.
18. On the basis of this information, Strain 1 animals are less resistant to melanoma-type cancers than either Strain 2 or 3 animals.
19. All three hosts produced more antibody at 60 days than they did at 40 days.
20. An Ag A phenotype containing three seems to be related to higher antibody production.
21. If it has a 1/3 Ag A phenotype, a mouse resulting from a cross of Strain 2 with one of Strain 3 would probably be a better antibody producer than a sibling having a 1/1 Ag A phenotype.

During wound healing, proliferation of cells in epithelial tissues, connective tissues, and vascular tissues occurs in order to fill in and resurface the defect caused by necrotic (dead) tissue. In experimental studies of the cellular kinetics of wound healing, it is often necessary to assess the amount of proliferation in various cell populations. Because cells replicate DNA within 8 to 12 hours before dividing, determination of the frequency of DNA synthesis at a particular time among cells in a population is a good index of the rate of cell division. DNA synthesis can be determined by tagging replicating DNA with radioactive thymidine. By the procedure of autoradiography, the nuclei of cells which have incorporated radioactive thymidine can be identified on histological sections. The percentage of cells labeled with radioactive thymidine is called the labeling index.

The following table includes data on the labeling index of endothelial cells which form the lining of blood vessels.

^{3}H-THYMIDINE INDEX IN WOUND HEALING

Wound Age	Amount of Epidermal Resurfacing	Endothelial Labeling Index
1 day	0%	3.5%
2 days	0%	13.3%
3 days	0-5%	10.5%
6 days	60-70%	5.6%
10 days	90-100%	2.5%

The following statements are related to the information presented. Based on the information given, select:

(A) if the statement is *supported by* the information given.
(B) if the statement is *contradicted by* the information given.
(C) if the statement is *neither supported nor contradicted by* information given.

22. The ^{3}H-thymidine labeling index, and hence the amount of endothelial proliferation, increased before epidermal resurfacing had become evident.

23. The endothelial labeling index, after day two, decreased both with advancing wound age and with advancing surface coverage.

24. The increased endothelial proliferation at two and three days led to the formation of new blood vessels, which then induced epidermal resurfacing.

25. Endothelial proliferation ceases when the wounds are 90-100% resurfaced with epidermis.

26. Synthesis of DNA may not lead to cell division, but rather may lead to an increase in the ploidy of the cell.

Androgen compounds are responsible for maintaining the secondary sex organs and characteristics of organisms. An endocrinology class was divided into 4 groups to conduct a blind experiment and at the end was asked to compare results. Each group received a compound and injected a similar amount. The experimental protocol in male animals was: 1) Unoperated control animals; 2) Unoperated control animals receiving vehicle only; 3) Bilaterally castrated (testes) animals; and 4) Bilaterally castrated animals receiving unknown. The results were summarized in table form.

	Prostate Weight-mg Student Groups				Seminal Vesicle Weight-mg Student Groups			
Experimental Groups	**1**	**2**	**3**	**4**	**1**	**2**	**3**	**4**
Unoperated Control	33	31	29	34	68	65	63	67
Unoperated Control and Vehicle	31	32	30	31	69	70	65	64
Bilaterally Castrated	10	9	7	8	12	14	10	15
Bilaterally Castrated and Unknown	37	33	28	31	70	64	61	59

The following statements are related to the information presented above. Based on the information given, select:

(A) if the statement is *supported by* the information given.
(B) if the statement is *contradicted by* the information given.
(C) if the statement is *neither supported nor contradicted by* information given.

27. Different compounds were used by the different groups.

28. The compounds used were in the androgen group.

29. The parameters used were not the proper ones.

30. The prostate gland is most sensitive to a lack of androgens.

31. These experiments were not properly controlled.

32. The results obtained are probably not statistically significant.

33. When these data are plotted on graph paper, it is found that the percentage of increase in organ weight corresponds to a dose relationship.

34. Bilateral castration removes a major source of sex hormones.

35. In the absence of the testes, the hypophysis exhibits an increased production of gonad stimulating hormones.

36. The absence of androgens affects the behavior of the animal.

In the laboratory experiment, red blood cells were placed into 0.5M solutions and the appearance of the solutions was observed two hours later with the naked eye.

Solution	Cells
0.5M glucose	no change
0.5M sucrose	no change
0.5M urea	hemolysis of RBCs
0.5M glycerol	hemolysis of RBCs

37. The solutions of urea and glycerol are _____________ to the red blood cells.
(A) isotonic
(B) hypotonic
(C) hypertonic
(D) none of the above

38. The reason for these results is that:
1. the number of particles in the urea and glycerol solutions is greater than that in the glucose and sucrose solutions.
2. glucose and sucrose form coatings around the red blood cells which prevent their breaking.
3. glucose and sucrose enter the cells but are immediately metabolized, therefore water does not enter the cells.
4. urea and glycerol can enter the cell, water follows them into the cell because it is then in greater concentration outside.

(A) 1 and 2
(B) 1 and 3
(C) 3 and 4
(D) 4

39. The property of the cell membrane that allows for this phenomenon to be demonstrated is called
(A) diffusion.
(B) osmosis.
(C) impermeability.
(D) semipermeability.

A 75-kg person and a 1-kg steel ball fall simultaneously from an airplane 5000 feet above ground level. The following graph and table summarize the kinetic data for the first few seconds of the fall.

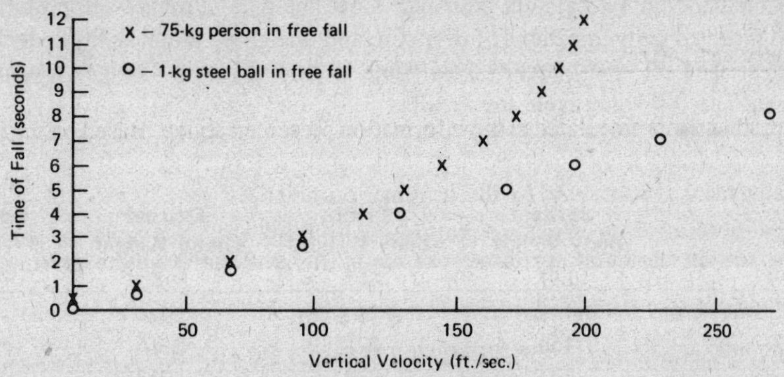

Time of Fall (sec.)	Vertical Velocity (ft./sec.) Person	Vertical Velocity (ft./sec.) Steel Ball	Distance of Fall (feet) Person	Distance of Fall (feet) Steel Ball
1	32	32	32	
2	64	64	96	
3	96	96	192	
4	115	128	307	
5	126	160	433	
6	141	192	574	
7	152	224	726	
8	159	256	895	
9	163		1058	
10	166		1224	
11	169		1393	
12	170		1563	

40. The greatest increase in downward velocity for the person occurs
(A) during the first 5 seconds of the fall.
(B) between 3 and 6 seconds of the fall.
(C) between 6 and 9 seconds of the fall.
(D) between 8 and 12 seconds of the fall.

41. Comparing the first 5 seconds with seconds 8-12 of the person's fall, the later velocity changes can be explained by
(A) the force of gravity being greater than atmospheric resistance.
(B) the force of gravity being less than atmospheric resistance.
(C) atmospheric resistance approaching the acceleratory force of gravity.
(D) none of the above.

42. After 7 seconds of the fall, how far is the steel ball from the person (vertical distance)?
(A) 96 feet
(B) 108 feet
(C) 144 feet
(D) 170 feet

43. Assuming the person's velocity does not change after 12 seconds (170 ft./sec.), the person will hit the ground
(A) 20 seconds after start of the fall.
(B) 24 seconds after start of the fall.
(C) 32 seconds after start of the fall.
(D) Cannot be calculated from data provided.

44. The person will hit the ground how many seconds after the steel ball? (Assume ball's velocity remains constant after 8 seconds of fall).
(A) 6 seconds
(B) 8 seconds
(C) 9 seconds
(D) 11 seconds

Gerbils were used for this experiment. One group served as a control; one group was thyroidectomized and maintained on 1% calcium gluconate since the parathyroids were probably removed also; one group received daily injections of thyroxin; and one group that was thyroidectomized and maintained as described above also received daily injections of thyroxin. Oxygen was measured in a standard manner. The following were the results.

Groups	Initial Body Weight gm	Final Body Weight gm	Thyroid Gland Weight mg	Liter of O_2 Consumed hour/ meter^2
Normal	143	150	5.0	1.54
Hypothyroid	160	174	0.0	0.16
Hyperthyroid	123	120	8.0	7.33
Hypothyroid + thyroxin	164	158	4.9	1.23

The following statements are stated on the information presented above. Based on the information given, select:
(A) if the statement is *supported by* the information given.
(B) if the statement is *contradicted by* the information given.
(C) if the statement is *neither supported nor contradicted by* information given.

45. The quantity of heat liberated by an organism as calculated on the basis of respiratory exchange is decreased by deficiencies and elevated by excesses of the active thyroid principle.

46. After total thyroidectomy the basal metabolic rate falls to 10% of its normal value.

47. Hypothyroid animals probably exhibited sluggishness.

48. Hypothyroidism is accompanied by a depression of the oxidative processes in the tissues and slight obesity probably due to the relatively slow burning of the consumed food.

49. Thyroxin probably is the active thyroid principle.

50. Animals can be made hyperthyroid if given thyroxin.

51. In thyroidectomized animals, glucose absorption is slower in the intestinal tract.

A manufacturer is testing a newly designed line of autoclaves that will be marketed. Calibration of timers and temperature controls are critical to insure destruction of bacteria.

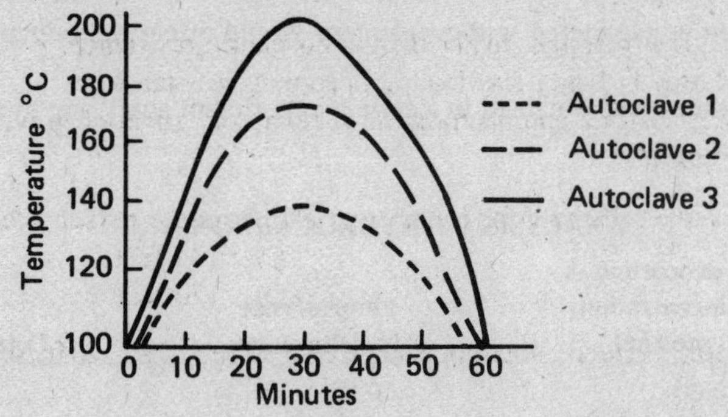

52. Bacteria X requires a minimum of 140°C for at least 20 minutes to be destroyed. Only ______________ could possible be used.
(A) autoclave 1
(B) autoclave 1 and 2
(C) autoclave 2 and 3
(D) autoclave 3

53. Virus Y requires 180°C or more. The technician would not place material in
(A) autoclave 1.
(B) autoclave 1 and 2.
(C) autoclave 2 and 3.
(D) autoclave 3.

54. Bacteria Z will only grow when the temperature is below 160°C. Therefore to be destroyed it can not be put into
(A) autoclave 1.
(B) autoclave 1 and 2.
(C) autoclave 2 and 3.
(D) autoclave 3.

The pineal complex is implicated in the modulation of reproductive functions of the golden hamster. Surgical removal of the eyes produced atrophy of the testes and seminal vesicles within four to six weeks, and simultaneous pinealectomy prevented the atrophy. In the following experiment the drug MTPH was injected subcutaneously daily for 30 days to learn if there was an enhancement of atrophy. The results are summarized below.

Treatment	Number of Hamsters Treated	Organ Weight (mg/100 g body weight) Testes	Seminal Vesicles
Untreated Control	6	2884	722
Blinding	6	1695[a]	396[a]
Pinealectomy	6	2600	544
Blinding, Pinealectomy	6	2580	577
MTPH, No Surgery	6	3069	699
MTPH, Blinding	6	1419[a]	398[a]
MTPH, Pinealectomy	6	2875	591
MTPH, Blinding, Pinealecomy	6	2635	577

[a]($P < 0.05$)

The following statements are related to the information presented above. Based on the information given, select:
(A) if the statement is *supported by* the information given.
(B) if the statement is *contradicted by* the information given.
(C) if the statement is *neither supported nor contradicted by* information given.

55. Drug MTPH increased the testicular atrophy in blinded hamsters when compared with blinded hamsters not receiving MTPH.

56. Drug MTPH increased the seminal vesicle atrophy in blinded hamsters when compared with blinded hamsters not receiving MTPH.

57. Drug MTPH had no effect on atrophy, either testicular or seminal vesicles.

58. Drug MTPH had no effect on the weights of testes or seminal vesicles.

59. Drug MTPH when administered without surgery would affect reproductive organ weight.

The table represents the results obtained in a certain experiment analyzing hydrocarbon A with a new fluorometric procedure.

ANALYSIS OF HYDROCARBON A

Sample	Hydrocarbon A Concentration, mole/ml	Fluorescence in delta units	Determinations
Blank	0.00	0.00	40
1	2.95×6^{-14}	1.26 ± 0.24	40
2	4.12×6^{-14}	2.21 ± 0.35	40
3	7.36×6^{-14}	3.48 ± 0.48	40
4	10.63×6^{-14}	4.84 ± 0.60	40
5	14.79×6^{-14}	6.67 ± 0.67	40
6	22.21×6^{-14}	10.14 ± 0.54	40
7	29.50×6^{-14}	13.42 ± 0.61	40

The following statements are related to the information presented above. Based on the information given, select:

(A) if the statement is *supported by* the information given.
(B) if the statement is *contradicted by* the information given.
(C) if the statement is *neither supported nor contradicted by* information given.

60. The table represents data for multiple analysis of hydrocarbon A exhibiting a range of 3×6^{-14} to 30×6^{-14} moles/ml.

61. Average deviations varied from 20% for the lowest concentration to 5% for the highest.

62. The variations in the blank obviously affected the reliability of the analysis more at the higher concentrations.

63. A fluorescence of 53.68 units corresponds to a hydrocarbon A concentration of 118 moles/ml.

Serum Vitamin K levels in the Tra-la bird of Upper Zulu were investigated. The following were the results.

SERUM VITAMIN K (μg/100 ml), PROTEIN (g/100 ml), AND BODY WEIGHT (g) FOR BIRDS

	Daytime		Nighttime		
Birds	Vitamin K	Protein	Vitamin K	Protein	Body Weight
Mature: Males	21.42	6.12	31.00	6.21	3370
Females	20.91	6.02	29.99	6.12	3200
Newborn: Males	14.97	5.71	17.79	5.69	1616
Females	14.19	5.49	17.46	5.71	1700

The following statements are related to the information presented above. Based on the information given, select:

(A) if the statement is *supported by* the information given.
(B) if the statement is *contradicted by* the information given.
(C) if the statement is *neither supported nor contradicted by* information given.

64. Mature males are about 5% heavier than females, while in the newborn the converse is true.

65. There is a definite correlation between body weight and the levels of Vitamin K and protein under investigation.

66. A diurnal rhythm is exhibited by Vitamin K levels.

67. Light influences protein synthesis.

68. After analysis of the table the reader comes to the conclusion that these experiments were well controlled.

STOP. If you finish before the time limit is up, go over your work for this section. DO NOT look at any other sections of the model examination. When your time limit is up, go on to the next section.

Model Test D Answers*

SCIENCE KNOWLEDGE

Biology

1. C	9. D	17. A	25. A	33. C
2. D	10. C	18. C	26. B	34. A
3. A	11. B	19. B	27. B	35. B
4. B	12. D	20. B	28. B	36. E
5. C	13. E	21. B	29. E	37. D
6. B	14. D	22. C	30. B	38. D
7. B	15. A	23. C	31. A	
8. E	16. C	24. A	32. B	

Chemistry

1. B	11. A	21. D	31. B	41. D
2. B	12. D	22. A	32. C	42. D
3. A	13. D	23. C	33. C	43. B
4. D	14. A	24. C	34. D	44. C
5. B	15. B	25. E	35. C	45. C
6. C	16. A	26. B	36. B	46. B
7. C	17. A	27. D	37. D	47. C
8. B	18. E	28. D	38. B	48. D
9. D	19. A	29. D	39. B	49. A
10. B	20. C	30. A	40. D	

Physics

1. A	9. A	17. B	25. D	33. E
2. B	10. C	18. E	26. A	34. A
3. C	11. E	19. E	27. C	35. B
4. A	12. D	20. B	28. D	36. D
5. D	13. D	21. B	29. D	37. D
6. D	14. C	22. E	30. C	38. A
7. C	15. A	23. A	31. D	
8. E	16. D	24. B	32. C	

*Explanations for science answers can be found on p. 316.

SCIENCE PROBLEMS

1. **B**	15. **D**	29. **E**	43. **A**	57. **C**
2. **B**	16. **E**	30. **D**	44. **A**	58. **A**
3. **B**	17. **D**	31. **D**	45. **C**	59. **A**
4. **E**	18. **A**	32. **C**	46. **D**	60. **E**
5. **E**	19. **E**	33. **A**	47. **A**	61. **E**
6. **A**	20. **D**	34. **E**	48. **A**	62. **D**
7. **C**	21. **E**	35. **A**	49. **D**	63. **E**
8. **B**	22. **D**	36. **A**	50. **D**	64. **A**
9. **D**	23. **D**	37. **D**	51. **E**	65. **A**
10. **B**	24. **D**	38. **E**	52. **E**	66. **A**
11. **A**	25. **A**	39. **A**	53. **D**	
12. **C**	26. **D**	40. **D**	54. **D**	
13. **B**	27. **B**	41. **C**	55. **A**	
14. **B**	28. **E**	42. **D**	56. **B**	

SKILLS ANALYSIS: READING

1. **B**	15. **C**	29. **C**	43. **C**	57. **B**
2. **B**	16. **B**	30. **A**	44. **A**	58. **C**
3. **A**	17. **A**	31. **B**	45. **C**	59. **B**
4. **A**	18. **B**	32. **B**	46. **A**	60. **A**
5. **C**	19. **A**	33. **A**	47. **A**	61. **C**
6. **B**	20. **A**	34. **B**	48. **A**	62. **C**
7. **C**	21. **B**	35. **C**	49. **C**	63. **A**
8. **B**	22. **A**	36. **C**	50. **A**	64. **C**
9. **A**	23. **A**	37. **A**	51. **B**	65. **B**
10. **A**	24. **C**	38. **B**	52. **B**	66. **A**
11. **A**	25. **C**	39. **A**	53. **A**	67. **A**
12. **C**	26. **A**	40. **C**	54. **C**	68. **A**
13. **B**	27. **A**	41. **B**	55. **A**	
14. **A**	28. **B**	42. **B**	56. **B**	

SKILLS ANALYSIS: QUANTITATIVE

1. **C**	15. **A**	29. **B**	43. **C**	57. **A**
2. **B**	16. **A**	30. **B**	44. **C**	58. **A**
3. **A**	17. **B**	31. **B**	45. **A**	59. **B**
4. **B**	18. **C**	32. **B**	46. **A**	60. **A**
5. **D**	19. **B**	33. **B**	47. **A**	61. **A**
6. **B**	20. **A**	34. **A**	48. **A**	62. **C**
7. **D**	21. **A**	35. **C**	49. **A**	63. **C**
8. **D**	22. **A**	36. **C**	50. **A**	64. **A**
9. **B**	23. **A**	37. **B**	51. **C**	65. **B**
10. **C**	24. **C**	38. **D**	52. **C**	66. **A**
11. **C**	25. **B**	39. **D**	53. **B**	67. **B**
12. **A**	26. **C**	40. **A**	54. **A**	68. **B**
13. **A**	27. **B**	41. **C**	55. **B**	
14. **A**	28. **A**	42. **D**	56. **B**	

Explanation of Answers for Science Questions-Model Test D

SCIENCE KNOWLEDGE

Biology

1. **(C)** Hyaluronidase is an enzyme carried by sperm, capable of hydrolysis of hyaluronic acid, promoting fertilization (penetration of sperm). Hyaluronidase is medically used to promote the diffusion and absorption of many injected medications.

2. **(D)** During meiosis in the female one functional gamete (egg) and three polar bodies are produced.

3. **(A)** Control of these functions is due to crossing of the fibers, and control of the right side is by the left cerebral hemispheres.

4. **(B)** The interstitial cells are stimulated be ICSH (interstitial cell stimulating hormone) a gonadotrophin of the pituitary to produce androgens. Testosterone is an androgen.

5. **(C)** Progesterone is produced by the corpus luteum.

6. **(B)** Between 3 to 4 ml of semen comprise one ejaculate which contains between 300-400 million sperm cells.

7. **(B)** The adrenal medulla can be considered to house the post ganglionic neurons for part of the sympathetic portion of the autonomic nervous system and is responsible for epi- and norepinephrine production.

8. **(E)** A mutation may be thought of as a sudden change in the genetic make up of the organism. It may be beneficial or harmful. It may occur spontaneously or may be experimentally produced with chemicals, X-rays, cosmic rays, etc. It may not be passed on to the next generation because, for example, it may be lethal or otherwise preclude reproduction.

9. **(D)** A sarcomere is the region between two Z bands. In simple terms we are dealing with this unit: ZIAHAIZ. Contraction of the sarcomere is due to the fine filaments (actin) sliding between the thick filaments (myosin) pulling the Z bands to which they are attached with them. This pulls the Z bands closer together, and so the sarcomeres are shortened.

10. **(C)** A bacteriophage is a virus that is a parasite of bacteria; sometimes lysis of the bacterial cell is a result.

11. **(B)** Hemophilia, a frequent disease of the royal houses of Europe, is a bleeding disorder transmitted through a sex-linked recessive gene. It results in abnormal coagulation; hemophilia A is the classical true hemophilia resulting from a deficiency of factor VIII.

12. **(D)** Genotype refers to the genetic makeup of the organism. The genotype is expressed via phenotypic characteristics that are visible and observable under normal circumstances.

13. **(E)** Humans are very well protected against the dangers of their surroundings. The external layer of skin is practically impermeable; it protects against trauma, bacteria, drying, water penetration, ultraviolet light, noxious agents, etc. White blood cells are influential in the mobilization of the immunological machinery of the body and also have the capability to engulf bacteria, etc., and destroy them. After an antigen enters the organism the immune system counters by producing antibodies to neutralize the effect and in many cases to protect the organism against susceptibility to the same agent in the future (the basis of immunization).

14. **(D)** An allele is one of a pair of genes that occupies the same locus on homologous chromosomes.

15. **(A)** The chemical mediator of cholinergic nerve impulses is acetylcholine and is released by the axon terminals.

16. **(C)** The ABO blood grouping system is explained on the basis of a single triallelic system with genes A, B, and O operating at a single genetic locus. Phenotypic and genotypic characteristics may be expressed as follows:

Phenotype	Genotype
A	A/A; A/O
B	B/B; B/O
O	O/O
AB	A/B

The A and B genes appear to be codominant; they are dominant over O, which is recessive.

17. **(A)** See explanation for question 16.

18. **(C)** The inferior vena cava empties into the right atrium, carries deoxygenated blood, and blood pressure is low at that point.

19. **(B)** Acromegaly is a result of pituitary oversecretion of growth hormone. Lack of iodine will result in goiter development of the thyroid gland. Rickets is due to a vitamin D deficiency. A skin rash is not a specific lesion that can be associated with only one specified cause as the others listed.

20. **(B)** Trypsin is the enzyme that is functional in protein digestion. Ptyalin (salivary amylase) acts on starches while pancreatic lipase (steapsin) acts on fats. Maltose is not an enzyme but a sugar.

21. **(B)** In skeletal muscle the nuclei are found peripherally. To complete the chart the speed of contraction should also be mentioned. Skeletal muscle is the fastest working, smooth the slowest, and cardiac muscle occupies an intermediate position.

22. **(C)** Identical twins arise from the same egg. One egg is fertilized by one sperm and a splitting (separation) occurs during the early cleavage divisions. Fraternal twins arise from the fertilization of two eggs, each by one sperm. Identical twins always are the same sex. Fraternal twins may be of either sex (50-50 proposition).

23. **(C)** While on the pill no new eggs are produced; the female is kept in the progestational phase (second half) of the menstrual cycle.

24. **(A)** Osmosis is a process in which solvent passes from an area of lower solute concentration to an area of higher solute concentration. In dialysis solvent and solute both pass through the membrane.

25. **(A)** Any substance that has the capability to elicit an immunological response, such as the production of antibody that is specific to that substance is considered an antigen.

26. **(B)** Vasectomy involves an interruption of the spermatic cords (vas deferens) in the male.

27. **(B)** After the secretion of sweat, evaporation of this product is the key to the cooling of the organism. In an environment of high humidity the effectiveness of this mechanism is decreased.

28. **(B)** Acromegaly and (or) giantism is due to overactivity of the alpha cells of the pituitary which secrete growth hormone. If a person is affected before puberty, he or she will develop into a fairly well proportioned giant. After maturity, an increase in the size of the hands and feet and massive development of the bones comprising the face are consequences. In the adult strictly speaking the term acromegaly must be applied to this condition.

29. **(E)** The question lists the most important features.

30. **(B)** Most researchers feel that the interstitial cells of Leydig of the seminiferous tubules are the source of androgen and possibly testicular estrogen. The most potent androgen is testosterone.

31. **(A)** Glucagon is released into the bloodstream in response to diminishing blood sugar levels. The main action of glucagon is to promote liver glycogenolysis; as a consequence glycogen stores of the liver diminish. Epinephrine secreted by the adrenal medulla has the same general effect. Epinephrine is an important factor in the normal organism for counteracting the hypoglycemic action of insulin.

32. **(B)** Impeded or sluggish venous blood flow, especially of the veins of the lower extremity, can lead to the formation of blood clots. The disease, thrombophlebitis, is characterized by an inflammation of veins with thrombosis.

33. **(C)** The releasing factors that have been isolated and identified to date are produced in hypothalamic areas.

34. **(A)** One of the main functions of the large intestine is the reabsorption of water.

35. **(B)** Hyperventilation is abnormally rapid, deep breathing resulting in a loss of CO_2 and an increase in blood pH. A person would be in the state of respiratory alkalosis since a decreased blood concentration of hydrogen ion is the result of pulmonary CO_2 elimination.

36. **(E)** Heart beat is initiated by the S-A (sino-atrial) node.

37. **(D)** A definition of resolution and the common resolving powers of the eye, light microscope, and electron microscope were stated. The ophthalmoscope provides a good light source and a little magnification but certainly does not help much to improve the resolving power of the eye.

38. **(D)** The question is self-explanatory.

Chemistry

1. **(B)** The equation is self-explanatory.

2. **(B)** $ØN_2^+ Br^- + H_2$ catalyst $Ø\text{-NH-NH}_2$

3. **(A)** In DNA there are principally 4 nitrogen bases: adenine, thymine, guanine, and cytosine. In RNA uracil is present instead of thymine. During transcription of RNA from DNA, the DNA bases of adenine, thymine, guanine, and cytosine will pair with the RNA bases of uracil, adenine, cytosine, and guanine, respectively.

4. **(D)** $CaC_2 + 2H_2O \rightarrow C_2H_2 + Ca(OH)_2$

5. **(B)** $H_2O + Na \rightarrow H_2 + NaOH$

6. **(C)** During the production of electricity the two half-cell reactions of the storage battery are
$Pb + SO_4^= \rightarrow PbSO_4 + 2e^-$
$PbO_2 + 4H + SO_4^= + 2e^- \rightarrow PbSO_4 + 2H_2O$
During recharging of the battery the two half-cell reactions are reversed.

7. **(C)** Silver ions will react with chloride ions and precipitate as AgCl.

8. **(B)** The four products of this Wurtz reaction are n-hexane, n-butane, and ethane. On the basis of probability only, the butane should represent 50% of the product on a molar basis.

9. **(D)** See explanation for question 8.

10. **(B)** $H_2S \rightleftarrows 2H^+ + S^=$. By the common ion effect, lowering the pH (increasing the H^+ concentration) will lower the $S^=$ concentration by displacing the reaction to the left. $K_i = \frac{(H^{+2})(S^=)}{(H_2S)}$. If H^+ increases, $S^=$ must decrease.

11. **(A)** Freezing point depression in water depends only on the number of solute particles per unit volume
1 M NaCl $= 2 \times 1 \times 6.02 \times 10^{23}$ particles per liter
0.3 M $NaSO_4 = 3 \times .03 \times 6.02 \times 10^{23}$ particles per liter
1.5 M glucose $= 1 \times 1.5 \times 6.02 \times 10^{23}$ particles per liter
0.5 M $BaSO_4 = 3 \times 0.5 \times 6.02 \times 10^{23}$ particles per liter
Dividing by 6.02×10^{23} we can see that the comparative figures are NaCl, 2; Na_2SO_4, 0.9; glucose, 1.5; and $BaSO_4$, 1.5. Thus, the NaCl solution has the greatest number of particles per unit volume (considering the ionization of NaCl, Na_2SO_4 and $BaSO_4$), and it will have the lowest freezing point.

12. **(D)** A reaction in which electrons (e^-) are removed is termed an oxidation reaction; the adding of electrons to an atom or molecule is termed a reduction reaction.

13. **(D)** A yellow precipitate of iodoform is produced in this reaction with methyl ketones, alcohols that may be oxidized to methyl ketones, or acetaldehyde.

14. **(A)** The hydronium ion, H_3O^+, is a protonated water molecule. $2H_2O \rightleftarrows H_3O^+ + OH^-$

15. **(B)** The alpha helix contributes to the secondary structure of proteins, but not all proteins (nor all regions of proteins) contain the alpha helix secondary structure.

16. **(A)** As long as the volume units are the same, $N_1V_1 = N_2V_2$

$$V_2 = \frac{N_1V_1}{N_2} = \frac{(50)(0.25)}{0.50} = 25 \text{ ml}$$

The fact that the acid produces two hydrogen ions per molecule does not enter into the calculations.

17. **(A)** Cyclopropane, containing 3 carbon atoms, is the smallest organic ring compound.

18. **(E)** Enzymes are influenced by:

temperature
1. inactivated usually above 60°C
2. rate of reaction is controlled as in any chemical reaction; the rate is approximately doubled by each 10°C increase
3. low temperatures slow the reaction

pH
there is an optimum pH for every reaction

poisons
some enzymes themselves can be harmful to the organism but they are also susceptible to compounds like cyanide, etc., which inactivate them

concentration
the rate of a reaction is directly proportional to the amount of enzyme present in relation to substrate. If a coenzyme or specific activator is required, that substance may control the overall rate of the reaction also

19. **(A)** This is a definition of the zwitterion; an example is the amino acid, glycine.

20. **(C)** Lye soap was produced in earlier days by boiling animal fat with lye. This process of forming the salt of fatty acids by treating a fat with alkali is called saponification.

21. **(D)** The different isomers are 1,1; 1,2; 1,3; 2,2; 1,4; and 2,3. There might appear to be other possi bilities; but 2,4 is more properly 1,3 and 3,4 is more properly 1,2.

22. **(A)** Markovnikov's rule predicts that in the absence of peroxides the addition of hydrogen halide across a double bond will occur with hydrogen being added to the carbon, which already contains the most hydrogen. In the presence of peroxides, however, a free radical mechanism results in hydrogen bromide being added in the opposite orientation.

23. **(C)** The starting compound may be pictured as

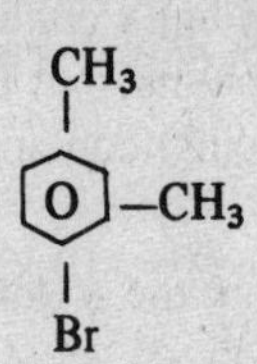

Monobromination in the 3, 5, or 6 position will produce different compounds. The identity of the alkyl groups is not important since ring monobromination was specified.

24. **(C)** $I_2 + 2S_2O_3^{=} \rightarrow 2I^- + S_4O_6^{=}$. Iodine is being reduced. Iodine (i.e., I_2) but not iodide (i.e., I^-) reacts with starch to form a blue complex.

25. **(E)** Hemoglobin is the oxygen carrier in red blood cells of all vertebrates. With carbon monoxide hemoglobin forms carboxyhemoglobin. The binding capacity (affinity) of hemoglobin for carbon monoxide is over 100 times that of the binding capacity for oxygen.

26. **(B)** Helium has a higher density and cost than hydrogen, but it is much safer. Hydrogen readily escapes through tiny holes, and if ignited, it reacts quite readily with oxygen. Helium is essentially inert chemically.

27. **(D)** The question states a fact and the information should be learned.

28. **(D)** Anaerobic oxidation is far less efficient than aerobic oxidation. Pasteur showed that fermentation can take place in the absence of air. The common equations are written in the following manner:
Aerobic respiration:
$C_6H_{12}O_6 + 6O_2 \rightarrow 6H_2O + 6\ CO_2$ + Energy (673 calories)
Anaerobic respiration (Alcoholic Fermentation):
$C_6H_{12}O_6 \rightarrow 2C_2H_5OH + 2CO_2$ + Energy (25 calories)

29. **(D)** Low molecular weight mercaptans have a very unpleasant odor even in low concentration. They are added to give an odor to the odorless natural gas. This is quite helpful in detecting leaks and thus avoiding explosions.

30. **(A)** Conversion of glycogen to glucose-1-phosphate is catalyzed by the enzyme, phosphorylase. Pancreatic amylase is usually not in contact with glycogen (except dietary glycogen); in any case it would not catalyze the formation of glucose-1-phosphate.

31. **(B)** This precipitate reacts with acid or base and, therefore, is amphoteric. It could be aluminum hydroxide.

$AL(OH)_3 + 3H^+ \rightarrow Al^{+++} + 3H_2O$
$AL(OH)_3 + OH^- \rightarrow AL(OH)_4$

32. **(B)** See explanation for question 31.

33. **(C)** Transuranium elements are those having more than the 92 protons of uranium. Several may be produced by neutron bombardment of lighter elements such as uranium.

34. **(D)** The electron is the negatively charged particle that forms part of an atom outside the nucleus.

35. **(C)** A compound can only be separated by chemical means and not by physical means. A mixture can, however, be separated by physical means.

36. **(B)** 2,4-D is applied to fields and lawns to eliminate weeds. Most of the weeds are dicotyledonous plants which are more sensitive to this potent stimulator of plant metabolism. The proper concentration must be carefully adhered to so that when the material is applied, the weeds will be stimulated to metabolize at such a great rate that they will consume their own protoplasm and die while the monocytyledonous grasses (or crops) will remain unharmed.

37. **(D)** The question lists the properties of a solid.

38. **(B)** The first reaction $CO_2 + H_2O \rightarrow H_2CO_3$ is a synthesis reaction.
The second reaction $2HgO \rightarrow 2Hg + O_2\uparrow$ is a decomposition reaction.
The third reaction $Zn + CuSO_4 \rightarrow ZnSO_4 + Cu$ is a single replacement reaction.
The fourth reaction $HCl + NaOH \rightarrow NaCl + H_2O$ is a double replacement reaction (as well as a neutralization or acid-base reaction).

39. **(B)** The more ions formed, the greater the electric current carried by an electrolyte solution.

40. **(D)** The compound whose structural formula was listed in the question was

Butane

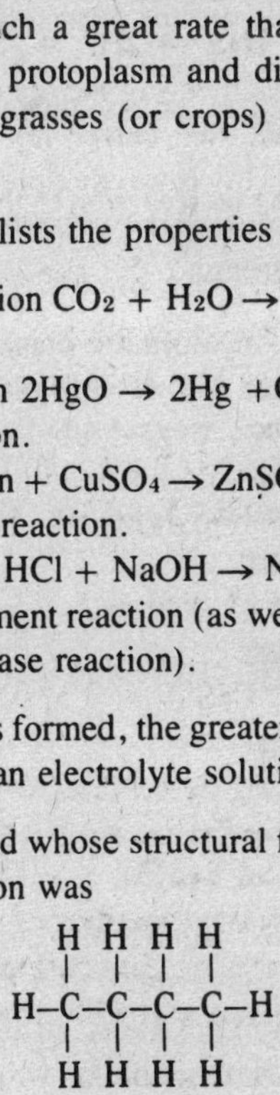

Pentane has the following structural formula

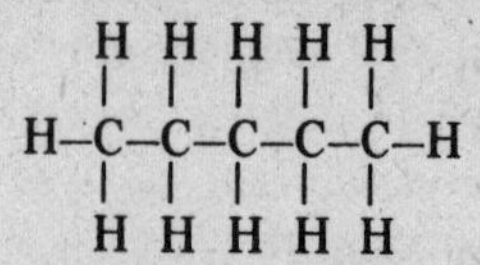

41. **(D)** The concentration of (OH^-) will decrease due to the common ion effect. Since (OH^-) × (H^+) = 10^{-14}, H^+ must increase, pH decreases and pOH increases.

42. **(D)** Light-catalyzed reduction of silver salts to produce elemental silver is the basis for black and white photographic film.

43. **(B)** The principle of LeChatelier, stated simply, says that a system, placed under stress, changes to relieve the stress. Four volumes of gas are on the left side of the equation, and only two volumes are on the right. A change of equilibrium toward the right would thus tend to relieve the stress brought about by higher pressure.

44. **(C)** James Chadwick discovered the neutron in 1932.

45. **(C)** This is a Friedel-Crafts acylation (similar to Friedel-Crafts alkylation). The acetyl group is substituted on the ring, producing a methylaryl ketone.

46. **(B)** Polyvinyl alcohol can be formed by polymerizing vinyl acetate and then removing the acetate groups (transesterification or saponification). Attempts to produce the monomer, vinyl alcohol, lead only to the production of acetaldehyde.

47. **(C)** This is an example of the aldol condensation. It requires an aldehyde or ketone possessing α-hydrogen.

48. **(D)** An aromatic diazonium salt, formed by an aromatic amine with nitrite and acid, will couple with an activated aromatic ring. Phenol is such an activated compound, and the result in this case (probably para) is ϕ—N=N—ϕ—OH.

49. **(A)**

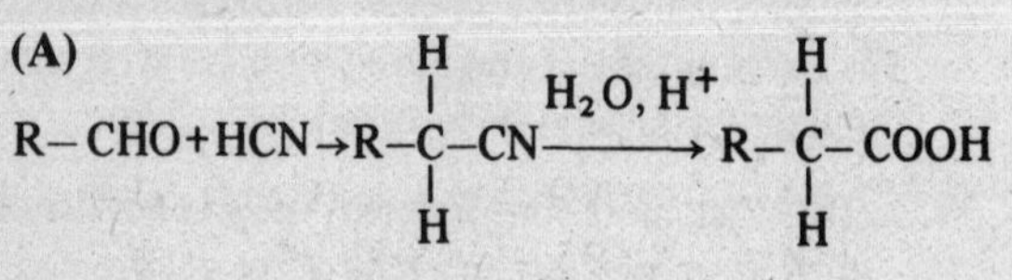

Physics

1. **(A)** At a uniform acceleration of 9.8 m/sec.^{2} the body goes from 0 to 9.8 m/sec. in the first second and from 9.8 m/sec. to 19.6 m/sec. at the end of the 2nd second of fall.

2. **(B)** The amount of heat needed to raise the temperature by 1 degree Celsius of 1 gram of substance is known as specific heat.

3. **(C)** Use $f = ma$ when m = 60 kg and f = 30.6 kg force (convert to newtons).
$f = (30.6)(9.8) = 300$ newtons
$a = f/m = 300$ kg/60
$a = 5$ m/sec.^{2}

4. **(A)** $F = ma$ if m = mass of body and a = constant. Since both m and a are constant, F must be constant.

5. **(D)** $PE = Wh$ when W = 10 kg and h = 9 m.
$PE = (10)(9.8)(9) = 10$ kg × 9.8 N × 9 m
$PE = 882$ joules

6. **(D)** $KE = \frac{1}{2}mv^2$
$KE_0 = \frac{1}{2}m_0v_0^2$
Increase m_0 to $3m_0$, increase v_0 to $3v_0$, then:
$KE = \frac{1}{2}(3m_0)(2v_0)^2$
$KE = \frac{1}{2}(12)(m_0v_0^2)$
Therefore KE will be multiplied by 12.

7. **(C)** The direction of the force exerted against a surface by a fluid at rest is normal or perpendicular to the surface.

8. **(E)** The statement is known as Boyle's law.

9. **(A)** $\text{Efficiency} = \dfrac{\text{useful work output}}{\text{work input}} \times 100\%$, by definition, or,
$\text{Efficiency} = \dfrac{\text{actual mechanical advantage}}{\text{theoretical mechanical advantage}}$ × 100%

10. **(C)** $\text{Speed of sound } (S) = \dfrac{\text{distance } (x)}{\text{time } (t)}$ when x = 1000 m and s = 333 m/sec.
$S = x/t$, therefore
$t = x/s$
$t = \dfrac{1000 \text{ m}}{333 \text{ m/sec.}} = 3$ seconds

11. **(E)** Energy of a wave is proportional to the square of its height.

12. **(D)** The umbra is that portion of a shadow which does not receive light from any part of the light source.

13. **(D)** W = force × distance when force = 100 kg × 9.8 N = 980 and distance = 3 m.
$W = (980)(3) = 2940$ joules

14-18. **(14-C) (15-A) (16-D) (17-B) (18-E)** The answers to questions *14-18* are self-explanatory.

19. **(E)** All of the above are true statements regarding the banking of a roadbed.

20. **(B)** Use $x = v_0 + ½at^2$ where x = distance of fall, v_0 = initial velocity = 0, a = acceleration, 9.8 m/sec.², and t = 1 second.
$x = 0 + ½at^2$
$x = (½)(9.8)(1)^2$
$x = 4.9$ m

21. **(B)** $F = ma$ where F = 45 kg force, m = ?, and a = 10 m/sec.²
1 kg force = 1 kg × 9.8 m/sec.²
45 kg force = 45 kg × 9.8 m/sec.²
F = 441 newtons
$m = F/a = \frac{441 \text{ kg m/sec.}^2}{10 \text{ m/sec.}^2}$
m = 44.1 kg

22. **(E)** All the statements are correct concerning the application and characteristics of Newton's law of universal gravitation.

23. **(A)** 45 kg-f · 40 kg-f
$\sum F_x = 45 - 40 = 5$ kg-f
(40 subtracted from 45 because the forces are in direct opposition to one another).

24. **(B)** Lowering the center of gravity increases the stability of the table lamp.

25. **(D)** The six devices known as simple machines are: inclined plane, lever, pulley, screw, wedge, and wheel-and-axle.

26. **(A)** $KE = \frac{mv^2}{2}$ when KE = 2500 joules, m = 50 kg, and v = ?
$2500 = \frac{50}{2}(v^2)$
$100 = v^2$
v = 10 m/sec.

27. **(C)** $v_1/v_2 = 1$ Bernoulli's equation holds here. Since the container is exposed to the atmosphere, the pressures at the surface and outlets are the same and the velocity at the outlet becomes a function of the heat and acceleration due to gravity making $v_1 = v_2$ therefore $v_1/v_2 = 1$.

28. **(D)** Specific gravity is numerically equal to density, so long as density is measured in gm/cm³.

29. **(D)** Definition of surface tension.

30. **(C)** The smoother the surface, the more regularly reflecting the surface is. Mirrors are smooth enough that they reflect in a regular fashion.

31. **(D)** A color disc as described induces the sensation of *white* by integrating its component colors.

32-36. **(32-C) (33-E) (34-A) (35-B) (36-D)** The answers to questions 32-36 are self-explanatory.

37. **(D)** Each 1590 years ½ of the remaining element would decay. Therefore, for the 6360 years $(½)^4$ of the original would remain or 1/16 would remain.

38. **(A)** Stable equilibrium.

SCIENCE PROBLEMS

1. **(B)** Choose the upward direction as negative and downward as positive. Then V_0 = −15 m/sec. and a = 9.8 m/sec.² at t = 3 seconds, X = ?
$X = V_0t + ½at^2$
$X = (-15)(3) + (½)(9.8)(3)^2$
$X = -45 + 44.1$
$X = -0.9$ m above ground

2. **(B)** What is V?
$V = V_0 + at$
$V = -15 + (9.8)(3)$
$V = -15 + 29.4$
V = 14.4 m/sec. downward

3. **(B)** At highest point $V = 0$, V_0 = −15 m/sec., a = 9.8 m/sec.², and t = ?
$V = V_0 + at$
$O = -15 + 9.8t$
$15 = 9.8t$
$1.53 = t$
$X = (-15)(1.53) + ½(9.8)(1.53)^2$
$X = -22.95 + (4.9)(2.34)$
$X = -22.95 + 11.47$
X = 11.48 m above the ground

4. **(E)** 1,4-dibromo-2-butene and 1,2-dibromo-3-butene would be the products.

5. **(E)** None of these are conjugated dienes.

6. **(A)** The diene removes Br^+ from the bromine molecule to form a 1-bromocarbonium ion. The double bond shifts to the 2 position and the positive charge primarily to the 4-position prior to reaction of the carbonium ion with Br^- to form the final product.

7. **(C)** $K = \frac{(1.0 - X)/50}{X/50}$

$$2 = \frac{1.0 - X}{X}$$
$$2X = 1.0 - X$$
$$3X = 1.0$$
$$X = 0.33 \text{ g}$$

8. **(B)** $K = \frac{(0.67 - X)/50}{X/50}$

$$2 = \frac{0.67 - X}{X}$$
$$2X = 0.67 - X$$
$$3X = 0.67$$
$$X = 0.22 \text{ g}$$

9. **(D)** $K = \frac{(1.0 - 0.8)/50}{0.8/X} = 2$

$$2 = \frac{0.2X}{(0.8)(5)}$$
$$X = \frac{(2)(0.8)(50)}{0.2} = 400 \text{ ml}$$

10-12. **(10-B) (11-A) (12-C)** The large spike encountered was probably due to an artifact since if the membrane is unimolecular and the same type of ions are present on the surface of the membrane, the same membrane potential should be existing and the spike should have the same height at all times. The normal impulse is due to an all or none response; there is no gradual (gradient) increase or decrease with respect to neural impulses. External increase in voltage will alter the height of the spike.

13. **(B)** A force diagram of this body would show the following when F_u = apparent weight, B = buoyant force, and F_d = weight.

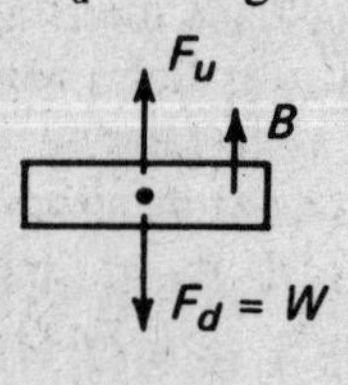

Since there is equilibrium $F_{up} = \Sigma F_{down}$ therefore $F_u + B = F_d$. Knowing F_u and F_d, B is easily established as $F_d - F_u$

$$B = 100 \text{ gm} - 800 \text{ gm}$$
$$B = 200 \text{ gm}$$

14. **(C)** In the metric system specific gravity is numerically equal to density. Here the B force = weight of the displaced fluid by definition

$$V = \frac{B}{d}$$
$$V = \frac{200}{1.25} \text{ cm}^3$$

$V = 160 \text{ cm}^3$ = volume of the body and the displaced liquid.

15. **(D)** To calculate density of body

$$p = \frac{m}{V} = \frac{1000}{160} = 6.25 \text{ gm/cm}^3$$

16. **(E)** By inspection of the graph, the largest number of molecules of a single velocity is at point C. The graph appears symmetrical and thus this would be also the average velocity.

17. **(D)** Both points A and C are improbable according to the graph. Very few molecules would achieve the high velocity represented by point C.

18. **(A)** The peak of the curve (i.e., the most probable velocity) would be shifted to the right, indicating a higher velocity.

19. **(E)** A change in concentration of any of the components of the equilibrium will not change the equilibrium constant for that temperature.

20. **(D)** As stated above, the equilibrium does not change. Thus the concentrations of the other components of the equilibrium must change in the stated directions.

21. **(E)** The equilibrium constant does not change.

22-24. **(22-D) (23-D) (24-D)** As can be seen from the table, there are four major blood types and the explanation as to universal donor and recipient is based on the following:

Type	Agglutinogens on Cells	Agglutinins in Serum and Plasma
AB — can receive A, B, AB, or O (universal recipient)	A, B	none
A — can receive A, O	A	anti b
B — can receive B, O	B	anti a
O — can receive only O, but can give to all; therefore, O is the universal donor	O	anti ab

25. **(A)** The answer is simple in that we know that $N_r = 1.5$ and $N_i = 1.0$, $\therefore \frac{N_r}{N_i} > 1.0$; therefore,

the ray of light slows down and bends towards the normal.

26. (D) $N = \frac{C}{S}$; $\therefore N_r = \frac{C}{S_r}$ and $N_i = \frac{C}{S_i}$. Substituting in the Snell's law given $\frac{\text{Sin } \theta_i}{\text{Sin } \theta_r} = \frac{\frac{C}{S_r}}{\frac{C}{S_i}}$ where C = speed of light in vacuum and S_i and S_r is speed of light in medium. Then $\frac{\text{Sin } \theta_i}{\text{Sin } \theta_r} = \frac{S_i}{S_r}$

27. (B) Using $\frac{\text{Sin } \theta_i}{\text{Sin } \theta_r} = \frac{S_i}{S_r}$ and knowing that
$S_i = 3 \times 10^8$ m/sec.
$S_r = S_i \left(\frac{\text{Sin } \theta_r}{\text{Sin } \theta_i}\right) = \left(3 \times 10^8\right)\left(\frac{0.500}{0.70}\right)$
$S_r = (3)(.7)(10^8)$
$S_r = 2.1 \times 10^8$ m/sec.

28. (E) $PV = nRT$ where P = pressure, V = volume, n = molecules (in the case of helium, atoms) of gas, R = universal gas constant, and T = temperature, °K. Since the volumes are equal, $\frac{P}{T}$ is proportional to the number of atoms.
$\frac{Px}{Tx} = \frac{760 \text{ torr}}{273°\text{K}} = 2.78$
$\frac{Py}{Ty} = \frac{1140 \text{ torr}}{410°\text{K}} = 2.78$
Without calculating the numbers of atoms, we can see that the numbers are equal. The average velocity will be higher in the container of the higher temperature.

29. (E) $\frac{PV}{T} = nR$. If n increases, both P and T will increase unless an attempt is made to control one or the other.

30. (D) $\frac{Px}{Tx}$ still equals $\frac{Py}{Ty}$ so the number of atoms is equal. There is insufficient information to allow a comparison of average velocities of the two gases.

31-33. (31-D) (32-C) (33-A) These questions essentially detail the activities carried out during a muscular contraction and are self-explanatory.

34. (E) To calculate the potential difference recall that V = potential difference, and $V = IR$ where I = current and R = resistance. In our case
$V = (10)(5)$
$V = 50$ volts

35. (A) To calculate the parallel resistance we can use the fact that $\frac{1}{R} = \frac{1}{R_2} + \frac{1}{R_3} + \frac{1}{R_4}$

Therefore, $\frac{1}{R} = \frac{1}{2} + \frac{1}{4} + \frac{1}{12} = \frac{6 + 3 + 1}{12}$
$10R = 12$
$R = 1.2$ ohms

36. (A) Again, $V = IR$ as above when $R = 1.2$ ohms and $I = 10$ amps.
$V = (10)(1.2)$
$V = 12$ volts

37. (D) The compound must be an aldehyde or ketone based on the first information. It must not be a ketone based on the second test.

38. (E) See explanation for question 37.

39. (A) Permanganate oxidation would oxidize the unsaturated 2-butene to a glycol. Periodic acid would oxidize the glycol to 2 molecules of acetaldehyde.

40. (D) pH $= -\log [H^+] = -\log (1 \times 10^{-4}) = 4$

41. (D) $1/10{,}000 = 1 \times 10^{-4}$
$1 \times 10^{-4} \times 1 \times 10^{-4} = 1 \times 10^{-8}$
$(1 \times 10^{-8}) + 1 \times 10^{-7}$ (from water ionization) $=$
1.1×10^{-7}
$-\log (1.1 \times 10^{-7}) = -(-6.96) = 6.96$
Although you could not make this complete calculation without logarithm tables, you should be aware that this small amount of acid would have a small effect on the pH of 7 in water.

42. (C) This is essentially a 1:10 dilution with water since the diluted solution (above) is essentially water and the volume of the second dilution is 10 ml to 90 + 10 ml.
$\frac{1 \times 10^{-4}}{10} = 1 \times 10^{-5}$
pH $= -\log [H^+] = -\log (1 \times 10^{-5}) = 5$

43-48. (43-A) (44-A) (45-C) (46-D) (47-A) (48-A) Let us identify the components of the neuron numbered: (2) nucleus with nucleolus, containing the genetic material of the cell and directing the synthetic activity of the cell; (3) Golgi apparatus (zone), the packaging and concentrating area of the cell's secretory activity; (4) dendrites; dendrites are the processes that pick up an impulse and carry it towards the cell body; (5) endoplasmic reticulum (rough in this case—ribosomes are attached), the synthetic machinery of the cell (proteins etc.,); (6) cell membrane, semipermeable and the protector of the cell from its environment; (7) cytoplasm (specifically the area here is called the axon hillock); (8) myelin sheath (Schwann cell covered by its neurilemma, the insulator of the axon; (9) direction of conduction of an impulse; axons (10a) conduct impulses away from the cell body to the function with the dendrites of another neuron. The junction point is known as the synaptic area; the impulse can cross the synapse only from the axon to the dendrite and no backflow is permitted; (11) terminal branches of the axon. In a lesion (cut) the process distal from the cell body would completely degenerate; retrograde degeneration would be detected in the proximal portion and the cell body, however, the proximal portion has the capacity and will regenerate.

49. **(D)** Using the general gas law $\frac{PV}{T} = \frac{P_0V_0}{T_0}$ when $0°C = 273°K = T_0$, $5\ m^3 = V_0$, $1\ atm = P_0$, $T_r = 293°K$, $V = ?$, and $P_r = 1$ atm.

$$\frac{V}{T} = \frac{V_0}{T_0}$$
$$\frac{V}{293} = \frac{5}{273}$$
$$273V = 1465$$
$$V = 5.36\ m^3$$

50. **(D)** Again using $\frac{PV}{T} = \frac{P_0V_0}{T_0}$ when $V_0 = 5\ m^3$, $P_0 = 1$ atm, $T_0 = 273°K$, $V = 2.5\ m^3$, $P = 4$ atm, and $T = ?$ Solving for T one gets

$$T = \frac{PVT_0}{P_0V_0} = \frac{(4)(2.5)(273)}{(1)(5)}$$
$$T = \frac{2730}{5} = 546°K$$

51. **(E)** All are correct statements and, combined, express Charles' law, Boyle's law, and the general gas law.

52. **(E)** To convert Fahrenheit to Celsius we can use the following formulas:

Celsius equals $\frac{5}{9} \times$ (Fahrenheit − 32)

Fahrenheit equals $\frac{9}{5}$ C + 32

104°F = 40°C = 313° Kelvin

$$\text{Celsius} = \frac{5}{9} \times (104 - 32)$$
$$C = \frac{5}{9} \times 72$$
$$C = 40°$$

53. **(D)** Now we take Kelvin 273° and add 40° and obtain a Kelvin temperature of 313°. 45°C will equal 113°F as calculated below.

$$°F = \frac{9}{5}(45) + 32$$
$$°F = 81 + 32$$
$$°F = 113°$$

54. **(D)** A normal body temperature on the Fahrenheit scale is 98.6° and on the Celsius scale it is 37°.

55. **(A)** $K_i = \frac{[H^+][X^-]}{[HX]} = 1 \times 10^{-7}$

$$\frac{[H^+][X^-]}{0.1} = 1 \times 10^{-7}$$

Since $[H^+] = [X^-]$ in the ionization,

$$[H^+][X^-] = [H^+]^2 = 0.1 \times 1 \times 10^{-7} = 1 \times 10^{-8}$$
$$[H^+] = \sqrt{1 \times 10^{-8}} = 1 \times 10^{-4}$$
$$pH = 4$$

56. **(B)** $1 \times 10^{-4} \times 0.1 = 1 \times 10^{-5}$
pH = 5

57. **(C)** Ionization constants are useful only at reasonably low concentrations.

58. **(A)** If we divide the percentage compositions by their respective atomic weights, we will have the relative atomic abundance of the elements in compound V.

$\frac{40}{12} = 3.33$ for carbon

$\frac{6.67}{1} = 6.67$ for hydrogen

$\frac{53.33}{16} = 3.33$ for oxygen (Oxygen analysis is usually only by difference from 100%.)

59. **(A)** Since the least abundant compound must be represented to the extent of at least one atom per molecule, divide the relative atomic abundance numbers by the smallest of them (3.33 in this case).

$$C = \frac{3.33}{3.33} = 1$$
$$H = \frac{6.67}{3.33} = 2$$
$$O = \frac{3.33}{3.33} = 1$$

The empirical formula is CH_2O.

60. **(E)** The empirical formula is correct for formadehyde, but the molecular weight and thus the molecular formula are wrong.

61. **(E)** $K_b = \frac{[Pyr^+][OH^-]}{[PyrOH]}$ Since $[Pyr^+] = [OH^-]$

$$[OH^-]^2 = K_b[PyrOH] = (1 \times 10^{-9})(0.1)$$
$$[OH^-] = \sqrt{1 \times 10^{-10}} = 1 \times 10^{-5}$$
$$pOH = -\log[OH^-] = 5$$
$$pH = 14 - pOH = 9$$

62. **(D)** Starting with a pH of 9, a hundredfold dilution will, by inspection, produce a pH of virtually 7.

63. **(E)** pH + pOH = 14. None of the other expressions is correct.

64. **(A)** Since pressure is measured in gauge, pressure and P_1 and P_2 are measured at surfaces exposed to the atmosphere, $P_1 = P_2 = 0$.

65. **(A)** $h_1 + \frac{P_1}{W} + \frac{V_1^2}{2a} = h_2 + \frac{P_2}{W} + \frac{V_2^2}{2a}$ at 1, the velocity in all practical purposes = 0 and $P_0 = P_2 = 0$ then the equation above can be written as

$$h_2 + \frac{V_2^2}{2a} = h_1$$
$$V_2^2 = (h_1 - h_2)\,2a$$
$$V_2 = [(h_1 - h_2)(2a)]^{1/2}$$

66. **(A)** The question is self-explanatory.

Appendix

LOGARITHMS AND EXPONENTS

Logarithms

The logarithm of any number is the exponent of the power to which 10 must be raised to produce the number. The logarithm X of the number N to the base 10 is the exponent of the power to which 10 must be raised to give N (for example, $\log_{10} N = X$). Logarithms consist of two parts. First, there is the "characteristic," which is determined by the position of the first significant figure of the number in relation to the decimal point. If we count leftwards from the decimal point as positive and rightwards as negative, the characteristic is equal to the count ending at the right of the first significant figure. Thus, the characteristic of the logarithm of 2340 is 3, and of 0.00234 is -3. Second, there is the "mantissa." It is always positive, is found in logarithm tables, and depends only on the sequence of significant figures. Thus, the mantissa for the two numbers is the same, namely 0.3692. The logarithm of a number is the sum of the characteristic and the mantissa. Thus, $\log 2340 = 3.3692$ while $\log 0.00234 = -3 + 0.3692 = -2.6308$.

The logarithms of the whole integers 1 to 10 are given below.

$\log 1.0 = 0.000$	$\log 6.0 = 0.778$
$\log 2.0 = 0.301$	$\log 7.0 = 0.845$
$\log 3.0 = 0.477$	$\log 8.0 = 0.903$
$\log 4.0 = 0.602$	$\log 9.0 = 0.954$
$\log 5.0 = 0.699$	$\log 10.0 = 1.000$

Useful Rules in Handling Logarithms

1. The logarithm of a product is equal to the sum of the logarithms of the factors:

$$\log ab = \log a + \log b$$

(Check this out by solving for log 6, using log 2 + log 3.)

2. The logarithm of a fraction is equal to the logarithm of the numerator minus the logarithm of the denominator:

$$\log \frac{a}{b} = \log a - \log b$$

Example:

$$\log \frac{10}{2} = \log 10 - \log 2 = \log 5$$

How about log 2.5? The answer from the log tables is 0.398.

3. The logarithm of the reciprocal of a number is the negative logarithm of the number:

$$\log \frac{1}{a} = \log 1 - \log a$$

Since $\log 1 = 0$, then

$$\log \frac{1}{a} = -\log a$$

Equally,

$$\log \frac{1}{2} = -\log 2 = -0.301$$

4. The logarithm of a number raised to a power is the logarithm of the number multiplied by the power:

$$\log a^b = b \log a$$

$$\log 2^2 = 0.603$$

Exponents

It is convenient to express large numbers as 10^x, where x represents the number of places that the decimal must be moved to place it after the first significant figure. This also represents $10 \cdot 10$ for x times. For example, 1,000,000 may be expressed as 1×10^6; 3663 as 3.663×10^3; and so on. To multiply, the exponents are added, but coefficients are multiplied. To divide, the exponents are subtracted, but coefficients are divided.

Multiplying: $(1 \times 10^x) \cdot (1 \times 10^y) = 1 \times 10^{x+y}$

$(4 \times 10^2) \cdot (2 \times 10^3) = 8 \times 10^5$

Dividing: $(1 \times 10^x) \div (1 \times 10^y) = 1 \times 10^{x-y}$

$(4 \times 10^2) \div (2 \times 10^3) = 2 \times 10^{-1}$

Numbers less than 1 are 10^{-x}. For example, 0.000001 is 1×10^{-6}.

Multiplying: $(1 \times 10^{-x}) \cdot (1 \times 10^{-y}) = 1 \times 10^{-(x+y)}$

$(4 \times 10^{-2}) \cdot (2 \times 10^{-3}) = 8 \times 10^{-5}$

A large number multiplied by a small number:

$$(4 \times 10^{-2})(2 \times 10^3) = 8 \times 10^1$$

(Logarithms and Exponents are reproduced through the courtesy of Dr. Richard B. Brandt, Dept. of Biochemistry, MCV, VCU, Richmond, Virginia, 23298).

Table of Common Logarithms

Numbers	0	1	2	3	4	5	6	7	8	9
10	0000	0043	0086	0128	0170	0212	0253	0294	0334	0374
11	0414	0453	0492	0531	0569	0607	0645	0682	0719	0755
12	0792	0828	0864	0899	0934	0969	1004	1038	1072	1106
13	1139	1173	1206	1239	1271	1303	1335	1367	1399	1430
14	1461	1492	1523	1553	1584	1614	1644	1673	1703	1732
15	1761	1790	1818	1847	1875	1903	1931	1959	1987	2014
16	2041	2068	2095	2122	2148	2175	2201	2227	2253	2279
17	2304	2330	2355	2380	2405	2430	2455	2480	2504	2529
18	2553	2577	2601	2625	2648	2672	2695	2718	2742	2765
19	2788	2810	2833	2856	2878	2900	2923	2945	2967	2989
20	3010	3032	3054	3075	3096	3118	3139	3160	3181	3201
21	3222	3243	3263	3284	3304	3324	3345	3365	3385	3404
22	3424	3444	3464	3483	3502	3522	3541	3560	3579	3598
23	3617	3636	3655	3674	3692	3711	3729	3747	3766	3784
24	3802	3820	3838	3856	3874	3892	3909	3927	3945	3962
25	3979	3997	4014	4031	4048	4065	4082	4099	4116	4133
26	4150	4166	4183	4200	4216	4232	4249	4265	4281	4298
27	4314	4330	4346	4362	4378	4393	4409	4425	4440	4456
28	4472	4487	4502	4518	4533	4548	4564	4579	4594	4609
29	4624	4639	4654	4669	4683	4698	4713	4728	4742	4757
30	4771	4786	4800	4814	4829	4843	4857	4871	4886	4900
31	4914	4928	4942	4955	4969	4983	4997	5011	5024	5038
32	5051	5065	5079	5092	5105	5119	5132	5145	5159	5172
33	5185	5198	5211	5224	5237	5250	5263	5276	5289	5302
34	5315	5328	5340	5353	5366	5378	5391	5403	5416	5428
35	5441	5453	5465	5478	5490	5502	5514	5527	5539	5551
36	5563	5575	5587	5599	5611	5623	5635	5647	5658	5670
37	5682	5694	5705	5717	5729	5740	5752	5763	5775	5786
38	5798	5809	5821	5832	5843	5855	5866	5877	5888	5899
39	5911	5922	5933	5944	5955	5966	5977	5988	5999	6010
40	6021	6031	6042	6053	6064	6075	6085	6096	6107	6117
41	6128	6138	6149	6160	6170	6180	6191	6201	6212	6222
42	6232	6243	6253	6263	6274	6284	6294	6304	6314	6325
43	6335	6345	6355	6365	6375	6385	6395	6405	6415	6425
44	6435	6444	6454	6464	6474	6484	6493	6503	6513	6522
45	6532	6542	6551	6561	6571	6580	6590	6599	6609	6618
46	6628	6637	6646	6656	6665	6675	6684	6693	6702	6712
47	6721	6730	6739	6749	6758	6767	6776	6785	6794	6803
48	6812	6821	6830	6839	6848	6857	6866	6875	6884	6893
49	6902	6911	6920	6928	6937	6946	6955	6964	6972	6981
50	6990	6998	7007	7016	7024	7033	7042	7050	7059	7067
51	7076	7084	7093	7101	7110	7118	7126	7135	7143	7152
52	7160	7168	7177	7185	7193	7202	7210	7218	7226	7235

53	7243	7251	7259	7267	7275	7284	7292	7300	7308	7316
54	7324	7332	7340	7348	7356	7364	7372	7380	7388	7396
55	7404	7412	7419	7427	7435	7443	7451	7459	7466	7474
56	7482	7490	7497	7505	7513	7520	7528	7536	7543	7551
57	7559	7566	7574	7582	7589	7597	7604	7612	7619	7627
58	7634	7642	7649	7657	7664	7672	7679	7686	7694	7701
59	7709	7716	7723	7731	7738	7745	7752	7760	7767	7774
60	7782	7789	7796	7803	7810	7818	7825	7832	7839	7846
61	7853	7860	7868	7875	7882	7889	7896	7903	7910	7917
62	7924	7931	7938	7945	7952	7959	7966	7937	7980	7987
63	7993	8000	8007	8014	8021	8028	8035	8041	8048	8055
64	8062	8069	8075	8082	8089	8096	8102	8109	8116	8122
65	8129	8136	8142	8149	8156	8162	8169	8176	8182	8189
66	8195	8202	8209	8215	8222	8228	8235	8241	8248	8254
67	8261	8267	8274	8280	8287	8293	8299	8306	8312	8319
68	8325	8331	8338	8344	8351	8357	8363	8370	8376	8382
69	8388	8395	8401	8407	8414	8420	8426	8432	8439	8445
70	8451	8457	8463	8470	8476	8482	8488	8494	8500	8506
71	8513	8519	8525	8531	8537	8543	8549	8555	8561	8567
72	8573	8579	8585	8591	8597	8603	8609	8615	8621	8627
73	8633	8639	8645	8651	8657	8663	8669	8675	8681	8686
74	8692	8698	8704	8710	8716	8722	8727	8733	8739	8745
75	8751	8756	8762	8768	8774	8779	8785	8791	8797	8802
76	8808	8814	8820	8825	8831	8837	8842	8848	8854	8859
77	8865	8871	8876	8882	8887	8893	8899	8904	8910	8915
78	8921	8927	8932	8938	8943	8949	8954	8960	8965	8971
79	8976	8982	8987	8993	8998	9004	9009	9015	9020	9025
80	9031	9036	9042	9047	9053	9058	9063	9069	9074	9079
81	9085	9090	9096	9101	9106	9112	9117	9122	9128	9133
82	9138	9143	9149	9154	9159	9165	9170	9175	9180	9186
83	9191	9196	9201	9206	9212	9217	9222	9227	9232	9238
84	9243	9248	9253	9258	9263	9269	9274	9279	9284	9289
85	9294	9299	9304	9309	9315	9320	9325	9330	9335	9340
86	9345	9350	9355	9360	9365	9370	9375	9380	9385	9390
87	9395	9400	9405	9410	9415	9420	9425	9430	9435	9440
88	9445	9450	9455	9460	9465	9469	9474	9479	9484	9489
89	9494	9499	9504	9509	9513	9518	9523	9528	9533	9538
90	9542	9547	9552	9557	9562	9566	9571	9576	9581	9586
91	9590	9595	9600	9605	9609	9614	9619	9624	9628	9633
92	9638	9643	9647	9652	9657	9661	9666	9671	9675	9680
93	9685	9689	9694	9699	9703	9708	9713	9717	9722	9727
94	9731	9736	9741	9745	9750	9754	9759	9763	9768	9773
95	9777	9782	9786	9791	9795	9800	9805	9809	9814	9818
96	9823	9827	9832	9836	9841	9845	9850	9854	9859	9863
97	9868	9872	9877	9881	9886	9890	9894	9899	9903	9908
98	9912	9917	9921	9926	9930	9934	9939	9943	9948	9952
99	9956	9961	9965	9969	9974	9978	9983	9987	9991	9996

Periodic Table of the Elements

Relative atomic masses are based on $^{12}C = 12.00000$

KEY

Atomic Mass (Weight)	12.01115
Symbol	C
Selected Oxidation States	+2 +4 −4
Atomic Number	6
Covalent Atomic Radius (Å)	0.77
Electron Configuration	2-4

Each cell: Atomic Mass, Oxidation States / Symbol / Atomic Number, Covalent Atomic Radius / Electron Configuration.

Transition Elements: Groups IIIB to IIB

Period	IA	IIA	IIIB	IVB	VB	VIB	VIIB	VIII	VIII	VIII	IB	IIB	IIIA	IVA	VA	VIA	VIIA	0
1	1.00797 +1 −1 **H** 1 0.32 1																	4.0026 0 **He** 2 0.31 2
2	6.939 +1 **Li** 3 1.23 2-1	9.0122 +2 **Be** 4 0.89 2-2											10.811 +3 **B** 5 0.82 2-3	12.01115 +2 +4 −4 **C** 6 0.77 2-4	14.0067 +1 +2 +3 +4 +5 −1 −2 −3 **N** 7 0.75 2-5	15.9994 −2 **O** 8 0.73 2-6	18.9984 −1 **F** 9 0.72 2-7	20.183 0 **Ne** 10 0.71 2-8
3	22.9898 +1 **Na** 11 1.54 2-8-1	24.312 +2 **Mg** 12 1.36 2-8-2											26.9815 +3 **Al** 13 1.18 2-8-3	28.086 +2 +4 −4 **Si** 14 1.11 2-8-4	30.9738 +3 +5 −3 **P** 15 1.06 2-8-5	32.064 +4 +6 −2 **S** 16 1.02 2-8-6	35.453 +1 +5 +7 −1 **Cl** 17 0.99 2-8-7	39.948 0 **Ar** 18 0.98 2-8-8
4	39.102 +1 **K** 19 2.03 2-8-8-1	40.08 +2 **Ca** 20 1.74 2-8-8-2	44.956 +3 **Sc** 21 1.44 2-8-9-2	47.90 +2 +3 +4 **Ti** 22 1.32 2-8-10-2	50.942 +2 +3 +4 +5 **V** 23 1.22 2-8-11-2	51.996 +2 +3 +6 **Cr** 24 1.18 2-8-13-1	54.9380 +2 +3 +4 +7 **Mn** 25 1.17 2-8-13-2	55.847 +2 +3 **Fe** 26 1.17 2-8-14-2	58.9332 +2 +3 **Co** 27 1.16 2-8-15-2	58.71 +2 +3 **Ni** 28 1.15 2-8-16-2	63.54 +1 +2 **Cu** 29 1.17 2-8-18-1	65.37 +2 **Zn** 30 1.25 2-8-18-2	69.72 +3 **Ga** 31 1.26 2-8-18-3	72.59 +2 +4 **Ge** 32 1.22 2-8-18-4	74.9216 +3 +5 −3 **As** 33 1.20 2-8-18-5	78.96 +4 +6 −2 **Se** 34 1.17 2-8-18-6	79.909 +1 +5 −1 **Br** 35 1.14 2-8-18-7	83.80 0 **Kr** 36 1.12 2-8-18-8
5	85.47 +1 **Rb** 37 2.16 2-8-18-8-1	87.62 +2 **Sr** 38 1.91 2-8-18-8-2	88.905 +3 **Y** 39 1.62 2-8-18-9-2	91.22 +4 **Zr** 40 1.45 2-8-18-10-2	92.906 +3 +5 **Nb** 41 1.34 2-8-18-12-1	95.94 +6 +3 **Mo** 42 1.30 2-8-18-13-1	98.9062 +4 +6 +7 **Tc** 43 1.27 2-8-18-14-1	101.07 +3 **Ru** 44 1.25 2-8-18-15-1	102.905 +3 **Rh** 45 1.34 2-8-18-16-1	106.4 +2 +4 **Pd** 46 1.28 2-8-18-18	107.870 +1 **Ag** 47 1.34 2-8-18-18-1	112.40 +2 **Cd** 48 1.48 2-8-18-18-2	114.82 +3 **In** 49 1.44 2-8-18-18-3	118.69 +2 +4 **Sn** 50 1.40 2-8-18-18-4	121.75 +3 +5 −3 **Sb** 51 1.40 2-8-18-18-5	127.60 +4 +6 −2 **Te** 52 1.36 2-8-18-18-6	126.9044 +1 +5 +7 −1 **I** 53 1.33 2-8-18-18-7	131.30 0 **Xe** 54 1.31 2-8-18-18-8
6	132.905 +1 **Cs** 55 2.35 2-8-18-18-8-1	137.34 +2 **Ba** 56 1.98 2-8-18-18-8-2	138.91 +3 **La** 57 1.69 2-8-18-18-9-2	178.49 +4 **Hf** 72 1.44 *-18-32-10-2	180.948 +5 **Ta** 73 1.34 -18-32-11-2	183.85 +6 **W** 74 1.30 -18-32-12-2	186.2 +4 +6 +7 **Re** 75 1.28 -18-32-13-2	190.2 +3 +4 **Os** 76 1.26 -18-32-14-2	192.2 +3 +4 **Ir** 77 1.27 -18-32-15-2	195.09 +2 +4 **Pt** 78 1.30 -18-32-17-1	196.967 +1 +3 **Au** 79 1.34 -18-32-18-1	200.59 +1 +2 **Hg** 80 1.49 -18-32-18-2	204.37 +1 +3 **Tl** 81 1.48 -18-32-18-3	207.19 +2 +4 **Pb** 82 1.47 -18-32-18-4	208.980 +3 +5 **Bi** 83 1.46 -18-32-18-5	(209) +2 +4 **Po** 84 1.46 -18-32-18-6	(210) **At** 85 1.45 -18-32-18-7	(222) 0 **Rn** 86 -18-32-18-8
7	(223) +1 **Fr** 87 -18-32-18-8-1	(226) +2 **Ra** 88 2.20 -18-32-18-8-2	(227) +3 **Ac** 89 2.0 -18-32-18-9-2															

Lanthanide Series

140.12 +3 +4 **Ce** 58 1.65	140.907 +3 **Pr** 59 1.64	144.24 +3 **Nd** 60 1.64	(145) +3 **Pm** 61 1.63	150.35 +2 +3 **Sm** 62 1.62	151.96 +2 +3 **Eu** 63 1.85	157.25 +3 **Gd** 64 1.62	158.924 +3 **Tb** 65 1.61	162.50 +3 **Dy** 66 1.60	164.930 +3 **Ho** 67 1.58	167.26 +3 **Er** 68 1.58	168.934 +3 **Tm** 69 1.58	173.04 +2 +3 **Yb** 70 1.70	174.97 +3 **Lu** 71 1.56

Actinide Series

232.038 +4 **Th** 90 1.65	231.036 +5 +4 **Pa** 91	238.03 +3 +4 +5 +6 **U** 92 1.42	237.048 +3 +4 +5 +6 **Np** 93	(244) +3 +4 +5 +6 **Pu** 94	(243) +3 +4 +5 +6 **Am** 95	(247) +3 **Cm** 96	(247) +3 +4 **Bk** 97	(251) +3 **Cf** 98	(254) **Es** 99	(257) **Fm** 100	(256) **Md** 101	(254) **No** 102	(257) **Lr** 103

Numbers in parentheses are mass numbers of most stable or most common isotope.

*Denotes the presence of (2–8–) for elements 72 and beyond.

DET 1309

LIST OF ELEMENTS WITH THEIR SYMBOLS

Element	Symbol	Element	Symbol
Actinium	Ac	Mendelevium	Md
Aluminum	Al	Mercury	Hg
Americium	Am	Molybdenum	Mo
Antimony	Sb	Neodymium	Nd
Argon	Ar	Neon	Ne
Arsenic	As	Neptunium	Np
Astatine	At	Nickel	Ni
Barium	Ba	Niobium	Nb
Berkelium	Bk	Nitrogen	N
Beryllium	Be	Nobelium	No
Bismuth	Bi	Osmium	Os
Boron	B	Oxygen	O
Bromine	Br	Palladium	Pd
Cadmium	Cd	Phosphorus	P
Calcium	Ca	Platinum	Pt
Californium	Cf.	Plutonium	Pu
Carbon	C	Polonium	Po
Cerium	Ce	Potassium	K
Cesium	Cs	Praseodymium	Pr
Chlorine	Cl	Promethium	Pm
Chromium	Cr	Protactinium	Pa
Cobalt	Co	Radium	Ra
Copper	Cu	Radon	Rn
Curium	Cm	Rhenium	Re
Dysprosium	Dy	Rhodium	Rh
Einsteinium	Es	Rubidium	Rb
Element 106		Ruthenium	Ru
Erbium	Er	Samarium	Sm
Europium	Eu	Scandium	Sc
Fermium	Fm	Selenium	Se
Fluorine	F	Silicon	Si
Francium	Fr	Silver	Ag
Gadolinium	Gd	Sodium	Na
Gallium	Ga	Strontium	Sr
Germanium	Ge	Sulfur	S
Gold	Au	Tantalum	Ta
Hafnium	Hf	Technetium	Tc
Helium	He	Tellurium	Te
Holmium	Ho	Terbium	Tb
Hydrogen	H	Thallium	Tl
Indium	In	Thorium	Th
Iodine	I	Thulium	Tm
Iridium	Ir	Tin	Sn
Iron	Fe	Titanium	Ti
Krypton	Kr	Tungsten	W
Lanthanum	La	Uranium	U
Lawrencium	Lr	Vanadium	V
Lead	Pb	Xenon	Xe
Lithium	Li	Ytterbium	Yb
Lutetium	Lu	Yttrium	Y
Magnesium	Mg	Zinc	Zn
Manganese	Mn	Zirconium	Zr